Ophthalmic
Diagnosis and Treatment

Ophthalmic Diagnosis and Treatment

Third Edition

Editor

Myron Yanoff MD
Professor and Chairman
Department of Ophthalmology
Drexel University College of Medicine
Philadelphia, Pennsylvania, USA

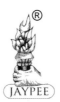

JAYPEE BROTHERS MEDICAL PUBLISHERS (P) LTD

New Delhi • London • Philadelphia • Panama

Jaypee Brothers Medical Publishers (P) Ltd

Headquarters

Jaypee Brothers Medical Publishers (P) Ltd
4838/24, Ansari Road, Daryaganj
New Delhi 110 002, India
Phone: +91-11-43574357
Fax: +91-11-43574314
Email: jaypee@jaypeebrothers.com

Overseas Offices

J.P. Medical Ltd
83, Victoria Street, London
SW1H 0HW (UK)
Phone: +44-2031708910
Fax: +02-03-0086180
Email: info@jpmedpub.com

Jaypee-Highlights.
Medical Publishers Inc
City of Knowledge, Bld. 237
Clayton, Panama City, Panama
Phone: +507-301-0496
Fax: +507-301-0499
Email: cservice@jphmedical.com

Jaypee Medical Inc.
The Bourse
111 South Independence Mall East
Suite 835, Philadelphia,
PA 19106, USA
Phone: + 267-519-9789
Email: jpmed.us@gmail.com

Jaypee Brothers
Medical Publishers (P) Ltd
17/1-B Babar Road, Block-B
Shaymali, Mohammadpur
Dhaka-1207, Bangladesh
Mobile: +08801912003485
Email: jaypeedhaka@gmail.com

Jaypee Brothers
Medical Publishers (P) Ltd
Shorakhute, Kathmandu
Nepal
Phone: +00977-9841528578
Email: jaypee.nepal@gmail.com

Website: www.jaypeebrothers.com
Website: www.jaypeedigital.com

Ophthalmic Diagnosis and Treatment

Third Edition: 2014

ISBN 978-93-5025-952-8

Printed at Replika Press Pvt. Ltd.

Section Editors

CATARACT AND SYSTEMIC AND ORBITAL DISORDERS

Myron Yanoff MD
Professor and Chairman
Department of Ophthalmology
Drexel University College of Medicine
Philadelphia, Pennsylvania, USA

CORNEAL AND EXTERNAL DISEASES

Prathima Thumma MD
Department of Ophthalmology
Drexel University College of Medicine
Philadelphia, Pennsylvania, USA

GLAUCOMA

Amanda Lehman MD
Department of Ophthalmology
Drexel University College of Medicine
Philadelphia, Pennsylvania, USA

NEURO-OPHTHALMOLOGY AND GENERAL OPHTHALMOLOGY

Yelena Doych MD
Department of Ophthalmology
Drexel University College of Medicine
Philadelphia, Pennsylvania, USA

PEDIATRIC OPHTHALMOLOGY

Robert Spector MD
Division of Ophthalmology
St. Christopher's Hospital for Children
Philadelphia, Pennsylvania, USA

WITH CONTRIBUTIONS FROM

Arjun Dirghangi MD and **Raza Shah** MD
Department of Ophthalmology
Drexel University College of Medicine
Philadelphia, Pennsylvania, USA

Preface

Ophthalmic Diagnosis and Treatment, Third Edition, provides in a simplified format, recommendations and treatments of conditions most often encountered by eye care providers. Entities are in alphabetical order for easy, rapid access of information for the eye care provider and student. Each entity has Diagnosis (definition, symptoms, differential diagnosis, etc.) on the left page and Treatment (diet and lifestyle, treatment aims, prognosis, pertinent references, etc.) on the right page. We have added new illustrations and have updated the material.

The same format is used throughout the book. The information, not intended to be encyclopedic, highlights the salient facts of each entity. Full-color illustrations are used throughout the book. As much as possible, each entity is followed by its diagnostic code, which is most helpful for billing purposes and for organizing patients' records.

We anticipate that the book will be used by eye care professionals and students as a quick reference guide of the significant points most commonly encountered and important entities pertaining to the eyes.

Myron Yanoff

Acknowledgments

The editors would like to acknowledge Joe Rusko and the staff of Jaypee Brothers Medical Publishers for their outstanding help in producing this book.

Contents

A

B

C

D

E

F

G

H

O

P

R

S

T

U

V

Contents by Specialty

Cataract and Systemic and Orbital Disorders

Corneal and External Diseases

Glaucoma

Neuro-ophthalmology

Pediatric Ophthalmology

Retinal and Vitreous Disorders

This book provides current expert recommendations in the form of tabular summaries on the diagnosis and treatment of all major disorders throughout ophthalmology. Essential guidelines on each of the topics have been condensed into two pages of vital information, summarizing the main procedures in diagnosis and management of each disorder to provide a quick and easy reference.

Each disorder is presented on facing pages: the main procedures in diagnosis on the left and treatment options on the right.

Listed in the main column of the **Diagnosis** page is the definition; other common names; the common symptoms, signs, and complications of the disorder; pearls and considerations; and referal information, with brief explaining their significance and probability of occurrence, together with details of investigations that can be used to aid diagnosis.

The **left shaded side column** contains information to help readers evaluate the probability that a patient has the disorder. It may also include other information that could be useful in making a diagnosis (e.g. classification or grading systems, comparison of different diagnostic methods).

The numbers that appear in parentheses next to disease names at the top of each page and scattered throughout the text are from *The International Classification of Diseases* (New York, 1995, McGraw-Hill). These numbers are used by physicians to organize their patients' medical records and to facilitate the timely reimbursement of their services.

On the **Treatment** page, the main column contains information on lifestyle management and nonspecialist medical therapy of the disorder, with general information on specialist management when this is the main treatment.

Whenever possible under "Pharmacologic treatment", guidelines are given on the standard dosage for commonly used drugs, with details of contraindications and precautions, main drug interactions, and main side effects. In each case, however, the manufacturer's drug data sheet should be consulted before any regimen is prescribed.

The main goals of treatment (e.g. to cure, to palliate, to prevent), prognosis after treatment, precautions that the physician should take during and after treatment, and any other information that could help the clinician to make treatment decisions (e.g. other nonpharmacologic treatment options, special situations or groups of patients) are given in the **right shaded side column**. The general references at the end of this column provide readers with further practical information.

Acute Posterior Multifocal Placoid Pigment Epitheliopathy (363.15)

DIAGNOSIS

Definition

An acquired, self-limited inflammatory disorder and vasculitis of the retina, retinal pigment epithelium (RPE), and choroid in otherwise healthy young adults.

Synonyms

None; often abbreviated AMPPE.

Symptoms

Rapid, painless loss of vision: in one or both eyes.

Signs

- Acute phase shows multiple circumscribed gray-white lesions at the level of the RPE located in the postequatorial retina (*see* Fig. 1)
- Late phase shows changes in the RPE similar to laser burns.
- Associated serous detachment: uncommon
- Perivenous exudation in the retina
- Slight dilation of the retinal veins
- Papilledema, papillitis, optic neuropathy
- Episcleritis
- Iridocyclitis.

Investigations

Fluorescein angiography, in the early phase, shows blockage of choroidal fluorescence (*see* Figs 2A to C), with mid-phase to late-phase diffuse staining of the acute lesions.

Complications

- *Choroidal neovascularization*: rare
- Cerebritis: has been reported.

Differential Diagnosis
Serpiginous choroidopathy

Cause
Unknown

Epidemiology
- Disease affects healthy young men and women
- One-third of patients give a history of a viral prodrome
- Recurrences are frequent.

Diagnosis continued on p. 4

TREATMENT

Diet and Lifestyle

No precautions are necessary.

Pharmacologic Treatment

Oral steroids should be instituted promptly if there are signs of associated cerebritis.

Treatment Aims

To observe a patient

Prognosis

Visual prognosis is good, and there is a low incidence of recurrence after treatment.

Follow-up and Management

Based on the severity of the symptoms, patients should be followed every few weeks until they are out of the acute phase.

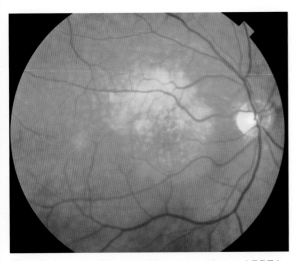

Fig. 1: Intense whitening of the outer retina and RPE in the macula of a patient with AMPPE.

Treatment continued on p. 5

Acute Posterior Multifocal Placoid Pigment Epitheliopathy (363.15)

DIAGNOSIS—cont'd

Pearls and Considerations

- Spontaneous visual recovery is expected with or without systemic therapy, with most eyes achieving 20/40 or better vision in 1–6 months from onset
- It is important to look for an underlying cause because the condition has been related to some antimicrobial agents, such as ampicillin and sulfonamides. If an antimicrobial agent is identified, it should be discontinued to prevent further recurrences.
- Associated cerebral vasculitis may occur as late as 3 months after presentation of AMPPE.

Referral Information

A computed tomography scan, magnetic resonance imaging or cerebral arteriogram is indicated in patients with severe headache to rule out cerebral vasculitis.

TREATMENT—cont'd

Nonpharmacologic Treatment

No nonpharmacologic treatment is recommended.

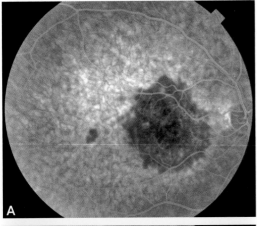

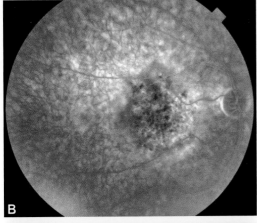

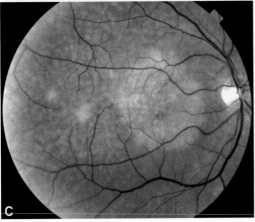

Figs 2A to C: (A) Red-free photograph as well as early and late phases of the fluorescein angiogram are seen; (B) There is early blockage of fluorescein in both the large central and the smaller temporal macular areas; (C) In the later frame, the temporal spot is no longer visible and there is hyperfluorescence of the central macular region. This early blockage and late hyperfluorescence is the hallmark of AMPPE.

GENERAL REFERENCES

Bird AC. Acute multifocal placoid pigment epitheliopathy. Retina, 4th edition. St Louis: Elsevier; 2006.

Glass D. Inflammatory diseases of the retina and choroid. In: Glass D (Ed). Stereoscopic Atlas of Diseases: Diagnosis and Treatment, 4th edition. St. Louis: Mosby; 1997.

Kooragayala LM, et al. (Eds). (2005). Acute multifocal placoid pigment epitheliopathy. [online]. Available from www.emedicine.com. [Accessed July, 2012].

Puilido JS, Blake CR. Inflammatory choroiditis. In: Tasman W et al. (Eds). Duane's Clinical Ophthalmology (CD-ROM). Philadelphia: Lippincott Williams & Wilkins; 2004.

Acute Retinal Necrosis (363.13)

DIAGNOSIS

Definition

Severe inflammation leading to necrosis of the retina starting in the periphery and progressing circumferentially and centripetally caused by one of the herpes viruses. Often referred to in the abbreviated form: ARN (acute retinal necrosis).

Synonyms

Necrotizing herpetic retinitis

Symptoms

- Blurry vision
- Ocular pain
- Photophobia
- Floaters.

Signs (Fig. 1)

White, confluent, retinal necrotic lesions affecting a large portion, if not the entire, peripheral retina is the hallmark of the condition. Panuveitis may be present, i.e. conjunctival inflammation, scleritis, vitreous and anterior chamber cells, obliterative retinal vasculitis as well as tenderness of the globe. There is a paucity of retinal hemorrhages compared to other conditions such as CMV retinitis. Patients are typically not immunocompromised. Most patients present unilaterally but progression to bilateral disease is common.

Investigations

- Fluorescein angiography shows staining of the peripheral vessels. Loss of peripheral circulation due to occlusive vasculitis is also seen. The posterior pole usually spared initially. If papillitis develops, leakage from the disk will be seen.
- Serial color fundus photos can document the progression of the disease.
- Labwork must include herpes 1, herpes 2 and varicella zoster titers. A vitreous biopsy to obtain polymerase chain reaction (PCR) of these DNA viruses may be done, as well.
- Labwork to rule out other conditions includes complete blood count (CBC), Lyme titer, human immunodeficiency virus (HIV), angiotensin converting enzyme (ACE) titer, toxoplasma titer, rapid plasma reagin (RPR) and fluorescent treponemal antibody absorption (FTA-ABS), purified protein derivative (PPD) skin testing, chest X-ray, and magnetic resonance imaging (MRI) of the brain and orbits.

Complications

Development of large retinal tears is common. These often lead to retinal detachment. Due to extensive retinal involvement, proliferative vitreoretinopathy with total retinal detachment often develops. Severe or even complete loss of vision may be the end result even with aggressive medical and surgical treatment.

Pearls and Considerations

Progressive outer retinal necrosis (PORN) has similar white lesions affecting the outer retina (i.e. beneath the retinal vessels) but without vitreous inflammation and without vasculitis. The cause is the same herpes viruses implicated in ARN. This is seen in immunocompromised individuals and is almost always bilateral. It frequently leads to retinal detachment and blindness in both eyes, even with treatment.

Referral Information

Retinal specialist to manage ocular complications and infectious disease specialist to manage systemic antiviral treatment

Differential Diagnosis

- Cytomegalovirus (CMV) retinitis which is seen in AIDS patients. Intraretinal blood is prominent.
- *Syphilis*: this requires lumbar puncture to rule out central nervous system (CNS) disease.
- *Toxoplasmosis*: has a much better prognosis.
- *Lyme disease*: may have other findings such as cranial nerve palsy.
- *Behcet's disease*: mouth ulcers in 90% of patients. HLA-B51 test often positive.
- *Ocular lymphoma*: diagnosed with vitreous biopsy and associated with CNS lymphoma
- *Fungal endophthalmitis*: need to do fungal blood cultures.

6

TREATMENT

Diet and Lifestyle

No special precautions are necessary.

Pharmacologic Treatment

- Immediate antiviral treatment with the goal of preventing disease in the fellow eye and preventing progression to retinal detachment. Oral valacyclovir 1 gram PO TID for 6 weeks. May substitute with acyclovir 600 mg five times a day.
- Systemic steroids are also given, although it is still controversial whether to initiate immediately or wait a week to give time for the antiviral medicine to work. Prednisone 60 mg PO daily for 1 or 2 weeks followed by a slow taper over the next month.
- May need to admit to hospital for intravenous antiviral and steroid medications.
- Topical prednisolone acetate one drop up to every 2 hours with a slow taper over the next month depending upon anterior chamber inflammation. Topical atropine 1% one drop BID for cycloplegia and to decrease ocular pain.

Nonpharmacologic Treatment

Peripheral laser retinopexy is recommended in order to prevent the development of retinal detachment. When retinal detachment develops vitrectomy and further laser with or without peripheral scleral buckling is done. Long-acting gas or even silicone oil is necessary to repair the complex rhegmatogenous/necrotic detachment.

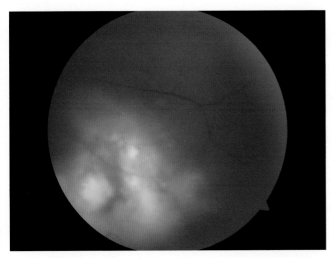

Fig. 1: Retina shows necrosis and detachment.

Treatment Aims

To prevent severe, irreversible visual loss by treating the underlying viral cause of the retinitis. In unilateral cases goal of antiviral medicine is to prevent bilateral disease.

Prognosis

If caught very early, may have good visual outcome. Most patients, however, suffer from some degree of both peripheral and central visual loss in spite of treatment.

Follow-up and Management

Must be followed daily while in hospital during acute phase of illness. As the retinitis stabilizes may be followed weekly, then monthly and as needed depending upon any surgery or complications.

GENERAL REFERENCES

Aizman A, Johnson MW, Elner SG. Treatment of acute retinal necrosis syndrome with oral antiviral medications. Ophthalmology. 2007;114: 307-12.

Luu KK, Missotten T, Salzmann J, et al. Acute retinal necrosis features, management and outcomes. Ophthalmology. 2007; 114:756-62.

Scott IU, Luu KM, Davis JL. Intravitreal antivirals in the management of patients with acquired immunodeficiency syndrome with progressive outer retinal necrosis. Arch Ophthalmol. 2002;120: 1219-22.

AIDS-Related Ocular Manifestations (042)

DIAGNOSIS

Definition

Any disease or condition of the eye or ocular adnexa that arises from a patient's underlying systemic acquired immunodeficiency syndrome (AIDS) infection or associated immunosuppression.

Synonyms

None

Symptoms

- Decreased vision, floaters, double vision
- Eye pain
- Facial rash
- Floaters
- Red eye
- Shadow.

Signs

Human immunodeficiency virus (HIV) retinopathy (noninfectious)

- Nerve fiber layer (NFL) and inner retinal hemorrhages
- Microaneurysms
- *Cotton-wool spot*: the most common manifestation of AIDS retinopathy.

Infectious Agents

Adnexa
- Herpes zoster ophthalmicus (HZO)
- Molluscum contagiosum.

Cryptococcus: papilledema, multiple choroiditis, meningitis, endophthalmitis.

Cytomegalovirus (CMV) retinitis: classic intraretinal hemorrhages with white infiltrates (*see* Fig. 1).

Granular form: "brush fire" appearance.

Hemorrhagic form: "tomato ketchup fundus".

Herpes retinitis [acute retinal necrosis (ARN) or progressive outer retinal necrosis (PORN)]: aggressive retinitis in which multiple white retinal infiltrates coalesce, leading to retinal detachment and visual loss (*see* retinal necrosis, acute).

Pneumocystis choroiditis: multiple, deep, yellow-orange lesions at the level of the choroid (*see* Fig. 2).

Toxoplasmosis: multifocal outer retinal lesions that spread quickly; normally, little vitreous inflammation is seen in immunocompetent patients; occurs in previously diagnosed patients (*see* Fig. 3).

Microsporidia: chronic keratoconjunctivitis.

Syphilis: plaque-like serous elevations in the posterior pole.

Diagnosis continued on p. 10

Differential Diagnosis

Cotton-wool spots: of diabetes, hypertension, ocular ischemia and vasculitis

Cause

HIV infection

TREATMENT

Diet and Lifestyle

Compliance with highly active antiretroviral therapy (HAART).

Pharmacologic Treatment

For Cytomegalovirus Infection

- Intravenous (IV) therapy with ganciclovir, foscarnet or cidofovir
- Intravitreal ganciclovir implant (sustained-release device) placed in the pars plana of the eye
- Intravitreal injections of ganciclovir or foscarnet.

For Pneumocystis sp. Infection

Bactrim, pentamidine.

For Herpes Simplex or Zoster Infection

Aggressive treatment with IV acyclovir.

For Toxoplasmosis

Pyrimethamine, sulfa drugs or clindamycin.

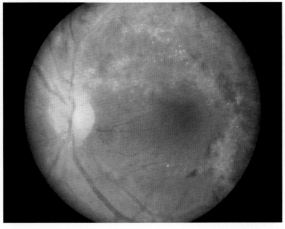

Fig. 1: Cytomegalovirus retinitis with the characteristic white perivascular retinal infiltrates and intraretinal hemorrhages or "pizza pie fundus".

Treatment continued on p. 11

DIAGNOSIS—cont'd

Tumors

- *Kaposi's sarcoma*: flat purplish lesion on the eyelid or conjunctiva similar to lesions seen on the skin; may be mistaken for subconjunctival hemorrhage
- Central nervous system (CNS) lymphoma
- Lymphomas
- Squamous cell carcinoma of the eyelid.

Neurologic Manifestations

- Cranial nerve palsies
- Papilledema
- Nystagmus
- Optic neuritis
- Visual field defects.

Investigations

Careful history: reviewing the patient's past medical history often gives clues to the cause.

CD4+ count: usually less than 50 cells/mm³ when patients develop CMV retinitis.

Cryptococcus: high risk of CNS infection.

Progressive outer retinal necrosis: CD4+ count greater than 50 cells/mm³.

Acute retinal necrosis: CD4+ count less than 50 cells/mm³.

Pneumocystis jiroveci (previously P. carinii): CD4+ count less than 200 cells/mm³.

Fluorescein angiography: helpful in differentiating retinal infections.

Computed tomography and magnetic resonance imaging scans: may be necessary for patients with CNS abnormalities.

Vitreous biopsy with analysis of polymerase chain reaction: helps distinguish herpes simplex from zoster and CMV when the clinical picture is not clear-cut.

Sequential fundus photographs: help monitor patients for response to therapy and evidence of disease progression.

Complications

- Visual loss
- Retinal detachment.

Medication-related

- *Cidofovir*: anterior uveitis and profound hypotony
- *Rifabutin (prophylaxis for atypical myobacterial infection)*: severe (sometimes bilateral) anterior uveitis.

Diagnosis continued on p. 12

TREATMENT—cont'd

For Syphilis

High-dose IV penicillin for 10–14 days.

Cryptococcus

Intravenous amphotericin, IV itraconazole, vitrectomy and intravitreal amphotericin for endophthalmitis.

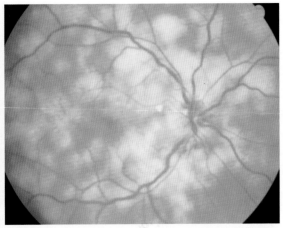

Fig. 2: *Pneumocystis* choroiditis showing deep choroidal, creamy yellow-orange infiltrates throughout the posterior pole.

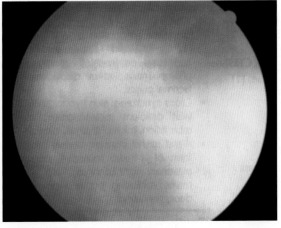

Fig. 3: Outer retinal toxoplasmosis in an AIDS patient showing the "brush fire" advancement of the infection.

Treatment continued on p. 13

DIAGNOSIS—cont'd

Pearls and Considerations

- Dilated fundus examination (DFE) should be performed every 3 months in patients with a CD4+ count less than or equal to 50 cells/mm^3 because of the potential for asymptomatic CMV retinitis. Once the CD4+ count rises above 100 cells/mm^3, the risk of retinitis is small.
- Acquired immunodeficiency syndrome patients' complications should be treated cautiously with steroids because of the potential for further immuno-suppression and infection
- Approximately 70–80% of AIDS patients will require treatment for an ocular complication at some time in their lives
- Cytomegalovirus is the most common severe and sight-threatening ocular infection in AIDS patients
- Infections of the cornea and adnexa are less common than intraocular infections in AIDS patients
- With HAART, many patients can reduce the detectable viral load to zero and can lead otherwise normal lives. Only when their immunity drops do they develop complications.

Referral Information

Variable and specific to the etiology of each complication.

TREATMENT—cont'd

Microsporidia

Topical fumagillin up to every 2 hours initially, and then taper slowly.

Nonpharmacologic Treatment

Regular periodic ocular examinations (e.g. CD4+ count < 50, every 3 months).

GENERAL REFERENCES

Copeland R, et al. (2006). Ocular manifestations of HIV. [online]. Available from www.emedicine.com. [Accessed July, 2012].

Holland GN, Levinson RD. Ocular infections associated with acquired immunodeficiency syndrome. In: Tasman W, Jaeger EA (Eds). Duane's Clinical Ophthalmology (CD-ROM). Philadelphia: Lippincott Williams & Wilkins; 2004.

Lightman S. HIV and the eye. London: Imperial College Press; 2000.

Moraes HV. Ocular manifestations of HIV/AIDS. Curr Opin Ophthalmol. 2002;13(6):397-403.

Rescigno R, Dinowitz M. Ophthalmic manifestations of immunodeficiency states. Clin Rev Allergy Immunol. 2001;20(2):163-81.

Rhee DJ, Pyfer MF (Eds). Acquired immunodeficiency syndrome (AIDS). The Wills Eye Manual. Philadelphia: Lippincott Williams & Wilkins; 1999. pp. 435-45.

Albinism (270.2)

DIAGNOSIS

Definition

The classification of a group of congenital diseases that result from defective pigment production (melanogenesis) can be ocular or oculocutaneous.

Synonyms

None; associated abbreviations: ocular albinism (OA) and oculocutaneous albinism (OCA), Chediak-Higashi syndrome (CHS), Hermansky-Pudlak syndrome (HPS), Griscelli syndrome (GS).

Symptoms

- *Painful photophobia*: In most patients
- *Decreased visual acuity (worse at distance than near)*: In most patients
- *Esthetic blemish from nystagmus*: In most patients
- *Poor binocular vision*: Because of near-total decussation of the optic nerves at the chiasm.

Signs

- *Horizontal nystagmus*: With possible null point and head posture to maximize visual acuity
- *Iris transillumination*: In patients with ocular albinism
- *Pink irides*: In patients with oculocutaneous albinism
- *Foveal hypoplasia or aplasia*: With retinal vascular presence in the foveal area
- *Decreased pigment in retinal pigment epithelium (RPE) and iris pigment epithelium (IPE)*: Figure 1
- *Esotropia*
- *Refractive errors*: Often myopia.

Investigations

- *Skin biopsy*: Patients with X-linked recessive ocular albinism have macroelanosomes
- *Testing for presence of tyrosinase*: Patients with tyrosinase-negative oculocutaneous albinism have no tyrosinase in hair bulbs; patients with tyrosinase-positive oculocutaneous albinism do
- Patients with Chediak-Higashi syndrome cannot opsonize certain bacteria
- Patients with Hermansky-Pudlak syndrome have platelet adherence abnormalities and capillary fragility.

Complications

- *Skin disorders, including melanomas*: Patients with oculocutaneous albinism are at risk for skin malignancies; protection is imperative
- *Photophobia*: It may disrupt outdoor activities
- *Chronic infections, including pneumonia*: In patients with Chediak-Higashi syndrome

Differential Diagnosis

Patients have depigmented skin or adnexal structures but no increased decussation of the optic nerves at the chiasm. Various albinoid forms exist:

- *Waardenburg syndrome*: Autosomal dominant association of white forelock (17%), piebald appearance, sensorineural deafness, synophrys, blepharophimosis, lateral displacement of lacrimal puncti.
- *Cross syndrome*: Skin hypopigmentation with deficient melanosomes, mental retardation, microphthalmia, cataracts.
- *Åland Island disease:* Believed to be a form of X-linked recessive, congenital stationary night blindness, with affected males exhibiting posterior-pole retinal depigmentation.

Cause

- Congenital, hereditary, stationary
- Oculocutaneous albinism segregates in most patients as an autosomal recessive; ocular albinism segregates in most affected patients as an X-linked recessive.

Associated Features

- *Tyrosinase negative*: White hair, pink skin.
- *Tyrosinase positive*: White hair as children; may become blond; may develop pigmented nevi.
- *Yellow mutant*: White hair and pink skin as infants; develop yellow hair at 6 months and normal skin pigmentation by 3 years.
- *Brown albinism*: Africans with reddish brown skin, red hair, freckles, brown irides.
- *Autosomal dominant oculocutaneous albinism*: White to cream skin, white hair, freckles, gray-blue irides.

Pathology

- Caucasian patients with ocular albinism have spotty areas of deficient melanin in the IPE melanosomes and generally no melanin in RPE melanosomes. Patients with oculocutaneous albinism have diffuse deficiency of IPE and RPE melanin; they also have varying amounts of absent dermal melanin.
- Patients with ocular and oculocutaneous albinism have absent foveal depressions, with vascular incursion into the area normally occupied by the fovea. They also have almost total decussation of the optic nerves at the chiasm.

Diagnosis continued on p. 16

TREATMENT

Diet and Lifestyle

Many patients will benefit from wearing sunglasses and sunscreen protection for the skin. Low-vision aids are recommended for elderly patients.

Pharmacologic Treatment

No pharmacologic treatment is recommended.

Treatment Aims

- To ensure patient comfort and safety
- To prevent bleeding diatheses in patients with Hermansky-Pudlak syndrome
- To treat infections early in patients with Chediak-Higashi syndrome.

Other Treatments

Glasses where appropriate; nystagmus prevents full benefit in many patients.

Prognosis

- Prognosis is stable in most patients; the nystagmus amplitude lessens with age, but visual acuity usually does not improve.
- Prognosis is guarded in patients with Hermansky-Pudlak or Chediak-Higashi syndrome.

Follow-up and Management

Yearly follow-up is sufficient for most patients. Those with Hermansky-Pudlak or Chediak-Higashi syndrome will require individualized follow-up and management of systemic problems. Many patients will want genetic counseling.

Treatment continued on p. 17

Albinism (270.2)

DIAGNOSIS—cont'd

- *Clotting abnormalities*: In patients with Hermansky-Pudlak syndrome
- Most patients with albinism and nystagmus cannot obtain a driver's license because their distance visual acuity is 20/100 to 20/200. Their near visual acuity, however, may be close to 20/20 if children are permitted to hold objects closely. Thus, children usually succeed in normal schooling environments if they are permitted to sit in front of the classroom and walk to the blackboard when necessary. Older children may require low-vision aids for near and distant work.

Classification

- Ocular albinism (X-linked recessive, rarely autosomal dominant or recessive)
- *Oculocutaneous albinism (autosomal recessive)*: Tyrosinase negative, brown albinism, tyrosinase positive, rufous albinism, yellow mutant, Hermansky-Pudlak, Chediak-Higashi.

Pearls and Considerations

- Ultraviolet-protective sunglasses are recommended for patients with any variant of ocular albinism or oculocutaneous albinism
- Patients affected by oculocutaneous albinism should be encouraged to be screened frequently for skin cancer
- Color vision remains normal in patients with albinism
- Clinicians should be mindful of the distinction between ocular albinism (with reduced acuity of 20/70 to 20/200) and *blond fundus,* associated with lightly pigmented individuals who have normal visual acuity.

Referral Information

Some variations of oculocutaneous albinism are potentially fatal; therefore, medical and hematologic referral should be considered to rule out these variants.

TREATMENT—cont'd

Nonpharmacologic Treatment

- Strabismus surgery
- *Eye muscle surgery*: To align the head in patients who adopt a posture resulting from the presence of a nystagmus-associated null point.

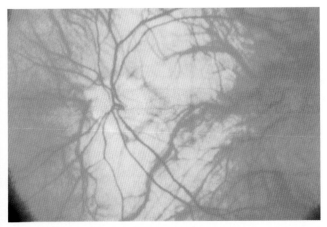

Fig. 1: Note pale fundus caused by lack of pigment in the retinal pigment epithelium and choroid.

GENERAL REFERENCES

Carr RE, Noble KG, Siegel IM. Disorders of the fundus. Albinism. Ophthalmology. 1981;88:377-8.

Cortin P, Tremblay M, Lemagne JM. X-linked ocular albinism: re*la*tive value of skin biopsy, iris transillumination and funduscopy in identifying affected males and carriers. Can J Ophthalmol. 1981; 16:121-3.

Creel DJ, Summers CG, King RA. Visual anomalies associated with albinism. Ophthalmic Pediatr Genet. 1990; 11:193-200.

Kasier PK, Friedman NJ. Albinism. The Massachusetts Eye and Ear Infirmary illustrated manual of ophthalmology, 2nd edition. Philadelphia: WB Saunders-Elsevier; 2004. pp. 407-8.

Kinnear PE, Jay B, Witkop CJ. Albinism. Surv Ophthalmol. 1985;30:75-101.

Mietz H, Green WR, Wolff SM, et al. Foveal hypoplasia in complete oculocutaneous albinism. A histopathologic study. Retina. 1992;12:254-60.

Mártinez-García M, Montoliu L. Albinism in Europe. J Dermatol. 2013; 40:319-24.

Seiving PA. Retinitis pigmentosa and related disorders. In: Yanoff M, Duker JS (Eds). Ophthalmology, 2nd edition. St Louis: Mosby Elsevier; 2006.

Amblyopia (368.0)

DIAGNOSIS

Definition

- Derived from Greek word meaning "dullness of vision"
- A functional reduction in the best-corrected visual acuity of an eye caused by "misuse" or "disuse" during the critical period of visual development not solely attributable to an organic abnormality.

Synonyms

"Lazy eye"

Symptoms

Decreased visual acuity from lack of use of an eye

Signs

- Decreased accommodative ability
- *Afferent papillary defect*: typically in patients of visual acuity less than 20/200
- Eccentric viewing may view with non-foveal retinal areas (abnormal retinal correspondence)
- *Enhanced crowding phenomenon*: single optotypes are discerned better than linear ones
- Loss of stereoscopic ability
- Strong fixation preferences in preverbal children.

Investigations

- *Visual acuity testing*: at least 2-line difference in visual acuity between eyes
- History of strabismus, anisometropia, or lens opacity
- Cycloplegic refraction
- Contrast sensitivity testing
- Electrodiagnostic testing and visual-evoked potentials.

Complications

- Permanent loss of visual acuity
- Loss of stereoscopic ability
- Loss of accommodative ability
- Occlusions or penalization may uncommonly cause visual loss (typically reversible) in the initially normal eye
- Patches can cause periocular skin rashes or abrasions.

Pearls and Considerations

- Prolonged use of atropine may lead to systemic reactions, hypersensitivity reactions of the lids, irritation, redness, edema, and follicular conjunctivitis or dermatitis
- Patients treated with atropine therapy should be monitored on a regular basis for these side effects
- Amblyopia should be suspected in any strabismic child who appears to have a preference for one eye over the other
- Amblyopia should be suspected in cases of reduced visual acuity in patients with greater than or equal to 2.00 diopters (D) of difference in hyperopic refractive error, or greater than or equal to 4.00 D difference in myopic refractive error.

Differential Diagnosis

- Incorrect refraction
- Central nervous system lesions
- Optic nerve dystrophies
- Keratoconus
- Subtle foveal lesions
- High refractive errors and dishabituation to clear retinal image.

Cause

- *Strabismus*: from foveal suppression in nonfixing eye
- *Anisometropia*: from persistently blurred image in eye with greater refractive error
- *Deprivation*: from media opacity (e.g. cataract, corneal lesion)
- *Isometropic (refractive)*: from persistent binocular image blurring caused by high refractive errors; controversial (many will respond to refractive correction alone).

Epidemiology

- Incidence 2–2.5% in general population
- No *de novo* development after 5.5 years of age. Earlier onset leads to more rapid development and deeper amblyopia.

Pathology

- Unequal visual competition causing: Atrophy of the lateral geniculate nucleus in the amblyopic eye. Loss of ability to respond to light within the primary visual cortex of either eye
- *Deprivation amblyopia*: axon bodies in lateral geniculate layers 2, 3, 5 (ipsilateral) decreased 18–25% in size; deprived-eye receptive bands in cortical layer IVc are narrower than normal-eye receptive bands
- *Anisometropic amblyopia*: no human specimens available; in monkeys, pathology is similar to deprivation amblyopia but at a slightly smaller effect
- *Strabismic amblyopia*: as with deprivation amblyopia, but in the lateral geniculate; body axons receiving input from the central 10° of fixation are affected.

Diagnosis continued on p. 20

TREATMENT

Diet and Lifestyle

No special precautions are necessary.

Pharmacologic Treatment

- No first line is indicated
- *Second line*: trials of oral levodopa and carbidopa suggest efficacy in temporarily improving acuity from an average of 20/121 to 20/96 in older amblyopic children and teenagers
- Penalization (atropinization of a highly hyperopic patient's better-sighted eye to switch fixation to the amblyopic eye) is recommended in some patients.

Treatment Aims

Equalizing and maintaining visual acuity between eyes without creating a contralateral amblyopia.

Other Treatments

- Anisometropic amblyopia patients will require refractive correction
- Patients who have media opacities will require surgery for these.

Prognosis

- Most children who have strabismic amblyopia will respond to treatment if initiated before 7 or 8 years of age; children as old as approximately 15 year deserve an attempt at treatment, and many will respond.
- Children who have anisometropic amblyopia are less responsive to treatment; those with media opacities are least responsive.

Follow-up and Management

- Close follow-up to ensure compliance and prevent occlusion amblyopia
- Check vision in both eyes during visits
- Patients who have aligned eyes and peripheral fusion should be patched no more than 5 hours/day. Patients who have constant strabismus can be patched all waking hours. Patients undergoing full-time occlusion should be re-examined weekly per year of age (e.g. q 3 week in a 3-year-old) until the acuity is equal.
- Taper occlusion following maximal improvement in visual acuity.

19

Treatment continued on p. 21

DIAGNOSIS—cont'd

- Patients with profound amblyopia are at increased risk for accidents because as much as one-fourth of their binocular visual field may be obscured or lost secondary to their reduced vision
- Microstrabismic amblyopia (or monofixation syndrome) is often detected later than other strabismic amblyopias because the small-angle esotropia is not obvious. Careful cover test analysis should be undertaken in all children to facilitate early detection
- Compliance with occlusive treatment is more important than the type of occlusion utilized.

Commonly Associated Conditions

- Anisometropia
- Strabismus
- High refractive error
- Asymmetric or unilateral lens opacities or visual pathway disruption.

Referral Information

- Refer for surgical correction of organic causes such as cataract (Fig. 1)
- Consider referring to appropriate pediatric specialists for implementation and monitoring of patching, orthoptic devices, and medical therapy.

TREATMENT—cont'd

Nonpharmacologic Treatment

- *Occlusion of the better-sighted eye*: either all waking hours or some fraction, followed by 1–2 hours/day occlusion until the patient's ninth birthday; this can be accomplished by a patch or occluding contact lens
- *Pleoptics*: dazzling of extrafoveal retina with bright light, followed by foveal stimulation; attempted in Europe on older patients with amblyopia
- *Game-format devices*: often used together with occlusion to stimulate amblyopic fovea
- *Red-glass treatment*: red filter placed over amblyopic eye to stimulate central fixation in patients with deep amblyopia having eccentric viewing; rarely used today.

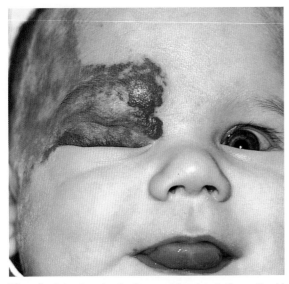

Fig. 1: Stimulus-deprivation amblyopia. A 6-month-old infant with infantile hemangioma of the right upper lid, completely covering the visual axis.

GENERAL REFERENCES

Diamond JR. Amblyopia. In: Yanoff M et al. (Eds). Ophthalmology. St Louis: Elsevier; 2006.

Eggers HM, Blakemore C. Physiologic basis of anisometropic amblyopia. Science. 1978;201:264-72.

Helveston EM. Relationship between degree of anisometropia and depth of amblyopia. Am J Ophthalmol. 1966;62:757-65.

Leguire LE, Rogers GL, Bremer DL, et al. Levodopa/carbodopa for childhood amblyopia. Invest Ophthalmol Vis Sci. 1993;34:3090.

Leske MC, Hawkins BS. Screening: relationship to diagnosis and therapy. In: Tasman W et al (Eds). Duane's Clinical Ophthalmology (CD-ROM). Philadelphia: Lippincott Williams & Wilkins; 2004.

Levi DM, Klein SA, Aitsebaomo AP. Vernier acuity, crowding and cortical magnification. Vision Res. 1985;25:963-72.

Mitchell DE, Sengpiel F, Hamilton DC, et al. Protection against deprivation amblyopia depends on relative not absolute daily binocular exposure. J Vis. 2011; 11(7). pii: 13. doi: 10.1167/11.7.13.

Rashad MA. Pharmacological enhancement of treatment for amblyopia. Clin Ophthalmol. 2012;6:409-16. Epub 2012 Mar 15.

Von Noorden GK, Crawford MLJ, Levacy RA. The lateral geniculate nucleus in human anisometropic amblyopia. Invest Ophthalmol Vis Sci. 1983;24:788-96.

Anatomically Narrow Angle (365.02)

DIAGNOSIS

Definition

A condition in which the anterior chamber angle is narrow or partially closed with an associated shallow anterior chamber, putting the patient at increased risk for angle-closure glaucoma.

Synonyms

None; associated abbreviations include ACG (angle-closure glaucoma) and CACG (chronic angle-closure glaucoma).

Symptoms

Patients are asymptomatic.

Signs

- *Hyperopia*: because these patients usually have smaller-than-average eyes, they will be hyperopic
- *Shallow peripheral anterior chamber*: generally with a van Herick grading of less than or equal to 2 when examined with the slit lamp (*see* Fig. 1)
- *Narrow angle on gonioscopy*: the anterior-chamber angle will appear quite narrow on gonioscopy, usually less than or equal to 20°; by definition, these patients do not have a closed angle or elevated intraocular pressure (IOP). However, the angle may appear optically closed, meaning that no angle structures are visible on gonioscopy, and the iris appears to be in contact with the peripheral cornea. An asymptomatic, anatomically narrow angle should open past the trabecular meshwork with pressure gonioscopy.

Investigations

Complete eye examination, including gonioscopy: in patients with critically narrow or optically closed angles, pupil dilation for funduscopy may provoke an attack of angle-closure glaucoma; such patients may be candidates for prophylactic peripheral iridectomy (*see* Nonpharmacologic Treatment).

A-scan ultrasound biometry: measurement of the anterior-chamber depth and axial length of the eye gives some indication of the risk of angle closure; an anterior-chamber depth of less than 2 mm is associated with a high risk of subsequent angle closure.

B-scan ultrasound biomicroscopy: this imaging technique allows a precise measurement of the width of the anterior-chamber angle and the relative positions of the iris root, angle structures and ciliary body.

Anterior segment OCT (optical coherence tomography): this is the most recently introduced option for imaging the anterior chamber and angle.

Complications

Angle-closure glaucoma: estimated lifetime risk is ~30% in patients with critically narrow angles.

Differential Diagnosis

Other conditions that may produce a narrow anterior-chamber angle on gonioscopy without elevated IOP or other signs of glaucoma include:
- Plateau iris configuration
- Phacomorphic angle narrowing: caused by a large lens
- Nanophthalmos
- Retinopathy of prematurity
- Subluxation of the lens
- Spherophakia.

Cause

Anatomically narrow angles result from the anatomy and configuration of the structures of the anterior segment of the eye. The eyes are smaller than average with a short axial length, shallow anterior chamber, small corneal diameter, anteriorly inserted iris root, and a normal or larger-than-normal crystalline lens. The result is an increase in the normal physiologic resistance to aqueous flow at the pupillary margin and a forward bowing and displacement of the peripheral iris toward the angle and peripheral cornea. The forward bowing of the iris may become great enough to cause the iris to adhere to the trabecular meshwork, obstruct the outflow of the aqueous, and cause angle-closure glaucoma (365.2).

Epidemiology

Population studies have found that anatomically narrow angles occur in 0.5–1.0% of the white and black American population. In some other ethnic groups (e.g. Koreans, North American Inuit), narrow angles are much more common.

Associated Features

- Hyperopia
- Small optic disks with very small or absent physiologic cups.

Diagnosis continued on p. 24

TREATMENT

Diet and Lifestyle

- Avoid drugs and activities that may dilate the pupil; such agents may provoke an attack of angle closure
- Many antihistamines and sympathomimetics found in proprietary cold and allergy medications should be avoided
- Phenothiazine and many other psychotropic drugs should be avoided
- Certain activities that cause the pupils to dilate, such as being in low-light situations (e.g. movie theater) or sexual intercourse, may cause pupillary dilation and angle-closure glaucoma in susceptible individuals.

Pharmacologic Treatment

Miotics

The use of miotics (e.g. pilocarpine) may reduce the risk of angle closure for a time. Studies have shown, however, that long-term use of pilocarpine does not prevent angle closure in high-risk individuals. With long-term use, miotics actually increase the likelihood of developing angle closure.

Treatment Aims

To widen the angle and eliminate the risk of angle closure

Prognosis

Studies have shown that the risk of angle closure in subjects with asymptomatic but very critically narrow angles is between 15% and 30%, a fairly high risk for a serious and potentially blinding disease. Many clinicians therefore advocate the use of prophylactic laser iridectomy in such patients, especially if pupil dilation is required regularly (e.g. diabetic patient at risk for retinopathy).

Follow-up and Management

Patients with critically narrowed angles should be advised of the risks and offered a laser iridectomy. Once an iridectomy has been done, the patient is no longer at risk for angle closure and may be followed as would any otherwise-normal individual. Patients who decline iridectomy should be advised of the symptoms of angle closure and instructed to seek medical attention immediately if any symptoms develop. In the absence of symptoms, patients declining iridectomy should be followed once or twice a year with gonioscopy and IOP measurements.

Treatment continued on p. 25

Anatomically Narrow Angle (365.02)

DIAGNOSIS—cont'd

Pearls and Considerations

- Anterior-chamber depth can be measured by ultrasound. A normal finding is generally ~3.5 mm. Anterior chambers less than or equal to 2.5 mm are considered at risk for angle closure
- Gonioscopy is contraindicated in patients with hyphema, compromised cornea or laceration of the globe
- Pilocarpine may result in severely blurred vision in patients with central lenticular opacities. A full ophthalmic examination should be performed to rule out such opacities before initiating pilocarpine therapy
- Pilocarpine should be used with caution in patients with cholelithiasis, biliary tract disease, cardiovascular disease, and pulmonary disease.

Referral Information

Referral should be considered for prophylactic peripheral iridotomy. Appropriate glaucoma workup should be obtained in patients with suspected acute or chronic angle-closure events; and in those with high IOP, referral for trabeculectomy or filtering surgery should be considered to lower pressure adequately.

TREATMENT—cont'd

Nonpharmacologic Treatment

Laser Iridectomy

Laser iridectomy is definitive treatment. By creating an alternative route for the aqueous from the posterior chamber to the anterior chamber, the relative pupil block and the forward bowing of the iris are eliminated. This allows the angle to widen and removes the risk of future angle closure. The treatment is almost 100% effective and very safe. Serious complications following laser iridectomy are extremely rare.

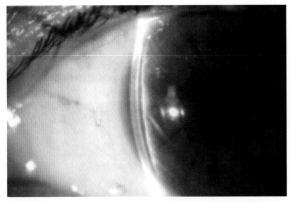

Fig. 1: Anatomically narrow angle. Van Herick test demonstrating shallow peripheral anterior chamber with the slit-lamp beam.

GENERAL REFERENCES

Alward WL. Color atlas of gonioscopy. London: Mosby-Year Book Europe; 1994.

Hom MM. Pilocarpine. Mosby's ocular drug consult. St Louis: Mosby-Elsevier; 2005. pp. 444-6.

Kasier PK, Friedman NJ. Angle closure glaucoma. The Massachusetts Eye and Ear Infirmary Illustrated Manual of Ophthalmology, 2nd edition. Philadelphia: Saunders-Elsevier; 2004. pp. 203-7.

Palmberg P. Gonioscopy. In: Ritch R, Shields MB, Krupin T (Eds). The Glaucomas, 2nd edition. St Louis: Mosby; 1996. pp. 455-69.

Panek WC, ChristEnsen RE, Lee DA, et al. Biometric variables in patients with occludable anterior chamber angles. Am J Ophthalmol. 1990;110:185-8.

Radhakrishnan S, See J, Smith SD, et al. Reproducibility of anterior chamber angle measurements obtained with anterior segment optical coherence tomography. Invest Ophthalmol Vis Sci. 2007;48(8): 3683-8.

Sawada A, Sakuma T, Yamamoto T, et al. Appositional angle closure in eyes with narrow angles: comparison between fellow eyes of acute angle-closure glaucoma and normotensive cases. J Glaucoma. 1997; 6:288-92.

Wilensky JT, Kaufman PL, Frohlichstein D, et al. Follow-up of angle-closure glaucoma suspects. Am J Ophthalmol. 1993; 115:338-46.

Wilensky JT, Ritch R, Kolker AE. Should patients with anatomically narrow angles have prophylactic iridectomy? Surv Ophthalmol. 1996;41:31-6.

Angioid Streaks (363.43)

DIAGNOSIS

Definition

Full-thickness breaks in calcified, thickened Bruch's membrane with disruption of overlying retinal pigment epithelium (RPE).

Synonyms

None

Symptoms

- Patients are usually asymptomatic in the early course
- Gradual decrease in vision: common with increase in age
- Loss of vision to legal blindness: seen in ~50% of patients
- Scotoma
- Metamorphosia.

Signs

- Radially oriented cracks in the pigment layer emanating from the optic nerve (*see* Fig. 1)
- "Peau d'orange" or mottled appearance of the RPE (*see* Fig. 2)
- Peripheral atrophic spots
- Disk drusen
- Subretinal crystalline deposits
- Subretinal hemorrhage: if associated with trauma or choroidal neovascularization
- Choroidal neovascular membrane (CNVM).

Investigations

Physical examination: to rule out systemic disorders, such as pseudoxanthoma elasticum (PXE), Ehlers-Danlos syndrome, Paget's disease and sickle cell disease.

Fluorescein angiogram: if choroidal neovascularization is suspected.

Serum alkaline phosphatase and urine calcium: if considering Paget's disease.

Sickle cell prep and hemoglobin electrophoresis: if considering sickle cell disease.

Complications

- High risk of subretinal bleeding secondary to blunt trauma
- Retinal pigment epithelium detachment
- Choroidal neovascularization
- Disciform scarring.

Differential Diagnosis

- Senile angioid streaks
- Choroidal rupture secondary to trauma
- Senile macular degeneration
- Idiopathic choroidal neovascularization
- Myopia with lacquer cracks
- Presumed ocular histoplasmosis.

Cause

- Idiopathic, 50%
- Pseudoxanthoma elasticum, 34%
- Paget's disease, 10%
- Sickle cell hemoglobinopathies, 6%
- Ehlers-Danlos syndrome
- Greenblad-Stranberg syndrome.

Epidemiology

- Fifty percent of patients with angioid streaks will have systemic associations.
- Eighty-five percent of patients with PXE have evidence of angioid streaks.
- Eight to fifteen percent of patients with Paget's disease have angioid streaks.

Associated Features

- Peau d'orange appearance
- Pseudoxanthoma elasticum "plucked-chicken skin" gastrointestinal tract bleeding, cardiac abnormalities.

Pathology

- Thickening, elastic degeneration, and calcification of Bruch's membrane
- Breaks in the elastic and collagenous layers of Bruch's membrane
- Fibrovascular ingrowth
- Secondary RPE atrophy, choriocapillaris damage, photoreceptor loss, RPE hypertrophy, serous retinal detachment, disciform scarring.

Diagnosis continued on p. 28

TREATMENT

Diet and Lifestyle

Safety glasses should be worn, because trauma precipitates hemorrhage.

Pharmacologic Treatment

A series of intravitreal anti-VEGF injections (Avastin or Lucentis) are performed if choroidal neovascularization is present. Due to the natural history of the RPE/Bruch's membrane pathology, patients do not experience as much visual improvement as seen in macular degeneration patients.

Treatment Aims

- To educate patients and detect secondary choroidal neovascularization early
- Low-vision aids may be useful
- Genetic counseling should be considered for hereditary conditions.

Prognosis

Long-term prognosis is guarded. Patients can lose vision to the level of legal blindness if the streaks involve the fovea or if secondary choroidal neovascularization in the fovea occurs.

Follow-up and Management

- Amsler grid testing daily
- Dilated fundus examination every 6 months.

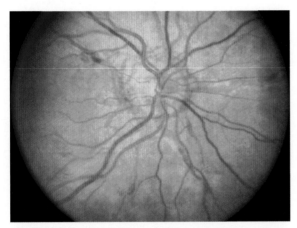

Fig. 1: An angioid streak is seen coursing radially from the disk into the inferior macula in a patient with pseudoxanthoma elasticum. The streak is grey and deep to the retina, in contrast to the normal red vessels within the inner retina.

Treatment continued on p. 29

Angioid Streaks (363.43)

DIAGNOSIS—cont'd

Pearls and Considerations

- In patients with angioid streaks, minor trauma can result in rupture of Bruch's membrane with resultant hemorrhage or choroidal neovascularization
- Patients with angioid streaks benefit from regular Amsler grid testing to monitor for visual changes associated with formation of CNVM
- The color of angioid streaks depends on natural fundus coloration and the amount of overlying RPE atrophy. Streaks appear red in blond fundi or medium to dark brown in more pigmented fundi.

Referral Information

- Patients who present with associated choroidal neovascularization should be referred for anti-VEGF injections (e.g. Avastin or Lucentis) or PDT as appropriate
- Patients identified with angioid streaks should have an appropriate medical referral to rule out underlying systemic disease. Evaluation should include skin biopsy and photographs
- Asymptomatic family members with inherited diseases such as pseudoxanthoma elasticum, may benefit from testing as well as monitoring for any ocular manifestations.

TREATMENT—cont'd

Nonpharmacologic Treatment

Amsler grid testing: for early detection of choroidal neovascularization.

Laser photocoagulation: of choroidal neovascularization.

- Thermal laser often causes further damage to the Bruch's/RPE complex, so it is no longer the treatment of choice even for extrafoveal lesions
- Prophylactic laser treatment should not be performed because it may induce choroidal neovascularization
- Photodynamic therapy (PDT) may be an option in certain cases, but it, too, can further damage the pigment epithelium and Bruch's membrane.

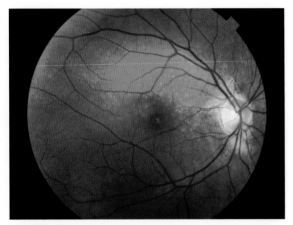

Fig. 2: Patient with pseudoxanthoma elasticum and "peau d'orange" appearance to the retinal pigment epithelium.

GENERAL REFERENCES

Abusamak M. (2005). Angioid streaks. [online]. Available from www.emedicine.com. [Accessed August, 2012].

Aessopos A, Famakis D, Loukopoulos D. Elastic tissue abnormalities resembling pseudoxanthoma elasticum in beta thalassemia and the sickling syndromes. Blood. 2002;99(1):30-5.

Atebara NH. Miscellaneous abnormalities of the fundus. In: Tasman W, et al. (Eds). Duane's Clinical Ophthalmology (CD-ROM). Philadelphia: Lippincott Williams & Wilkins; 2004.

Kaiser PK, Friedman NJ. Angiod streaks. The Massachusetts Eye and Ear Infirmary Illustrated Manual of Ophthalmology, 2nd edition. Philadelphia: Saunders-Elsevier; 2004. pp. 333-5.

Landy J, Brown GC. Update on photodynamic therapy. Curr Opin Ophthalmol. 2003;14(3):163-68.

Anterior Ischemic Optic Neuropathy, Arteritic (Giant Cell Arteritis, Temporal Arteritis) (377.30)

DIAGNOSIS

Definition

Ischemia of the anterior optic nerve head secondary to underlying systemic granulomatous vasculitis of the large- and medium-sized blood vessels; a sight-threatening medical emergency.

Synonyms

Giant cell arteritis (GCA), temporal arteritis; abbreviated as AAION.

Symptoms

Acute unilateral or bilateral blindness: 2–9 weeks after onset of headaches.
Premonitory amaurosis fugax: May present in 10% of patients.
Amaurosis: Induced by bright light.
Painful diplopia: May present in 6% of patients.

Systemic Symptoms

- Recent headache in temple, occipital region, neck, eye, or ear; jaw claudication; tongue pain and numbness; toothache; intermittent fevers; night sweats; anorexia, weight loss; malaise; depression
- Proximal muscle pain, myelopathy, polymyalgia rheumatica.

Note: Many patients may have no constitutional complaints and will present only with the eye sign (occult GCA).

Headache

- Headache is the initial manifestation of GCA in 50–90% of patients
- Head pain is a "different kind of headache" that can be severe and boring
- Headache is worse at night and with exposure to cold
- There is tenderness of the scalp overlying the greater superficial temporal arteries. These arteries may appear enlarged, nodular, and erythematous. Patients may complain of sensitivity when brushing hair or placing head on pillow because of scalp and temple tenderness.
- Pain may involve neck, face, jaw, tongue, ear, or throat. Jaw claudication and neck pain have a high specificity.

Signs

- Afferent pupillary defect (APD), if unilateral
- Anterior ischemic optic neuropathy (AION) with pallid disk swelling (Figs 1A and B), bilateral AION, central retinal artery occlusion (CRAO), branch retinal artery occlusion (rare), combined CRAO and AION, cilioretinal artery occlusion (combined with any of the above) (Figs 1A and B).
- Choroidal ischemia, infarcts of the nerve fiber layer, pupil-sparing third-nerve paresis, sixth- and seventh-nerve palsies, ischemic ocular syndrome.

Differential Diagnosis

- Idiopathic anterior ischemic optic neuropathy
- Acute angle-closure glaucoma
- Herpes zoster sine eruptione
- Aneurysm
- Temporomandibular joint syndrome
- Pituitary apoplexy
- Carotid artery dissection
- Wegener's granulomatosis
- Systemic cholesterol microembolization syndrome
- Carotid-cavernous fistula.

Cause

Autoimmune vasculitis of the elderly of unknown cause.

Epidemiology

- Overall incidence, 2.9:100,000; 50–59 years of age, 1.7:100,000; more than 80 years of age, 55.5:100,000.
- Mean age of presentation is 75 years with lower limit of 50 years.
- More common in white women; less common in black and Asian populations.

Associated Features

- Polymyalgia rheumatica. (Ret. 4)
- Giant cell arteritis may be the cause of death (myocardial infarction, dissecting aortic aneurysm, cerebral infarction).

Immunology

- An autoimmune syndrome develops from the immunologic response directed toward antigens residing in the wall of medium-sized arteries
- Genetic risk is supported by a sequence motif in the *HLA-DRBI* gene
- T lymphocytes undergoing clonal expansion have been demonstrated infiltrating the temporal artery wall
- A small number of tissue-infiltrating T cells produce interferon-γ, an important cytokine governing the disease process
- Circulating macrophages secrete interleukin-6, the major inducer of acute-phase reactants.

Pathology

- Active disease is characterized by fragmentation and destruction of the internal elastic lamina and inflammatory infiltrate in the vessel wall.
- Healed vasculitis shows a diffuse intimal thickening, intimal and medial fibrosis and fragmentation or loss of internal elastic lamina.

Diagnosis continued on p. 32

TREATMENT

Diet and Lifestyle

No special precautions are necessary.

Pharmacologic Treatment

- Protect the unaffected eye
- Patient should be hospitalized immediately and pulse steroids administered.

Standard Dosage

Solu-Medrol, 250 mg IV every 6 hour for 3 days, then oral prednisone, maximum of 60–80 mg/day.

Special Points

- After 1 month, taper by 5 mg/week using the patient's symptoms and ESR as a guide (< 20 mm/hr)
- Slow reduction to about 20 mg by 8th week is typical
- A maintenance dose of 10–15 mg may be needed for up to 2 years.

Other Drugs

Immunosuppressive drugs, including cyclophosphamide, methotrexate and azathioprine.

Note: There are no data to support a therapeutic advantage to immunosuppressive drugs.

Treatment Aims

- To preserve the vision in the remaining eye
- To prevent systemic complications of the disease, such as stroke.

Prognosis

- If left untreated, 30–40% of patients may go bilaterally blind, with the highest risk of vision loss within 10 days
- Despite treatment, 5–10% go blind
- Risk of vision loss remains high up to 2 months
- Vision loss after 4 months is unlikely
- A slight improvement with treatment occurs in 15–34%.

Follow-up and Management

- Because there is a 26% relapse rate in patients under age 2 years, these patients must be meticulously monitored
- Erythrocyte sedimentation rate and symptoms should decline with effective treatment.

Treatment continued on p. 33

DIAGNOSIS—cont'd

Investigations

- *Westergren erythrocyte age-adjusted sedimentation rate (ESR) of 47–107 mm/hr*: In about 9% of patients, ESR will be normal
- *C-reactive protein*: More than 2.45 mg/dL
- *Complete blood count*: Normochromic, normocytic anemia
- *Reactive thrombocytosis*
- *Fluorescein angiography*: With an abnormal choroidal filling time more than 18 seconds that carries a 93% sensitivity and a 94% specificity for GCA
- *Biopsy of greater superficial temporal artery (GSTA)*: Bilateral GSTA biopsies increase yield by 5–14%
- *Ocular pneumoplethysmography*.

Complications

Permanent bilateral visual loss (in 40% of patients), myocardial infarction, transient ischemic attacks, stroke.

Classification

1990 criteria for the classification of giant cell (temporal) arteritis:
- Age at disease onset more than or equal to 50 years
- New headache
- Temporal artery abnormality
- Elevated ESR
- Abnormal artery biopsy.

Note: If three of the five criteria are present, patient is said to have GCA.

Pearls and Considerations

- Temporal artery biopsy (TAB) remains the only confirmatory test for AAION
- On confirmation of AAION, high-dose corticosteroid treatment is mandatory
- High-dose corticosteroid therapy has a high incidence of undesirable side effects in this patient population because of advanced age and comorbidity. Complications of high-dose corticosteroid therapy include diabetes mellitus, hypertension, Cushing's syndrome, osteoporosis, muscle wasting, gastrointestinal disturbance, avascular necrosis of the femoral head and mental disturbances. Patients must be monitored for these side effects, and the beneficial effects of treatment must be balanced against the side effects.
- In general, the life expectancy of patients with GCA is reportedly similar to that of the general population; however, the risk for death from cardiovascular disease in the first year after diagnosis, if patient is inadequately treated, is significantly higher than in the general population.

Referral Information

- On presentation, refer to laboratory for complete blood workup and TAB
- On confirmation, refer for hospitalization and systemic treatment.

TREATMENT—cont'd

Nonpharmacologic Treatment

Trendelenburg's position: Patient is supine on the bed with the head tilted downward 30–40° and the bed is angulated beneath the knees.

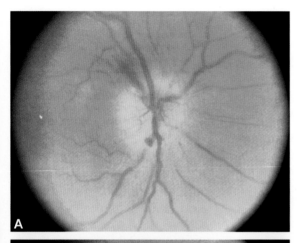

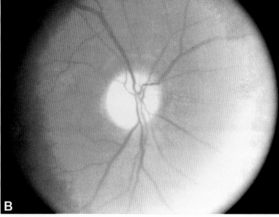

Figs 1A and B: (A) Arteritic anterior ischemic optic neuropathy. There is pallid swelling of a right optic disk with a flame-shaped hemorrhage. This 76-year-old patient had no constitutional signs or symptoms but had an ESR of 110 mm/hr and a positive temporal artery biopsy; (B) Optic atrophy 2 months later.

GENERAL REFERENCES

Diaz VA, DeBroff BM, Sinard J. Comparison of histopathologic features, clinical symptoms, and erythrocyte sedimentation rates in biopsy-positive temporal arteritis. Ophthalmology. 2005;112(7):1293-8.

Hunder GG, Bloch DA, Michel BA, et al. The American College of Rheumatology 1990 criteria for the classification of giant cell arteritis. Arthritis Rheum. 1990;33:1122-8.

Niederkohr RD, Levin LA. Management of the patient with suspected temporal arteritis: a decision-analytic approach. Ophthalmology. 2005;112(5):744-56.

Nordborg E, Nordborg C. Giant cell arteritis: strategies in diagnosis and treatment. Curr Opin Rheumatol. 2004;16(1):25-30.

Rahman W, Rahman FZ. Giant cell (temporal) arteritis: an overview and update. Surv Ophthalmol. 2005;50:415-28.

Salvarani C, Cantini F, Boiardi L, et al. Polymyalgia rheumatica. Best Pract Res Clin Rheumatol. 2004;18(5):705-22.

Anterior Ischemic Optic Neuropathy, Nonarteritic (Idiopathic) (377.41)

DIAGNOSIS

Definition

Ischemia of the anterior optic nerve head caused by underlying vasculopathy or disruption of blood flow within the optic nerve head and often associated with hypertension and diabetes.

Synonyms

None; abbreviated NAION.

Symptoms

Acute (hours) and subacute (days) monocular visual loss: May worsen over weeks; visual nadir is ~3–4 days.

Bilateral NAION: Extremely unusual and suggests an alternative diagnosis.

The patient usually has no pain and often notices the condition on awakening in the morning.

Signs

- *Hyperemic, edematous optic nerve head*: With segmental infarction, flame-shaped hemorrhages, and luxury perfusion (Fig. 1)
- Small optic disk without a physiologic cup
- Relative afferent pupillary defect
- Inferior altitudinal, inferior nasal, or central scotoma
- *Vision better than 20/200*: In ~50% of patients.

Investigations

- Blood pressure measurement
- Westergren erythrocyte sedimentation rate (ESR)
- C-reactive protein
- Complete blood count
- Fluorescein angiography
- Biopsy of greater superficial temporal artery (GSTA).

Pearls and Considerations

- Clinical features that help differentiate NAION from AAION include a relatively younger age at onset, less severe vision loss, and relatively little or no reported pain with NAION
- Full clinical workup is still indicated to rule out the arteritic form of the disease.

Referral Information

Referral to laboratory for full clinical workup, including blood tests and temporal artery biopsy.

Differential Diagnosis

- Giant cell arteritis
- Papillitis.

Cause

- Unknown, but thought to result from the occlusion of posterior ciliary arteries providing the laminar, prelaminar, and retrolaminar blood supply to the optic nerve.
- Risk factors include hypertension; diabetes mellitus; cigarette smoking; and elevated fibrinogen, cholesterol and triglyceride levels.

Associated Features

- Systemic hypertension (35–50% of patients)
- Nocturnal arterial hypotension (10–25% of patients)
- Favism
- Diabetes mellitus
- Systemic vasculitis
- Migraine
- After cataract extraction (within 2 weeks)
- Elevated intraocular pressure
- Coagulopathies (e.g. anticardiolipin antibody syndrome, protein S and protein C deficiencies)
- Acute blood loss, anemia, hypotension.

Pathology

Unknown

TREATMENT

Diet and Lifestyle

- Patients should stop smoking
- If patient takes blood pressure medication at bedtime, consider different medication schedule.

Pharmacologic Treatment

Although controversial, aspirin may offer a short-term benefit (1–2 year) in reducing the incidence of second-eye NAION. Long-term benefit (5 years) has not been established.

Nonpharmacologic Treatment

No nonpharmacologic treatment is recommended.

Other Treatments

Optic nerve fenestration has been shown ineffective in treating patients and produces a poorer visual outcome than the natural course of the disease.

Treatment Aims

To treat the underlying vasculopathy; if none present, no treatment will be effective.

Prognosis

- Approximately 24% of patients will have a significant improvement in visual acuity and visual field
- There is less than 5% chance of recurrence in the same eye
- There is a 25–50% chance that the fellow eye will be involved within 5 years
- No concrete relationship has been established between NAION and cerebrovascular disease.

Follow-up and Management

Serial testing of visual fields should be performed over 12 months to monitor improvement.

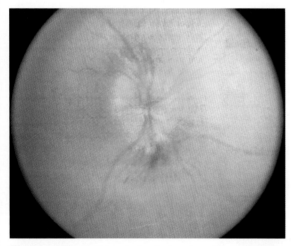

Fig. 1: Nonarteritic anterior ischemic optic neuropathy (NAION) of right eye in 60-year-old woman with hypertension. There is diffuse disk edema and flame-shaped hemorrhages at the 6 and 12 o'clock positions. Note the absence of a physiologic cup.

GENERAL REFERENCES

Hayreh SS. Posterior ischaemic optic neuropathy: clinical features, pathogenesis, and management. Eye (Lond). 2004;18(11):1188-206.

Rucker JC, Biousse V, Newman NJ. Ischemic optic neuropathies. Curr Opin Neurol. 2004;17(1):27-35.

Yanoff M, Duker J. Ophthalmology, 2nd edition. St Louis: Elsevier; 2003.

Anterior Uveitis: Iritis (Acute 364.0, Chronic 364.1), Iridocyclitis (Acute 364.0, Chronic 364.1)

DIAGNOSIS

Definition

Inflammation of the uveal tract.

Synonyms

Iritis, uveitis, pars planitis.

Symptoms

- Pain
- Redness
- Photophobia
- Increased lacrimation
- Blurry vision.

Note: Pain, decreased vision, and redness may be minimal in subacute cases.

Signs

Acute

- Ciliary injection of conjunctiva (hyperemia around limbus), posterior synechiae, iris bombé; shallow anterior chamber (Fig. 1)
- Fine to large keratic precipitates (granulomatous) and fibrin dusting of corneal endothelium
- Anterior chamber shows many cells, variable flare, and in rare cases, a hypopyon
- Dilated iris vessels and rarely a hyphema
- Posterior synechiae (adhesion of pupillary iris to lens)
- Iris nodules
- Anterior vitreous cells
- Cystoid macular edema and rarely a disk edema; peripheral anterior synechiae on gonioscopy
- Low intraocular pressure (IOP) (low aqueous production): With cyclitis
- *High IOP*: Trabeculitis or obstruction of trabecular meshwork by inflammatory debris; partial or complete pupillary block caused by posterior synechiae.

Chronic

- Variable conjunctival redness as well as anterior-chamber reaction
- Secluded/occluded pupil.

Differential Diagnosis

- Rhegmatogenous retinal detachment (pigment cells in the anterior chamber)
- Leukemia
- *Retinoblastoma*: In children
- Intraocular foreign body
- Malignant melanoma
- Juvenile xanthogranuloma.

Cause

- *Idiopathic*: Most common
- *HLA-B27*–positive iridocyclitis
- Juvenile rheumatoid arthritis [most cases pauciarticular or oligoarticular arthritis, rheumatoid factor (−), ANA (+), young girls].
- Fuchs' heterochromic iridocyclitis
- Herpes simplex keratouveitis
- Syphilis
- Traumatic, sarcoid, and tuberculosis iridocyclitis.

Associated Features

Iris heterochromia, corneal band keratopathy.

Immunology

Mostly type III hypersensitivity reaction, but also type II.

Pathology

Neutrophils, eosinophils, and lymphocytes in anterior chamber and on corneal endothelial and iris surfaces: large keratic precipitates and iris nodules are granulomas.

Diagnosis continued on p. 38

TREATMENT

Diet and Lifestyle

No special precautions are necessary.

Pharmacologic Treatment

Cycloplegia

Standard dosage:

- Cyclopentolate 1–2%, three times daily for mild to moderate inflammation
- Atropine 1%, two or three times daily for moderate to severe inflammation
- Prednisolone acetate 1%, every 1–6 hours.

Special points:

- Consider subtenons injection of steroid or systemic steroid if patient unresponsive to topical therapy
- Treat secondary glaucoma with topical antiglaucoma medication
- If an infectious cause is determined, the specific management should be added to the above regimen
- Consider a rheumatology consult.

Treatment Aims

To lessen or obviate inflammatory response in anterior chamber and anterior vitreous.

Other Treatments

Other immunosuppressive therapy may be necessary to control inflammation.

Prognosis

- Prognosis is usually good with therapy
- There is a high complication rate with cataract surgery in patients with juvenile rheumatoid arthritis but not with Fuchs' heterochromic iridocyclitis.
- Patients with sarcoid, tuberculosis (TB), and syphilis do well with appropriate therapy.
- Make sure anti-TB systemic treatment is addressed before initiating prednisone.

Follow-up and Management

- Patients should be followed every 1–7 days in the acute phase and every 1–6 months when stable. Complete ocular examination should be performed at each visit.
- If the anterior-chamber reaction is improving, the steroid should be tapered slowly. In some patients, chronic low-dose steroids may be needed to prevent recurrence.

Treatment continued on p. 39

DIAGNOSIS—cont'd

Investigations

- *Histories*: Onset and duration of symptoms, systems review (especially of arthritic, gastrointestinal, and genitourinary disorders), insect bite, rash, sexual, drug, family back disorders (e.g. ankylosing spondylitis).
- Visual acuity testing
- Slit-lamp examination (SLE)
- IOP
- Dilated fundus examination
- If uveitis is bilateral, granulomatous, associated with positive review of systems, poorly responsive to usual dose of topical steroids, significant flare, or recurrent: complete blood count, erythrocyte sedimentation rate (ESR), antinuclear antibody (ANA), rapid plasma reagin, Lyme disease titers, angiotensin-converting enzyme (ACE), fluorescent treponemal antibody (FTA) absorption, purified protein derivative (PPD, tuberculin) with anergy panel. Obtain a chest radiograph and *HLA-B27*.

Complications

- Cataract
- Glaucoma
- Corneal edema
- Cystoid macular edema.

Classification

Acute: Signs and symptoms appear suddenly and last for up to 6 weeks.

Chronic: Onset is gradual, and inflammation lasts longer than 6 weeks.

Granulomatous: Insidious onset; chronic course; eye almost white; iris nodules and large keratic precipitates (mutton fat) present; posterior segment often involved.

Nongranulomatous: Acute onset; shorter course; red eye and intense flare present; no iris nodules.

Infectious: Viruses, bacteria, rickettsiae, fungi, protozoa, parasites.

Noninfectious: Exogenous (trauma, chemical injury), endogenous (immunologic types 1–4 hypersensitivities).

Pearls and Considerations

- On second presentation of idiopathic iridocyclitis, patients should be referred for full systemic workup
- Anterior-chamber cells and flare are best observed at SLE, with a bright conic section and room lights very dim.

Referral Information

See Pearls and Considerations.

TREATMENT—cont'd

Nonpharmacologic Treatment

Glaucoma surgery (e.g. tube-shunt devices): To control IOP.

Cataract surgery: Usually not undertaken until the eye is quiet for at least 6 months.

Laser peripheral iridectomy: For posterior synechiae with iris bombé to prevent acute angle-closure glaucoma (AACG). Multiple iridectomies may be needed because they can close by inflammation.

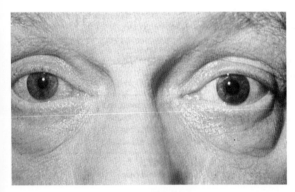

Fig. 1: Injected conjunctiva and constricted pupil of right eye in patient with acute iritis.

GENERAL REFERENCES

Albert DM, Jakobiec FA (Eds). Principles and Practice of Ophthalmology, vol I. Philadelphia: WB Saunders; 1994.

American Academy of Ophthalmology. Basic and Clinical Science. San Francisco: American Academy of Ophthalmology; 1994-1995.

Menezo V, Lightman S. The development of complications in patients with chronic anterior uveitis. Am J Ophthalmol. 2005; 139(6):988-92.

Monnet D, Breban M, Hudry C, et al. Ophthalmic findings and frequency of extraocular manifestations in patients with HLA-B27 uveitis: a study of 175 cases. Ophthalmology. 2004;111(4):802-9.

Smith JR. HLA-B27-associated uveitis. Ophthalmol Clin North Am. 2002;15(3): 297-307.

Wright K. Textbook of ophthalmology. Baltimore: Lippincott Williams & Wilkins; 1997.

Asteroid Hyalosis and Synchisis Scintillans (379.22)

DIAGNOSIS

Definition

Asteroid Hyalosis

White refractile crystals composed of calcium soaps that float in the vitreous and do not settle with gravity.

Synchisis Scintillans

Brown refractile crystals composed of cholesterol that float in the vitreous and do settle with gravity.

Synonyms

None

Symptoms

* Patients are usually asymptomatic
* Floaters.

Signs

Asteroid Hyalosis

* Small, white refractile particles made up of calcium soap; float in the vitreous; do not settle with gravity (*see* Fig. 1)
* Monocularity in 75% of cases
* Asteroid hyalosis occurs more often in diabetic patients.

Synchisis Scintillans

Numerous yellow-white or gold particles made up of cholesterol; located in the vitreous and anterior chamber; settle to the bottom of the eye with gravity (*see* Fig. 2).

Investigations

Asteroid Hyalosis

Fluorescein angiogram can be performed to view the macula clearly if patients present with decreased vision and if the view of the posterior pole is obscured by the asteroid.

Synchisis Scintillans

Careful history to determine if there was previous surgery or trauma to the eye.

Pearls and Considerations

* Asteroid hyalosis has no clinical association, whereas synchisis scintillans is often found after vitreous hemorrhage, uveitis or trauma
* Color fundus photography gives a poor view of the retina, but fluorescein angiography gives an excellent view of the retina due to the fact that the light is being emitted from the fluorescein in the blood vessels rather than being reflected from the retina back to the camera.

Referral Information

None

Differential Diagnosis

* Past vitreous hemorrhage
* Uveitis
* Pigment floating in the vitreous.

Causes

Asteroid Hyalosis

* An innocuous degenerative disease of unknown origin
* Usually diagnosed in patients more than 60 years of age.

Synchisis Scintillans

History of severe, accidental, or surgical trauma associated with a large intraocular hemorrhage

Epidemiology

Asteroid hyalosis

* More common in older individuals
* Overall incidence, 1:200

Associated Features

Synchisis Scintillans

Posterior vitreous detachment; this often allows the crystals to settle interiorly.

Pathology

Asteroid Hyalosis

Calcium and lipid particles ranging from 0.01–0.10 mm in diameter

Synchisis Scintillans

Cholesterol particles

TREATMENT

Diet and Lifestyle

Asteroid Hyalosis

No special precautions are necessary.

Synchisis Scintillans

Safety glasses should be worn to protect the better eye.

Pharmacologic Treatment

None

Nonpharmacologic Treatment

- Treatment is generally not indicated unless an unrelated cause of decreased vision must be treated, in which case a pars plana vitrectomy should be performed to clear out the vitreous cavity.
- Conditions often associated with the need for vitrectomy include diabetic macular edema and choroidal neovascularization.

Prognosis

Asteroid Hyalosis

Good, because it is asymptomatic and does not affect vision.

Synchisis Scintillans

Good, but often associated with trauma or inflammation; in such patients, vision may be decreased from structural changes to the eye caused by the trauma or inflammation, in addition to the cholesterol found in the vitreous cavity.

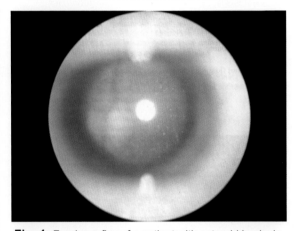

Fig. 1: Fundus reflex of a patient with asteroid hyalosis.

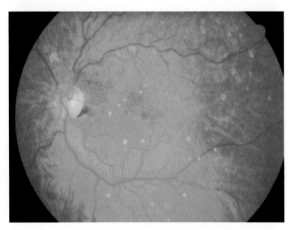

Fig. 2: Small, round, yellow dots floating in the vitreous in a patient with diabetic retinopathy.

GENERAL REFERENCES

Yazar Z, Hanioglu S, Karakoc G, et al. Asteroid hyalosis. Eur J Ophthalmol. 2001;11(1):57-61.

Kaider PK, Friedman NJ. Synchysis scintillans. The Massachusetts Eye and Ear Infirmary Illustrated Ophthalmology, 2nd edition, Philadelphia: Saunders; 2004. p. 287.

Spraul CW, Grossniklaus HE. Vitreous hemorrhage, Surv Ophthalmol. 1997;421 (1):3-39.

Mitchell P, Wang MY, Wang JJ. Asteroid hyalosis in an older population: the Blue Mountain Eye Study. Ophthalmic Epidemiol. 2003;10(5):331-5.

Komatsu H, Kamura Y, Ishi K, et al. Fine structure and morphogenesis of asteroid hyalosis, Med Electron Microscopy. 2003;36(2):112-9.

Bacterial Endophthalmitis (360.0)

DIAGNOSIS

Definition

An intraocular infection caused by microbial organisms.

Synonyms

None

Symptoms

- Rapid visual loss
- Pain (usually an ache, as opposed to a foreign body sensation)
- Redness
- Tearing.

Signs

- Conjunctival injection
- Chemosis
- Hypopyon
- Severe vitritis.

Investigations

- Careful measurement of visual acuity
- Full slit-lamp and dilated eye examinations
- *Gonioscopy*: to look for a microhypopyon
- *B-scan ultrasound*: if the view of the vitreous and retina is obscured by the anterior-chamber inflammation (Check for vitreous opacities)
- *Gram stain, culture, and sensitivity*: both the anterior-chamber fluid and the vitreous fluid.

Complications

- Loss of vision
- Secondary retinal detachment
- *Loss of the eye*: if severe pain or phthisis develops.

Classification

- Endogenous bacterial endophthalmitis (usually acute or subacute)
- Exogenous bacterial endophthalmitis (usually acute or subacute)
- Fungal endophthalmitis (usually chronic).

Differential Diagnosis

- Sterile endophthalmitis
- Panuveitis
- Viral retinitis (e.g. acute retinal necrosis)

Cause

Exogenous after Intraocular Surgery

Occurs after any type of eye surgery; patients usually present 48–72 hours after initial surgery with complaints of pain and decreased vision; common organisms include *Staphylococcus epidermidis* (most common) and *S. aureus. Streptococcus pneumoniae* and *Haemophilus influenzae* occur more often after filtering blebs; *Propionibacterium acnes* infection presents as a persistent low-grade anterior uveitis with white plaques on the posterior capsule (*see* Fig. 1).

Endogenous Endophthalmitis

Systemic infection seeds the eye; patient workup for endocarditis; can also occur in patients with indwelling catheters; immunocompromised patients are at higher risk.

Post-traumatic Endophthalmitis

Can follow penetrating eye injuries; it is important to rule out retained intraocular foreign bodies; more serious pathogens, such as *Bacillus cereus* or a polymicrobial inoculum, can occur in rural settings.

Endogenous Fungal Endophthalmitis

Usually secondary to indwelling catheters and long-term parenteral nutrition; patients are often immunocompromised and usually present with gradual decrease in vision and increasing floater formation; most common organism is *Candida albicans*. Less common forms (e.g. *Aspergillus, Cryptococcus*, and *Fusarium* spp.) are seen in severely immunosuppressed patients.

Diagnosis continued on p. 44

TREATMENT

Diet and Lifestyle

No precautions are necessary.

Pharmacologic Treatment

For Endogenous Endophthalmitis

Systemic antibiotic therapy will usually be sufficient treatment for bacterial and fungal organisms.

For Exogenous Endophthalmitis

Topical fortified antibiotics (e.g. ancef, vancomycin, aminoglycoside); once response to antibiotics evident, administer steroids and cycloplegics (e.g. atropine).

Inject intravitreal antibiotics tailored to the organism involved. Most patients receive combination therapy (e.g. vancomycin and amikacin with or without steroids) at the time of diagnosis to cover both Gram-positive and Gram-negative organisms until the Gram stain and cultures are available. Additional intravitreal injections may be necessary for more virulent strains or fungi. One exception is the treatment for *Propionibacterium acnes*. Patients require clindamycin intravitreally, and often the capsular bag must be removed to eradicate the infection.

Treatment Aims

- To eradicate the infection
- To decrease inflammation
- To restore vision

Prognosis

Visual prognosis is poor even with prompt treatment.

Follow-up and Management

- Once the diagnosis of endophthalmitis has been made and treatment instituted, patients need to be followed daily, looking for improvement, a poor response to the chosen antibiotics, or a secondary complication of retinal detachment.
- Once culture results have provided sensitivity information on which antibiotics are effective in treating the offending organism, the antibiotic therapy may have to be augmented or changed.
- Virulent Gram-negative organisms may need repeated intravitreal antibiotic injections within 48 hours of the initial therapy.
- Subjectively, a decrease in pain usually correlates with response to treatment, even though ocular examination may not change initially.

Treatment continued on p. 45

Bacterial Endophthalmitis (360.0)

DIAGNOSIS—cont'd

Pearls and Considerations

- Endophthalmitis is considered a sight-threatening ophthalmic emergency
- Infection rarely spreads outside the confines of the sclera to surrounding tissue
- The endophthalmitis vitrectomy study (EVS) determined that up to one quarter of patients did not initially report pain with endophthalmitis. Rather, the nearly universal presenting symptom was *blurred vision*. This should therefore be considered a critical symptom when triaging postcataract patients.

Referral Information

A patient with endophthalmitis should be referred immediately to a vitreoretinal surgeon.

Epidemiology

- Postoperative exogenous endophthalmitis occurs in 0.04% of patients after cataract extraction.
- A reported 10.7% of patients with intraocular foreign bodies will develop endophthalmitis.
  - The incidence of *Candida* endophthalmitis in association with documented candidemia is reported at 9%.
  - The incidence of endophthalmitis following intravitreal injections has been reported as low as 0.02%.

Pathology

Polymorphonuclear leukocytic infiltration into the involved tissues

TREATMENT—cont'd

Nonpharmacologic Treatment

Pars plana vitrectomy may be necessary if: (1) the patient presents with vision worse than hand motions (HM); (2) there is evidence of retinal detachment; or (3) if the patient is getting worse after initial intravitreal antibiotic therapy. Follow EVS guidelines:

- *If visual acuity (VA) light perception (LP) or worse*: vitrectomy + intravitreal antibiotics
- *If VA HM or better*: vitreous tap + intravitreal antibiotics.

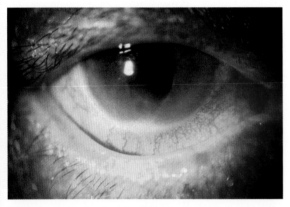

Fig. 1: Patient who developed endophthalmitis after glaucoma filtering surgery. Note the conjunctival injection and the layered hypopyon in the anterior chamber.

GENERAL REFERENCES

Bialasiewicz AA. Therapeutic indications for local anti-infectives: bacterial infections of the eye. Dev Ophthalmol. 2002;33:243-9.

Das T, Sharma S. Current management strategies of acute post-operative endophthalmitis. Semin Ophthalmol. 2003;18(3): 109-15.

Donahue SP, Greven CM, Zuravleff JJ, et al. Intraocular candidiasis in patients with candidemia: clinical implications derived from a prospective multicentered study. Ophthalmology. 1994;101:1302-9.

Endophthalmitis Vitrectomy Study Group. Results of the Endophthalmitis Vitrectomy Study: a randomized trial of immediate vitrectomy and of intravenous antibiotics for the treatment of postoperative bacterial endophthalmitis. Arch Ophthalmol. 1995;113:1479-96.

Fintak DR, Shah GK, Blinder KJ, et al. Incidence of endophthalmitis related to intravitreal injection of bevacizumab and ranibizumab. Retina. 2008;28(10):1395-9.

Flynn HW, Scott IU, Brod RD, et al. Current management of endophthalmitis. Int Ophthalmol Clin. 2004; 44(4):115-37.

Graham RH, Wong DT, Lakosha H. (2006). Bacterial endophthalmitis; [Online]. Available from www.emedicine.com.

Jackson TL, Eykyn SJ, Graham EM, et al. Endogenous bacterial endophthalmitis: a 17-year prospective series and review of 267 reported cases. Surv Ophthalmol. 2003;48(4):403-23.

Kowalski RP, Dhaliwal DK. Ocular bacterial infections: current and future treatment options. Expert Rev Antiinfect Ther. 2005;3(1):131-9.

Miller JJ, Scott IU, Flynn HW, et al. Acute-onset endophthalmitis following cataract surgery (2000–2004): incidence, clinical settings, and visual acuity outcomes after treatment. Am J Ophthalmol. 2005; 139(6):983-7.

DIAGNOSIS

Definition
Failure of the eyes to work together efficiently for any reason, including extraocular muscle imbalance, accommodative insufficiency, and anisometropia.

Synonyms
"Lazy eye," "crossed eyes," "walleyed," and "double vision".

Symptoms
- *Diplopia*: perception that an object is located in two different positions in space
- *Visual confusion*: perceptions that two objects are located in the same position in space
- *Asthenopia*: visual discomfort—can be caused by diplopia and visual confusion
- *Suppression*: creating an absolute scotoma under binocular viewing to prevent diplopia for the object of the fixating eye
- *Abnormal retinal correspondence (ARC)*: reordering of visual cortical directional values to prevent sensations of diplopia and visual confusion for peripheral objects
- *Convergence insufficiency*: inability to converge the eyes smoothly and effectively from distance to near.

Signs
- Squinting and rubbing of the eyes (possible asthenopia)
- Visual comfort in a patient with strabismus (possible suppression and ARC)
- Headaches and difficulty reading.

Investigations
- *Sensory test*: determining the presence or absence of sensory adaptations to strabismus in patients who developed strabismus before age 7
- *Motor test*: determining eye alignment
- Measuring near point of convergence and ability to maintain near fixation.

Complications
- Suppression and ARC prevent stereopsis, and if the resulting scotoma is large enough, it may prevent monocular input from the strabismic eye
- Diplopia and visual confusion cause difficulty locating objects in space, especially when acuity is similar in each eye. This may result in difficulty walking, driving, and reading.

Pearls and Considerations
Topic too broad for specific recommendations.

Commonly Associated Conditions
Strabismus is commonly associated with disorders of binocular vision, but the eye misalignment may be so small as to be undetectable except by careful sensory and motor tests.

Referral Information
Varies depending on the etiology of the binocular vision disorder.

Differential Diagnosis
Monocular diplopia can occur in patients with cataracts, corneal lesions, or other media abnormalities. These patients do not have strabismus, and the diplopia persist when the other eye is covered. This may be obviated by viewing through a pinhole or by bringing a card up from below until if covers one of the images.

Cause
- Diplopia and visual confusion are caused by sensory inputs from eyes that do not have the same visual directions.
- The adaptations of suppression and ARC occur spontaneously in patients who initially develop strabismus before age 7. Suppression is caused by a cordial phenomenon in which the retinal locus [on which falls the foveae image in the other (straight) eye] is not viewed. The suppression scotoma is absolute and facultative (it exists only under binocular viewing conditions). ARC is a cortical phenomenon in which peripheral directional values arising in the strabismus eye are altered. This prevents peripheral diplopia and visual confusion.

Epidemiology
- Sensory adaptations of suppression and ARC occur in children who initially develop strabismus before 7–9 years of age.
- Diplopia and visual confusion occur in older children and adults who initially develop strabismus after 7–9 years of age.

Associated Features
Strabismus is associated with disorders of binocular vision, but the eye misalignment may be so small as to be undetectable except by careful sensory and motor tests.

TREATMENT

Diet and Lifestyle

No special precautions are necessary.

Pharmacologic Treatment

No pharmacologic treatment is recommended.

Nonpharmacologic Treatment

- Orthoptic therapy/computer orthoptics
- Pencil push-ups/accommodative target therapy
- Alignment of the visual axis in strabismic eyes will treat diplopia and visual confusion. Children will revert to normal retinal correspondence, and suppression will disappear over time
- Treatment may require glasses, fusional training exercises, prisms, or surgery.

Treatment Aims

In Adults
- To ensure disappearance of diplopia and visual confusion
- To recover peripheral fusion and stereopsis.

In Children
- To achieve normal retinal correspondence
- To recover peripheral fusion and stereopsis.

Prognosis

- Sensory cure prognosis is better in younger children and worse in older adults. It is also likely better in patients who are not neurologically impaired.
- The duration of time in which the eyes were strabismic and whether this change was constant will also affect prognosis.
- Adults with diplopia and visual confusion may learn over time to ignore the displaced image. It is often less distinct than the image seen by the fixating eye.

Follow-up and Management

Please refer "Nonpharmacologic Treatment".

GENERAL REFERENCES

Burian HM. The sensorial retinal relationships in comitant strabismus. Arch Ophthalmol. 1947;37:336-40.

Diamond G. Strabismus and pediatric ophthalmology. In: Yanoff M, Podos S (Eds). Textbook of Ophthalmology, vol. 5. London: Mosby-Wolfe; 1993.

Huang CB, Zhou J, Lu ZL, et al. Deficient binocular combination reveals mechanisms of anisometropic amblyopia: signal attenuation and intraocular inhibition. J Vis. 2011;11(6). pii: 4. doi:10.1167/11.6.4.

Jampolsky A. Characteristics of suppression in strabismus. Arch Ophthalmol. 1947;37:336-40.

Parks MM. Stereoacuity as an indicator of bifixation. In: Knapp P (Ed). Strabismus Symposium. New York: Karger; 1968. pp. 361-4.

Travers T. Suppression of vision in squint and its association with retinal correspondence and amblyopia. Br J Ophthalmol. 1938;22:557-604.

Wensveen JM, Smith EL, Hung LF, et al. Brief daily periods of unrestricted vision preserve stereopsis in strabismus. Invest Ophthalmol Vis Sci. 2011;52(7):4872-9.

Blepharitis (373.0) and Blepharoconjunctivitis (372.2)

DIAGNOSIS

Definition

Blepharitis: A family of inflammatory processes of the eyelids.

Blepharoconjunctivitis: Inflammation of the conjunctiva secondary to blepharitis.

Synonyms

None

Symptoms

- Itching, burning, tearing
- Mild pain
- Foreign body sensation
- Crusting around the eyes on awakening.

Signs (Figs 1A and B)

- Crusty, red, thickened eyelid margins with prominent blood vessels
- Inspissated oil gland at the eyelid margins (meibomianitis)
- Conjunctival injection with papillary reaction and/or papillofollicular reaction
- Swollen eyelids
- Mild mucus discharge
- Superficial punctate keratitis (SPK), marginal infiltrates
- *Phlyctenules*: Elevated milky whitish nodules on the conjunctiva or rarely the cornea.

Investigations

- *History*: Chronic history of eye irritation, often worse in the morning
- *Complete external examination*: Noting health of the periorbital region and facial skin [e.g. telangiectasia and rhinophyma (acne rosacea), scaling (seborrhea), vesicles (herpes simplex or zoster), umbilicated nodules (molluscum contagiosum)]
- *Visual acuity test*: May be decreased because of tear-film abnormalities and SPK
- Intraocular pressure (IOP)
- *Slit-lamp examination*: Eyelash debris and collerates (flat crusted rings surrounding the eyelash base) may be seen in infectious blepharitis
- *Dilated fundus examination*: Usually normal
- For persistent inflammation despite therapy, consider swab culture of the eyelids and conjunctiva.

Complications

- Corneal pannus and scarring
- *Peripheral keratitis*: Occurs more often with bacterial infection
- *Phlyctenule*: Often related to *Staphylococcus aureus*.

Pearls and Considerations

Long-term use of topical steroid may result in steroid-related complications such as cataract or elevated IOP because of the potential for corneal penetration. Patients should be closely monitored for such complications.

Referral Information

Referral not required in most cases. Consider referral to dermatologist for underlying rosacea or other skin disease.

Differential Diagnosis

- Preseptal cellulitis
- Sebaceous gland carcinoma
- Discoid lupus.

Cause and Classification

Infectious

- Bacterial (*Staphylococcus aureus, S. epidermidis, Streptococcus pneumoniae, Haemophilus influenzae, Moraxella lacunata*).
- Viral (herpes simplex, herpes zoster, molluscum contagiosum).

Noninfectious

- Acne rosacea
- Eczema
- Seborrhea
- Meibomian gland dysfunction.

TREATMENT

Diet and Lifestyle

- Lid hygiene is crucial in the treatment and prevention of blepharitis and blepharoconjunctivitis
- Scrub the eyelid margins twice daily with mild shampoo on a cotton-tipped applicator
- Apply warm compresses for 15 minutes two to four times daily; most effective when used before eyelid scrubs.

Pharmacologic Treatment

For Bacterial and Seborrheic Blepharitis

- Administer artificial tears four to eight times daily
- Apply topical antibiotic ointment (erythromycin, bacitracin, gentamicin, or sulfacetamide) to the eyelids two or three times daily. Seborrheic blepharitis may have an infectious component
- If significant inflammatory component, consider topical corticosteroid (loteprednol or fluorometholone) three or four times daily with rapid taper, and/or topical cyclosporine 0.05% twice daily
- Consider systemic treatment (especially when seen with rosacea) with doxycycline, 100–200 mg daily.

For Herpetic Blepharitis and Conjunctivitis

Standard dosage

Trifluridine 1% solution, five times daily.

Special points

Chronic trifluridine therapy may produce a toxic superficial keratitis and conjunctivitis. May apply topical antibiotic ointment on the skin lesions to prevent bacterial superinfection (erythromycin or bacitracin ophthalmic ointment).

For Recurrent Meibomianitis

Standard dosage

- Doxycycline, 100 mg PO daily or twice daily
- Tetracycline, 250 mg PO four times daily.

Contraindications

Pregnancy; can be deposited in a fetus' growing teeth, discoloring them.

Special points

Patients taking doxycycline or tetracycline may develop skin photosensitivity and should avoid skin sun exposure.

Nonpharmacologic Treatment

No nonpharmacologic treatment is recommended.

Treatment Aims
- To reduce bacterial count
- To prevent corneal complications (pannus, scarring).

Prognosis
- Patients do well with appropriate therapy
- Lid hygiene and chronic therapy are often necessary to maintain ocular health.

Follow-up and Management

Every 3–4 weeks as needed; if steroid is being used, need to follow up every 2 weeks to monitor IOP.

GENERAL REFERENCES

Albert DM, Jakobiec FA (Eds). Principles and practice of ophthalmology, vol I. Philadelphia: WB Saunders; 2000.

American Academy of Ophthalmology. Basic and Clinical Science. San Francisco: The Academy; 2006- 2007.

Wright K. Textbook of ophthalmology. Baltimore: Williams & Wilkins; 1997.

Blepharophimosis Syndrome (374.46)

DIAGNOSIS

Definition

Severe, bilateral ptosis with poor levator function in which the palpebral fissures are horizontally shortened (blepharophimosis) with resulting telecanthus (increased distance between the medial canthi of the eyes).

Synonyms

None

Symptoms

Chin-up posture with severe ptosis

Signs (Figs 1A and B)

- Bilateral telecanthus
- Ptosis
- Commonly epicanthus inversus
- Greatly reduced horizontal fissure size
- Occasionally, true hypertelorism
- Flattened supraorbital rides with eyebrow arching
- Variable vertical lid shortening can lead to ectropion of lateral lower half of lids.

Investigations

Ptosis and epicanthus inversus can be variable. Each patient should be carefully studied prior to surgery.

Complications

- Stimulus-deprivation amblyopia
- Astigmatism depending on placement of lids on ocular surface
- Lacrimal sac puncture may occur during repair of telecanthus.

Pearls and Considerations

Treatment usually requires a staged approach.

Commonly associated conditions

In some family lines, associated with amenorrhea.

Referral Information

Oculoplastics referral for repair with medial canthal tendon and local skin flaps, bilateral frontalis suspension, and possibly skin grafting as appropriate

Differential Diagnosis

Each feature of the syndrome may occur without the others

Cause

Unknown

Epidemiology

- Found in 6% of children with congenital ptosis
- Most cases are autosomal dominant
- Predominantly males.

Associated Features

- Flattened supraorbital ridges with eyebrow arching
- Vertical lid shortening
- Antimongoloid lid-fissure slant.

TREATMENT

Diet and Lifestyle

No special precautions are necessary.

Pharmacologic Treatment

No pharmacologic treatment is recommended.

Nonpharmacologic Treatment

- Surgery is often deferred until after 18 months of age.
- Epicanthus and telecanthus are repaired first, then ptosis. Transnasal wiring is usually required to repair telecanthus because of the strong tension on medial canthal tendons.
- Levator resections are often initially effective, but lids fall with time, and most patients will eventually require bilateral sling procedures.
- Many surgeons wait 1 year after telecanthus repair to perform ptosis surgery.

Treatment Aims

To obviate telecanthus and epicanthal folds

Prognosis

- Excellent for stable telecanthus and epicanthal folds
- Ptosis tends to ultimately require bilateral frontalis sling suspension.

Follow-up and Management

- The uncommon patient with amblyopia and anisometropia should be managed in the usual manner with typical surgical postoperative care
- Note symmetric bilateral ptosis, telecanthus, and epicanthal folds.

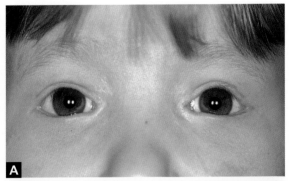

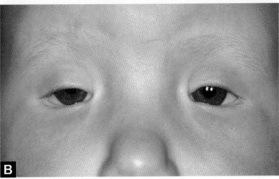

Figs 1A and B: Blepharophimosis syndrome. (A) With symmetric bilateral ptosis, telecanthus, and epicanthal folds; (B) Postoperative appearance following bilateral canthoplasty and frontalis suspension.

GENERAL REFERENCES

Callahan A. Ptosis. In: Troutman RC, Converse JM, Smith B (Eds). Plastic and Reconstructive Surgery of Eye and Adnexae. London: Butterworth; 1962. pp. 361-85.

Custer PL. Blepharoptosis. In: Yanoff M, Duker JS (Eds). Ophthalmology. St Louis: Elsevier; 2006.

De Baere E. Blepharophimosis, Ptosis, and Epicanthus Inversus. 2004 Jul 8 [Updated 2009 Nov 12]. In: Pagon RA, Bird TD, Dolan CR, et al. (Eds) GeneReviews™ [Internet]. Seattle (WA): University of Washington, Seattle; 1993.

Hu S, Guo J, Wang B, et al. Genetic analysis of the FOXL2 gene using quantitative real-time PCR in Chinese patients with blepharophimosis-ptosis-epicanthus inversus syndrome. Mol Vis. 2011;17:436-42.

Mustarde JC. Ptosis. Repair and Reconstruction in the Orbital Region, 2nd edition. Edinburgh: Churchill Livingstone; 1980. pp. 952-62.

Roveda JM. Epicanthus et blepharophimosis: notre, technique de correction. Ann D'oculist. 1967;200:551-62.

Cataract, Congenital (743.30)

DIAGNOSIS

Definition
Any opacity of the crystalline lens that is present from birth (Figs 1 to 3).

Synonyms
None

Symptoms
- Decreased visual acuity
- Glare

Signs
- Leukokoria
- Strabismus
- Nystagmus
- Squinting in sunlight
- Microphthalmos.

Investigations
- Evaluation of red reflex in every newborn, preferably before discharge from nursery
- Cycloplegic refraction
- Determination of the cataract's visual significance
- Examination of optic nerve and retina
- Evaluation for TORCH titers (toxoplasmosis, other infections, rubella, cytomegalovirus infection, and herpes simplex), serum glucose, urea nitrogen, galactose enzymes, urine glucose, and protein.

Complications
- Posterior capsule/anterior vitreous face opacification and aphakic glaucoma (40%) after cataract extraction
- *Nystagmus*: untreated cases typically develop irreversible nystagmus at 2–3 months
- Infection/hemorrhage after surgery
- Toxic anterior segment syndrome (TASS) causing postoperative corneal edema.

Pearls and Considerations
Congenital cataracts can be caused by ocular developmental dysgenesis, intrauterine infections, metabolic syndromes, gene mutation, or as a part of a systemic syndrome. Congenital cataract is of particular concern because of the potential for deprivation amblyopia and secondary glaucoma. Early detection and intervention are keys to a desirable visual outcome. All cataracts are not visually significant. Cataracts not visually significant should be monitored regularly because of the potential for progression.

Differential Diagnosis
Leukokoria: Retinoblastoma, toxocariasis, Coats' disease, persistent fetal vasculature, retinal astrocytoma, retinochoroidal coloboma, retinal detachment, myelinated nerve fibers, uveitis, incontinentia pigmenti, toxoplasmosis

Cause
Most commonly autosomal dominant with variable penetrance.

Epidemiology
1.6–6 cases per 10,000

Pathology
- Pathology of nuclear, cortical, and posterior subcapsular cataracts is similar to that in adults.
- Posterior lenticonus opacities show a thin posterior lens capsule with posteriorly bulging cortex with abnormal lens epithelial cells.

Diagnosis continued on p. 54

TREATMENT

Diet and Lifestyle

Patients with galactosemia and galactose-kinase deficiency should be placed on a galactose-free diet. The cataracts may improve.

Pharmacologic Treatment

No pharmacologic treatment is recommended.

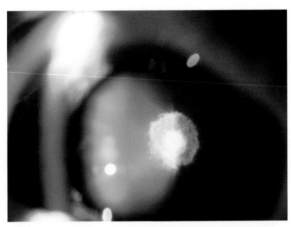

Fig. 1: Slit beam (front of eye toward left side of beam) shows an opaque plaque on the back part of the lens in a young adult, characteristic of a congenital posterior polar cataract.

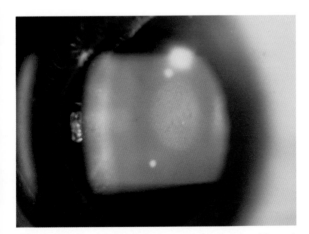

Fig. 2: Slit beam (front of eye toward left side of beam) shows central granular opacity in the center of the lens, characteristic of a congenital nuclear cataract.

Treatment continued on p. 55

Cataract, Congenital (743.30)

DIAGNOSIS—cont'd

Commonly Associated Conditions

Microphthalmia is often associated with congenital cataracts. This is also found in the following conditions:

- *Intrauterine infections*: Rubella, vermicelli, toxoplasmosis, herpes simplex, bacterial, or fungal endophthalmitis, cytomegalovirus
- *Metabolic disorders*: Galactosemia, hypocalcemia, hypoglycemia, diabetes mellitus, hyperferritinemia, Wilson syndrome, Fabry's syndrome, Refsum syndrome, homocystinuria, myotonia dystrophy, pseudohypoparathyroidism
- *Chromosomal*: Trisomy 21, Turner syndrome, Trisomy 13, Trisomy 18, Cri du chat syndrome
- *Renal disease:* Lowe syndrome, Alport syndrome, Hallermann-Streiff-Francois syndrome
- *Central nervous system diseases*: Marinesco-Sjögren syndrome, Sjögren syndrome
- *Mandibulofacial syndromes*: Pierre Robin syndrome, Treacher Collins syndrome
- *Dermal syndromes*: Incontinentia pigmenti, congenital ectodermal dysplasia, Werner syndrome, Rothmund-Thomson syndrome
- *Others:* Norrie disease, aniridia, retinitis pigmentosa, persistent fetal vasculature, retinopathy of prematurity, endophthalmitis.

Referral Information

Cataract surgeon when visually significant or causing ocular complications

TREATMENT—cont'd

Nonpharmacologic Treatment

- Lensectomy should be performed as soon as possible in all children with visually significant congenital cataracts (axial opacities > 3.0 mm in diameter)
- Unilateral congenital cataracts should be removed when discovered, preferably before 3 weeks of age
- Bilateral congenital cataracts should be removed before 8 weeks of age, either simultaneously or within 3 days of one another
- After lensectomy, the refractive power of the lens must be replaced with either an intraocular lens (reserved for children more than 2 or 3 years of age), contact lens, or glasses (generally, bilateral aphakes with contraindications to intraocular lens or contact lens treatment).

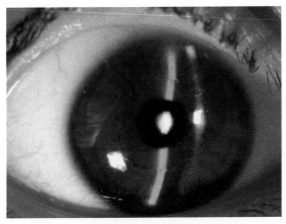

Fig. 3: Slit beam shows congenital anterior subcapsular cataract.

GENERAL REFERENCES

Birch EE, Cheng C, Vu C, et al. Oral reading after treatment of dense congenital unilateral cataract. J AAPOS. 2010; 14(3):227-31.

Haargaard B, Wohlfahrt J, Fledelius HC, et al. A nationwide Danish study of 1027 cases of congenital/infantile cataracts: etiological and clinical classifications. Ophthalmology. 2004;111(12): 2292-8.

Junk AK, Stefani FH, Ludwig K. Bilateral anterior lenticonus: Scheimpflug imaging system documentation and ultrastructural confirmation of Alport syndrome in the lens capsule. Arch Ophthalmol. 2000;118(7):895-7.

Kramer PL, LaMorticella D, Schilling K, et al. A new locus for autosomal dominant congenital cataracts maps to chromosome 3. Invest Ophthalmol Vis Sci. 2000; 41(1):36-9.

Lambert SR, Drack AV. Infantile cataracts. Surv Ophthalmol. 1996;40(6): 427-58.

Zhang L, Zhang Y, Liu P, et al. Congenital anterior polar cataract associated with a missense mutation in the human alpha crystallin gene CRYAA. Mol Vis. 2011;17:2693-7. Epub 2011 Oct 15.

Cataract, Secondary to Ocular and Other Complications (366.3)

DIAGNOSIS

Definition

Opacity of the lens secondary to ocular inflammation or disease process.

Synonyms

None

Symptoms

- *Obscuration of vision*: depending on the underlying condition, the onset of decreased vision may be *rapid* (e.g. sudden, usually reversible osmotic cataract of juvenile diabetes) or insidious (e.g. posterior subcapsular cataract of retinitis pigmentosa); the patient may perceive obscuration of vision as blurred, dim, or hazy vision.
- *Halos at night*: in low light when the pupils are condensely dilated or fully dilated, nuclear cataracts ankle is halos to appear around lights; it is important to differentiate this phenomenon and from the same symptom that occurs with angle-closure glaucoma (with nuclear cataract, the eye is white, painless, and has a normally reactive pupil, whereas with angle-closure glaucoma, the eye is red and painful and the pupil is dilated and fixed).
- *Red eye*: depending on the underlying course of the cataract (e.g. uveitis, acute angle-closure glaucoma, Stevens-Johnson syndrome) the eye may be red secondary to ciliary injection.
- *Painful eye*: depending on the underlying course of the cataract, the eye may be painful; usually associated with those entities that course ciliary injection.

Note: Some patients may be asymptomatic, and cataract may be detected during a routine eye examination.

Signs

- Opacification within the lens cortex [*cortical cataract* (366.15)] and/or nucleus [*nuclear cataract* (366.16)]
- Opacification just posterior to the anterior lens capsule: [*anterior subcapsular cataract* (366.13)] were just anterior to the posterior lens capsule [*posterior subcapsular cataract* (366.14)]
- Completely white (mature) cataract (366.17): As the cortex undergoes cataractous change, it becomes liquefied (*Morgagnian degeneration*; seen with the slit lamp as cortical spokes); the cortex then becomes more and more milky until finally it becomes opaque (*mature cataract*); the liquefied cortex and this gave to the intact lens capsule, closing capsular folds [hypermature cataract (366.18)].
- *Elshnig's pearls*: remaining lens epithelial cells form new lens "fibers" (*see* Cataract, after)
- *Soemmerring's ring*: (366.51): Lens cortex tract and equatorial port of "lens capsular bag" (*see* Cataract, after)
- *Subluxation*: (Within posterior chamber but not in normal position) or dislocation (in the anterior chamber or vitreous compartment)
- *Ciliary injection*: If the eye is inflamed.

Differential Diagnosis

- Primary cataracts unrelated to a secondary process
- Other causes of decreased vision (e.g. diabetic retinopathy).

Cause

See Boxes 1 and 2.

Epidemiology

- Although all the entities listed in Boxes 1 and 2 may be associated with cataracts, the exact frequency is not known.
- Cataracts often complicate chronic intraocular inflammation.
- Degenerative disorders (especially retinitis pigmentosa and Wilson's disease) have a high frequency of associated cataracts.

Classification

Cataracts can be classified as:
- Cortical (366.15)
- Nuclear (366.16)
- Anterior subcapsular (366.13)
- Posterior subcapsular (366.14)
- Mature (366.17).

Pathology

The pathology depends on the type of cataract.

Complications

- Decreased vision
- Retinal detachment
- Uveitis
- Infrequently, a swollen mature cataract can cause a secondary angle-closure glaucoma
- Rarely, a hypermature cataract can "leak" fluid, leading to a secondary open-angle glaucoma called *phacolytic glaucoma* (*see* Cataract, infantile, juvenile, and presenile).

Diagnosis continued on p. 58

TREATMENT

Diet and Lifestyle

In the vast majority of patients, no specific precautions are necessary.

Pharmacologic Treatment

For Cataracts Secondary to Ocular Complications

- Appropriate pharmacologic treatment is indicated for the relevant underlying conditions
- In most of these cases, however (although the underlying condition may be brought under control), the cataract is not reversible, and cataract surgery must be performed.

Box 1: Causes of cataracts secondary to ocular complications

Cataracta complicata (366.30)

Acute angle-closure glaucoma

   Glaukomflecken (366.31)

Intraocular inflammation

   Chronic choroiditis (363.0)

   Iridocyclitis (364.1)

Degenerative disorders

   Retinitis pigmentosa (362.74)

Box 2: Cataracts secondary to systemic and other entities

Diabetic (366.41)

   Secondary to diabetes mellitus (250.5)

   Sunflower cataract of Wilson's disease (366.34)

Tetanic (366.42)

   Secondary to calcinosis (275.4)

   Hypoparathyroidism (252.1)

Myotonic (366.43)

   Secondary to myotonic dystrophy (359.2)

Other systemic syndromes

   Craniofacial dysostosis (756.0)

   Galactosemia (271.1)

Toxic or drug-induced (366.45)

   Posterior subcapsular cataract secondary to corticosteroids or radiation-induced (366.46)

Other entities

   Acquired immunodeficiency syndrome (AIDS)

   Stevens-Johnson syndrome

   Vitamin A deficiency

Treatment Aims

To improve vision: Patients who have cataracts secondary to ocular and systemic problems often do not achieve 20/20 vision. Many of these patients, however, usually appreciate any improvement in vision. For example, removing a cataract from an incapacitated patient with hand-motions vision can give the patient 20/200 or 20/400 vision, which can increase mobility and independence.

Other Treatments

Other treatments are aimed at the underlying conditions. Unfortunately, this generally does not reverse the cataractous lens changes, and if visual incapacity results from the cataract, surgery is required.

Prognosis

The prognosis depends on the underlying ocular or systemic condition; by the time the underlying condition is controlled, however, irreversible cataractous changes may have occurred in the lens.

Follow-up and Management

- Long-term follow-up is needed to ensure proper visual rehabilitation and treatment of the underlying ocular or systemic condition.
- Cataract extraction and lens implantation in this group of patients is fraught with complications. The patient must be followed to diagnose the early stages of glaucoma, recurrence of intraocular inflammation, retinal tear and detachment, and other conditions.

57

Treatment continued on p. 59

Cataract, Secondary to Ocular and Other Complications (366.3)

DIAGNOSIS—cont'd

Investigations

- *History*: A meticulous history of past episodes of red eye (e.g. previous iridocyclitis), metabolic defects (e.g. secondary to hypoparathyroidism), and inherited conditions (e.g. retinitis pigmentosa) is extremely important in establishing the course of the cataract.
- Visual acuity testing
- Refraction
- Intraocular pressure
- On dilated and dilated slit-lamp examination
- Dilated fundus examination
- *Appropriate evaluation of any underlying cause*: as indicated.

Pearls and Considerations

Vision worsens, refer to an eye care physician.

Referral Information

Varied and dependent on the suspected cause of the disease.

TREATMENT—cont'd

For Cataracts Secondary to Systemic Diseases

- Appropriate pharmacologic treatment is indicated for the relevant underlying conditions
- In rare cases (e.g. osmotic cataract of juvenile diabetes, tetanic cataract of calcinosis secondary to hypoparathyroidism) coma cataract may be reversible when the underlying condition can be brought under control. In most of these patients, however (although the underlying conditions may be managed), the character is not reversible and cataract surgery must be performed.

Nonpharmacologic Treatment

If visual potential exists in the eye, surgical treatment is indicated. Extracapsular cataract extraction (ECCE), either by nuclear expression or phacoemulsification (usually with intraocular lens implantation), is performed.

Some conditions have surprisingly better results than would be expected for the clinical data. For example, patients with advanced retinitis pigmentosa who are legally blind because of the restrictive visual field become even more disabled by the characteristic subcapsular cataract and develops in this condition. Cataract extraction and lens implantation often greatly benefit these patients. Another example is heterochromic iridocyclitis (Fuchs), which might indicate chart surgery on an inflamed dye. Experience, however, shows that these patients tolerate intraocular surgery quite well, and active inflammation here is not a contraindication to surgery.

GENERAL REFERENCES

Cumming RG. Use of inhaled corticosteroids and the risk of cataracts. N Engl J Med. 1997;337(1):8-14.

Garbe E, Suissa S, LeLorier J. Exposure to allopurinol and the risk of cataract extraction in elderly patients. Arch Ophthalmol. 1998;116(12):1652-6.

Stambolian D, Scarpino-Myers V, Eagle RC, et al. Cataracts in patients heterozygous for galactokinase deficiency. Invest Ophthalmol Vis Sci. 1986;27(3):429-33.

Toogood JH, Markov AE, Baskerville J, et al. Association of ocular cataracts with inhaled and oral steroid therapy during long-term treatment of asthma. J Allergy Clin Immunol. 1993;91 (2):571-9.

Yanoff M, Sassani JW. Ocular Pathology, 6th edition. St Louis: Mosby; 2009. pp. 380-4.

Cataract, Traumatic (366.22)

DIAGNOSIS

Definition

Opacity of the linens secondary to blunt trauma or penetrating injury.

Synonyms

None

Symptoms

Obscuration of Vision

The onset of decreased vision depends on the underlying cause: e.g. following blunt trauma, a typical petal-shaped cataract may take years to progress to the point where vision is decreased; on the other hand, perforating trauma may injure the lens and cause instant loss of vision; the patient may describe obscuration of vision is blurred, dim, or hazy vision.

Halos at Night

Blunt trauma may cause nuclear cataracts, which, when the pupils are semi-dilated or fully dilated, can cause halos to appear around lights; it is important to differentiate this phenomenon from the same symptom that occurs with angle-closure glaucoma (with nuclear cataract, the eye is white, painless, and has a normal reactive pupil, whereas with angle-closure glaucoma, the eye is red and painful and the pupil is dilated and fixed).

Red and/or Painful Eye

Depending on the underlying cause of the cataract (e.g. traumatic uveitis, endophthalmitis, secondary angle-closure glaucoma), the eye may be red secondary to ciliary injection, which often also causes pain.
- *Note*: Some patients may be asymptomatic
- A traumatic cataract, usually following blunt trauma, may take years to develop the point at which vision is affected.

Signs

- Opacification within the lens cortex [*cortical cataract* (366.15)] and/or nucleus [*nuclear cataract* (366.16)]. Often a petal-shaped cortical cataract is seen (Fig. 1)
- Opacification just posterior to the anterior lens capsule [*anterior subcapsular* cataract (366.13)] or just anterior to the posterior lens capsule [posterior subcapsular cataract (366.14)]
- Completely white cataract [*mature cataract* (366.17)]
- Completely white but shrunken cataract [*hypermature cataract* (366.18)]
- Subluxated or dislocated lens (Fig. 2).

Investigations

Visual acuity testing: It is extremely important to test visual acuity after ocular trauma, especially after penetrating ocular trauma in which uveal prolapse occurs; if after 1 week to 10 days no useful vision is present, the eye should be enucleated to avoid the development of *sympathetic uveitis* (see Uveitis, sympathetic).

Differential Diagnosis

- Primary (presenile or "senile") or secondary cataracts unrelated to trauma.
- Other causes of decreased vision include:
  - Cystoid macular edema
  - Age-related macular degeneration
  - Diabetic retinopathy
  - Glaucoma
  - Retinal detachment
  - Vitreous hemorrhage
  - Corneal edema.

Cause

Most often caused by blunt trauma to the eye; also, can be secondary to penetrating trauma to the eye; may not become apparent or symptomatic for months to years after blunt trauma.

Epidemiology

Although the majority of cataracts are caused by the aging process, a significant percentage is traumatic.

Classification

Traumatic cataracts (366.2) also can be classified as:
- Cortical (366.15)
- Nuclear (366.16)
- Anterior subcapsular (366.13)
- Posterior subcapsular (366.14)
- Mature (366.17)
- Completely white but shrunken, i.e. hypermature (366.18).

Associated Features

The trauma that caused the cataract can also cause corneal problems, glaucoma, Berlin's edema, retinal detachment, vitreous hemorrhage, intraocular foreign bodies, endophthalmitis, and traumatic chorioretinopathy.

Pathology

The pathology depends on the type of cataract. In general, degenerative changes are found in the nucleus, cortex, or anterior or posterior subcapsular areas. Globe pathology depends on the associated injury and its consequences.

Diagnosis continued on p. 62

TREATMENT

Diet and Lifestyle

In the vast majority of patients, no special precautions are necessary.

Pharmacologic Treatment

Pharmacologic treatment has no effect on the cataracts but may be extremely important in some of the consequences of the trauma. For example, perforating trauma may introduce into the eye pathogenic organisms that must be treated vigorously (usually by topical and intravenous antibiotics and often along with vitrectomy and intraocular antibiotics). The type and dosage of the antibiotic depend on the particular protocol in use by the surgeon.

Nonpharmacologic Treatment

- If visual potential exists in the eye, surgical treatment may be indicated. Visual acuity potential can be measured by a variety of methods (e.g. potential acuity measurement instrument, laser interferometry, color discrimination).
- Extracapsular cataract extraction (ECCE), either by nuclear expression or phacoemulsification (usually with intraocular lens implantation), is performed. Often, with perforating trauma, a vitrectomy is combined with a lensectomy and intraocular lens insertion. Other problems, such as traumatic retinal detachment, can be repaired at the same time.
- If a cataractous lens is *subluxated* (i.e. in posterior chamber but not in its normal location) poor *dislocated* (i.e. not in posterior chamber but in vitreous or anterior chamber), special precautions need to be taken during surgery. An intracapsular cataract extraction right pars plana lensectomy may be warranted.
- José subluxated or dislocated lens, vitreous usually is present in the anterior chamber. ECCE by nuclear expression or phacoemulsification may be extremely difficult. Sometimes the safest method is a pars plana lensectomy or an intracapsular cataract extraction with an anterior-chamber lens implant or a scleral-fixated, sewn-in posterior-chamber lens implant.

Treatment Aims

To improve vision

Other Treatments

Other ocular problems secondary to the trauma should be dealt with as indicated. Often the traumatic cataract is the least of the vision-threatening complications that can occur after ocular trauma (e.g. secondary glaucoma, anterior-chamber hemorrhage, retinal tears or detachment, vitreous hemorrhage, endophthalmitis).

Prognosis

Prognosis depends on other associated ocular injuries. If no other vision-threatening ocular injuries are present, cataract extraction and intraocular lens implantation result in ~95% visual improvement to a visual acuity of 20/40 or better.

Follow-up and Management

Long-term follow-up is needed to ensure proper visual rehabilitation and to check for postoperative complications, such as corneal edema, opacification of the posterior lens capsule ("after cataract"), glaucoma, intraocular inflammation, cystoid macular edema, and retinal detachment. Also, any other ocular injuries resulting from the trauma need to be appropriately managed.

A delayed type of glaucoma can result from blunt injury, especially when the injury causes an anterior-chamber hemorrhage.

61

Treatment continued on p. 63

Cataract, Traumatic (366.22)

DIAGNOSIS—cont'd

- *Refraction*
- *Intraocular pressure*: A clue to an occult rupture of the globe may be a reduced pressure in the injured eye, especially when accompanied by a deeper-than-normal anterior chamber or a vitreous hemorrhage
- *Undilated and dilated slit-lamp examination*
- *Dilated fundus examination.*

Complications

- Decreased vision
- Glaucoma, secondary open-angle. E.g. contusion deformity of the anterior-chamber angle (*angle-recession glaucoma*)
- Glaucoma, secondary angle-closure. E.g. iris neovascularization (*neovascular glaucoma*); infrequently, a mature cataract can cause secondary angle-closure glaucoma
- Ocular complications closed by the trauma. E.g. vitreous hemorrhage, retinal tears and detachment, choroidal rupture, perforation of the globe, intraocular foreign bodies
- Rarely, a swollen, hypermature cataract can "leak" fluid trauma leading to a secondary open-angle glaucoma called *phacolytic glaucoma.*

Pearls and Considerations

Infrared energy, electric shock, and ionizing radiation are other, less common causes of traumatic cataract.

Referral Information

Surgical referral for cataract extraction as appropriate.

TREATMENT—cont'd

When the eye cannot be salvaged by surgical or medical means, enucleation may be necessary. This needs to be carefully explained to the patient before surgery; however, the patient may not be alert enough to comprehend the impact of enucleation. In such cases, therefore, surgical and medical care should be performed. Postoperatively, when the patient is aware that no useful vision is present, enucleation can be discussed. In any event, if no useful vision is present and if ocular perforation with uveal prolapse occurred at the time of the injury, the eye should be enucleated within 5–10 days after the trauma to prevent sympathetic uveitis.

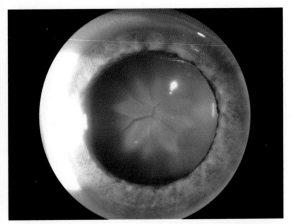

Fig. 1: Some months after blunt trauma to the eye—a typical petal-shaped cataract developed.

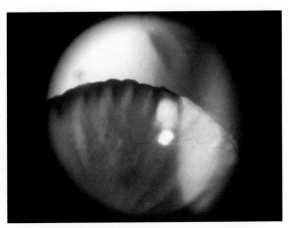

Fig. 2: Lens is traumatically subluxated inferiorly. The lens zonules can be seen superiorly.

GENERAL REFERENCES

Finkelstein M, Legmann A, Rubin PAD. Projectile metallic foreign bodies in the orbit: a retrospective study of epidemiologic factors, management, and outcomes. Ophthalmology. 1997;104(1):96-103.

Giovinazzo VJ, Yannuzzi LA, Sorenson JA, et al. The ocular complications of boxing. Ophthalmology. 1987;94(6): 587-96.

Mulrooney BC, Allinson RW, et al. (2006). Traumatic cataract. [online]. Available from www.emedicine.com.

Portellos M, Orlin SE, Kozart DM. Electric cataracts. Arch Ophthalmol. 1996;114(8): 1022-3.

Wong TY, Seet B, Ang CL. Eye injuries in twentieth century warfare: a historical perspective. Surv Ophthalmol. 1997; 41(6):433-59.

Yanoff M, Sassani JW. Ocular Pathology, 6th edition. Philadelphia: Mosby; 2009. pp. 115-7.

Cataract, After (366.53)

DIAGNOSIS

Definition

A late complication of extracapsular cataract extraction (ECCE) in which the capsular epithelium proliferates and opacifies the posterior lens capsule.

Synonyms

Secondary cataract; posterior capsular opacification (PCO).

Symptoms

- Symptoms follow ECCE, either nuclear expression or phacoemulsification
- *Obscuration of vision*: (366.53; if vision is not obscured. 366.52) may occur as early as a few weeks after ECCE, but usually occurs months to years later
- Blurred vision
- *Dim vision*: patients often complain of a combination of dim vision (vision used to be brighter) and blurred vision
- Hazy vision
- Halos at night.

Note: Some patients may be asymptomatic. Reduced vision may first be detected during a routine eye examination, because if the vision is normal in the other eye, patients generally do not notice reduced vision in the eye with increased PCO.

Signs

- *Opacification of posterior lens capsule*: the posterior lens capsule initially appears mildly translucent (rather than transparent); with progression, the translucency advances to a watery, milky color and finally, in the end stage, to white and opaque; generally the loss of transparency is diffuse, but the posterior lens capsule usually contains islands of differing density (Figs 1A and B).
- *Cellular reaction on anterior surface of intraocular lens implant*: the reaction is one of large foreign body giant cells that are often admixed with pigment; this usually occurs weeks to months after an ECCE.
- *Fibrinous reaction on anterior surface of intraocular lens implant*: generally the fibrinous reaction is seen in the early postoperative period. Rarely the anterior capsular opacification can become severe so as to interfere with vision.
- *Elschnig's pearls*: remaining lens epithelial cells form new lens "fibers"; Elschnig's pearls are seen on slit-lamp examination as tiny balls of new lens fibers resembling fish eggs.
- *Soemmerring's ring (366.51)*: lens cortex trapped in equatorial part of "lens capsular bag"; because Soemmerring's ring cataract occurs in the equatorial (peripheral) portion of the "lens bag," it may not be observed until the pupil is dilated widely and does not interfere with vision.

Differential Diagnosis

Other courses of decreased vision after cataract surgery include:

- *Refractive change*: probably most common cause of postoperative change in visual acuity.
- *Cystoid macular edema*: occurs in approx. 5% of post-ECCE patients
- *Age-related macular degeneration*: usually predates cataract surgery but may not have been visualized because of the cataract.
- *Corneal edema*: Occurs in approx. 1% of post-ECCE patients
- *Intraocular inflammation*: extremely rare and may be sterile or infectious
- *Retinal detachment*: occurs in <1% of patients after ECCE.

Cause

Proliferation of residual anterior lens capsular epithelial horn to the posterior lens capsule.

Epidemiology

Occurs in approx. 25% of patients after ECCE and lens implantation.

Classification

Grade I: diaphanous haze
Grade II: mild haze (has a watery, milky appearance)
Grade III: moderate haze (often has geographic areas of differing densities)
Grade IV: white, capsular haze

Pathology

The proliferated lens epithelium undergoes fibers metaplasia, which results in the formation of scar tissue over the posterior lens capsule. The proliferated metaplastic cells are both fibroblasts and myofibroblasts and, therefore, have the potential for contraction.

Diagnosis continued on p. 66

TREATMENT

Pharmacologic Treatment

- No medical treatment is available to prevent, stabilize, or reverse posterior capsular lens opacities
- An early fibrinous inflammatory reaction on the anterior surface of the lens implant usually responds well to 1% corticosteroid solutions given topically, one drop every 2–4 hours daily.

Nonpharmacologic Treatment

Neodymium:Yttrium-Aluminum-Garnet (Nd:YAG) Laser (668.21)

- Inflammatory membranes on the anterior surface of the lens implant that do not respond to corticosteroid therapy can be removed easily by the use of the Nd:YAG laser, using an energy level of 0.8–1.0 millijoule (mJ).
- Before treatment, the undilated pupil is examined to make certain that it is centered or, if not, to see where the pupil is in relation to the lens opacity so that an opening in the posterior lens opacity can be made in the appropriate location. The pupil is dilated. One drop of apraclonidine 1% sterile ophthalmic solution (Iopidine; Alcon Laboratories, Randburg, South Africa) is instilled in the eye. YAG laser capsulectomy (either direct or with special posterior capsulectomy contact lens) is performed at the minimum energy level that can be used to dissolve the posterior lens opacity (start at 0.8 mJ and increase energy in increments of 0.1–0.2 mJ). After an adequate opening in the proper anatomic location is obtained, another drop of Iopidine is instilled. The patient is asked to wait for a few hours to make certain that the IOP does not rise above normal (if a persistent IOP rise occurs, it should be treated appropriately with antiglaucoma medications). The patient is then discharged with no medication or perhaps a mild corticosteroid eyedrop to be used four times daily. Follow up with patient in about a week.
- Because the YAG energy is propagated anteriorly, when performing the YAG laser capsulectomy on the posterior lens capsule, the helium-neon (HeNe) aiming beam should be focused slightly posterior to the posterior lens capsule to avoid "pinging" the lens implant. If no dissolution of the posterior capsule occurs, the aiming beam can be moved cautiously, by tiny increments, anteriorly until capsular dissolution results. Conversely, when performing the YAG laser on a membrane on the anterior lens capsule (YAG laser membranectomy), again because the YAG energy is propagated anteriorly, the focusing of the HeNe aiming beam is not nearly as critical as when focusing on the posterior capsule.

Other Treatments

- *Surgical incision of posterior capsule*: rarely performed since the advent of Nd:YAG laser treatment.

Treatment Aims

- To produce an adequate opening in the opacified posterior lens capsule for clear vision within the visual axis.
- To avoid placing energy anterior to the posterior lens capsule by carefully aligning and aiming for the HeNe being suicidal to "ping" the lens implant (fortunately, if this happens, it is rarely clinically significant).
- To avoid post-Nd:YAG complications, which include glaucoma (used preoperative and postoperative pressure-lowering drops); cystoid macular edema (wait at least 4–6 weeks after cataract surgery before performing Nd:YAG anterior surgical treatment).

Prognosis

After successful Nd:YAG laser treatment, approx. 100% of patients are cured (meaning that the opening created in the posterior lens capsule is permanent). In extremely rare cases, the opening may close (usually in an eye that has an anterior uveitis).

Follow-up and Management

Patients should be checked a few days to a few weeks after Nd:YAG laser treatment to make certain that (1) visual acuity has improved; (2) an adequate opening is present in the posterior lens capsule; (3) IOP is normal; (4) cystoid macular edema has not developed; and (5) a retinal tear or detachment is not present.

Treatment continued on p. 67

DIAGNOSIS—cont'd

Investigations

- *Visual acuity testing*: usually the best visual acuity is reduced over the last visit; however, sometimes the patient sees the same as the last visit but notes that the visual acuity screen is less bright
- *Refraction*: reduced vision may be secondary to a refractive change rather than to PCO
- Intraocular pressure (IOP)
- Undilated and dilated slit-lamp examination
- *Dilated fundus examination*: with the use of a high plus in the direct ophthalmoscope, the red reflex is less bright than normal and also uneven; when focused on the retina, the image is blurred.

Complications

- *Decreased vision*: patient may note the decreased vision as an actual decrease in clarity of vision, a darkening of vision, or a combination of both
- Subluxation or dislocation of intraocular lens implant (secondary to capsular contraction)
- *Delayed infection*: usually caused by *Staphylococcus epidermidis* or *Propionibacterium acnes* trapped in the lens capsule at cataract surgery; this infection tends to be indolent and may not appear until many months after surgery.

Pearls and Considerations

Frequency of "after cataract" is age-related, with almost all children developing PCO and the incidence decreasing in adults.

Referral Information

Referral for yttrium-aluminum-garnet (YAG) laser capsulotomy is indicated.

TREATMENT—cont'd

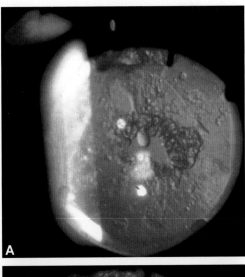

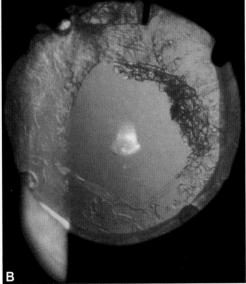

Figs 1A and B: Posterior lens capsule opacification after cataract extraction and lens implantation.

GENERAL REFERENCES

Awasthi N, Guo S, Wagner BJ. Posterior capsular opacification: a problem reduced but not yet eradicated. Arch Ophthalmol. 2009;127(4):555-62.

McLeod SD. Risk factors for posterior capsule opacification. Br J Ophthalmol. 2005;89:1389-90.

Werner L. Secondary cataract. In: Yanoff M, Duker JS (Eds). Ophthalmology, 3rd edition. St Louis: Mosby; 2009. pp. 497-502.

Yoshida S, Senoo T, Fujikake F, et al. Clinical evaluation of posterior capsule opacification in eyes with different small-incision intraocular lenses. Ophthalmic Surg Lasers. 2002;33(6): 450-5.

Cataract, Age-Related (Senile) (366.15)

DIAGNOSIS

Definition

"Senescent lens changes related, in part, to ultraviolet B (UVB) radiation"

Synonym

Senile cataract

Symptoms

Obscuration of vision: The onset of decreased vision tends to be insidious, usually over many years; occasionally, however, the onset may be rapid (perception of rapidity may be brought on when, for the first time in a long time, patient covers the good eye and notes decreased vision in the cataractous eye, which may have been present for some time; true rapidity of decreased vision occurs rarely, with some rapidly developing posterior subcapsular cataracts and mature cataracts); patient may describe obscuration of vision as blurred, dim, or hazy vision.

Haloes at night: In low light when the pupils are semidilated or fully dilated; nuclear cataracts can cause haloes to appear around lights; it is important to differentiate this phenomenon from the same symptom that occurs with angle-closure glaucoma (with nuclear cataract, the eye is white, painless, and has a normally reactive pupil, whereas with angle-closure glaucoma, the eye is red, painful, and the pupil is dilated and fixed).

Note: Many patients may be asymptomatic, and cataract may first be detected during a routine eye examination.

Signs

Opacification within the lens cortex [cortical cataract (366.15) and/or nucleus (nuclear cataract (366.16)]: See Figures 1A and B.

Opacification just posterior to the anterior lens capsule [anterior subcapsular cataract (366.13) or just anterior to the posterior lens capsule (posterior subcapsular cataract (366.14)]: See Figure 2.

Completely white (mature) cataract (366.17): As the cortex undergoes cataractous change, it becomes liquefied (morgagnian degeneration; seen with the slit lamp as cortical spokes); the cortex then becomes more and more milky until finally it becomes opaque (mature cataract); the liquefied cortex can escape through the intact lens capsule, causing capsular folds [*hypermature cataract (366.18)*]; *see* Figure 3.

Investigations

Visual acuity testing: In moderate or advanced cataracts, testing visual acuity with the Snellen chart gives a reasonable estimate of the patient's vision.

Note: Some patients with normal or near-normal visual acuity can be quite symptomatic. For example, a posterior subcapsular cataract may be small, dense, and centrally located, but with the pupil at a normal size, the patient can see around the cataract, and the vision may be normal. However, when the patient goes outside into bright sunlight and the pupil constricts, the patient's vision may fall precipitously because the cataract now occupies the entire pupil. Special testing for brightness (brightness acuity tester) and glare is often indicated in the evaluation of a patient who has a cataract.

Refraction; intraocular pressure; undilated and dilated slit-lamp examination; dilated fundus examination.

Differential Diagnosis

- Cataracts may not be primary (senile) and may be related to a secondary process (e.g. neoplasm).
- Other causes of decreased vision include:
  - Cystoid macular edema
  - Age-related macular degeneration
  - Diabetic retinopathy
  - Glaucoma
  - Retinal detachment
  - Vitreous hemorrhage
  - Corneal edema.

Cause

Risk factors include heredity, age, diabetes mellitus, oral or inhaled corticosteroid therapy, exposure to UVB radiation, poor nutrition and smoking.

Epidemiology

- Cataracts are common, and cataract surgery is the most frequently performed surgery in the elderly patient.
- Cataracts can occur at any age. The two peaks are in patients less than 10 years old (congenital cataracts) and those more than 65 years old, but cataracts occur in every decade of life.

Classification

Cataracts can be classified as cortical (366.15), nuclear (366.16), anterior subcapsular (366.13), posterior subcapsular (366.14), or mature (366.17).

Pathology

- The pathology depends on the type of cataract. In general, degenerative changes are found in the nucleus, cortex, or anterior or posterior subcapsular areas.
- Early cataractous changes in the cortex appear as tiny areas of liquefaction called "morgagnian degeneration", seen clinically as cortical spokes. The liquefaction can progress to involve the entire cortex, which then appears milky white. The cataractous nucleus loses its artifactitious clefts and appears homogeneous in microscopic sections.

Diagnosis continued on p. 70

TREATMENT

Diet and Lifestyle

Diet and lifestyle have no effect on most cataracts. Avoidance of excess UVB radiation exposure may be helpful.

Pharmacologic Treatment

No pharmacologic treatment is recommended.

Nonpharmacologic Treatment

- If visual potential exists in the eye, surgical treatment may be indicated.
- Even if the vision is reduced significantly and testing shows an excellent chance for good vision after cataract surgery, the patient may not want surgery. The benefits and risks of cataract surgery and lens implantation and the patient's lifestyle and expectations must be discussed thoroughly with the patient. For example, a taxi driver who has a posterior subcapsular cataract and a visual acuity of 20/30 may choose cataract surgery before a retired individual who mainly reads and watches television and has a nuclear cataract that reduces visual acuity to 20/60. Only through a comprehensive discussion with the patient and other involved family members or friends can a mutual decision for cataract surgery be reached.
- Some patients who have a nuclear cataract note that they are able to read for the first time in years without glasses. This increased ability for near vision, known as "second sight", is caused by the increased index of refraction of the nuclear cataract, which induces nearsightedness. Despite that the nuclear cataract may reduce distance vision, patients who spend most of their time using near vision (reading, watching television) will be most unhappy with cataract surgery if they now need glasses to read. Again, a full discussion, including the patient's expectations, is mandatory.

Treatment Aims

- To improve vision
- To rehabilitate the patient as rapidly as possible.
- With modern small-incision, no-stitch, outpatient phacoemulsification ECCE surgery, wound stability is rapid and rehabilitation is minimal. The patient generally can resume normal activities the day after surgery. Glasses, if needed, may be prescribed in 2–8 weeks.
- With the larger incision needed for nuclear expression ECCE, the time course is somewhat delayed. Glasses, if needed, generally are not prescribed for 4–10 weeks after surgery.

Other Treatments

In the rare instances of phacolytic glaucoma or secondary angle-closure glaucoma, cataract removal usually alleviates the problem.

Prognosis

Cataract surgery results in about 95% visual improvement to a visual acuity of 20/40 or better.

Follow-up and Management

Long-term follow-up is needed to ensure proper visual rehabilitation and to check for postoperative complications, such as corneal edema, opacification of the posterior lens capsule (after cataract), glaucoma, intraocular inflammation, cystoid macular edema, and retinal detachment.

Treatment continued on p. 71

Cataract, Age-Related (Senile) (366.15)

DIAGNOSIS—cont'd

Complications

Decreased vision: Infrequently a swollen, mature cataract can cause a secondary angle-closure glaucoma; rarely a hypermature cataract can "leak" fluid, leading to a secondary open-angle glaucoma called "phacolytic glaucoma".

Pearls and Considerations

• A diagnosis of exclusion; secondary causes should be ruled out
• Potential acuity meter (PAM) is a useful tool in predicting postextraction visual acuity
• Success rate for routine cataract surgery is more than 95%.

Referral Information

Refer for cataract extraction and intraocular lens implantation once the cataract becomes visually significant.

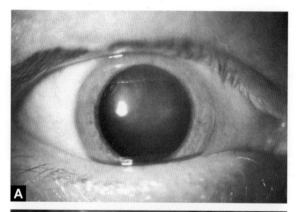

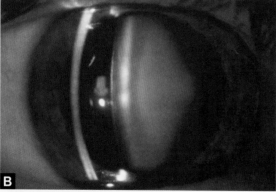

Figs 1A and B: (A) Pupil has a dull, yellowish reflex secondary to a nuclear cataract (nuclear sclerosis); (B) Slit beam demonstrates the yellow nuclear cataract and white cortical cataract.

TREATMENT—cont'd

Extracapsular Cataract Extraction

An extracapsular cataract extraction (ECCE), either by nuclear expression or phacoemulsification, usually with intraocular lens implantation, can be performed. The decision of whether to perform nuclear expression ECCE or phacoemulsification ECCE depends on several factors. First and foremost is the skill of the individual surgeon and the type of procedure with which the surgeon is most comfortable. In general, the type of surgery depends on the hardness of the nuclear component of the cataract (all cortical cataracts are soft). If the nuclear cataract is soft to moderately hard, most surgeons will perform phacoemulsification ECCE. If the nuclear cataract is very hard, some surgeons will perform nuclear expression ECCE. Most surgeons perform phacoemulsification ECCE on almost all cataracts.

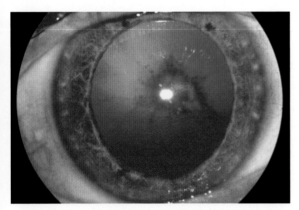

Fig. 2: A density can be seen toward the back of the lens in this posterior subcapsular cataract.

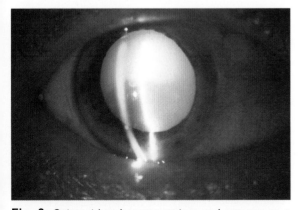

Fig. 3: Cataract has become mature and appears as a milky reflex in the pupil. Note yellow-brown nucleus has been displaced inferiorly in milky, liquid cortex.

GENERAL REFERENCES

Hiller R, Sperduto RD, Podgor MJ, et al. Cigarette smoking and the risk of development of lens opacities. The Framingham Studies. Arch Ophthalmol. 1997;115:1113-8.

Kasier PK, Friedman NJ. Lens. The Massachusetts Eye and Ear Infirmary illustrated manual of ophthalmology, 2nd edition. Philadelphia: WB Saunders; 2004. p. 268.

Klein BE, Klein R, Lee KE, et al. Socioeconomic and lifestyle factors and the 10-year incidence of age-related cataracts. Am J Ophthalmol. 2003;136(3): 506-12.

Sachdev NH, Di Girolamo N, Nolan TM, et al. Matrix metalloproteinases and tissue inhibitors of matrix metalloproteinases in the human lens: implications for cortical cataract formation. Invest Ophthalmol Vis Sci. 2004;45(11):4075-82.

The Italian-American Cataract Study Group. Incidence and progression of cortical, nuclear, and posterior subcapsular cataracts. Am J Ophthalmol. 1994;118(5): 623-31.

Vrensen G, Willekens B. Biomicroscopy and scanning electron microscopy of early opacities in the aging human lens. Invest Ophthalmol Vis Sci. 1990;31(8):1582-91.

Cataract, Infantile, Juvenile, and Presenile (366.0)

DIAGNOSIS

Definition

Acquired opacity of the lens found in children and young adults

Synonyms

None

Symptoms

- *Decreased vision*: in infants or very young children, decreased vision is difficult to evaluate; the parent often will notice that the infant or child is not focusing on objects or that the eyes are wandering aimlessly.
- *Strabismus*: often in an infant or young child who has a unilateral cataract will develop strabismus to remove the blurred image caused by the cataractous eye from the macular portion of the retina.
- *Leukokoria (white pupil)*: noted by parent; this type of presentation is rare that occurs with the cataract becomes "mature" and has a white, milky appearance; the leukokoria (cat's eye reflex) may mimic that which is seeing with retinoblastoma.

Note: Some patients may be asymptomatic, and cataract may be detected during a routine eye examination.

Signs

- Opacification within the lens cortex (366.03) and/or nucleus (366.04) or at the junction of the nucleus and cortex [*zonular cataract* (366.03)]
- Opacification just posterior to the anterior lens capsule [*anterior subcapsular or polar cataract* (366.01)] or just anterior to the posterior lens capsule [*posterior subcapsular or polar cataract* (366.02)]: an opacification caused by an abnormal anterior curvature of the lens (*anterior polar or anterior pyramidal cataract*); an "oil globule" reflex is seen within the pupillary red reflex.
- Completely White (Mature) Cataract (366.17).

Investigations

- *History*: Important because congenital and infantile cataracts may be orders normal dominant (most common), autosomal recessive, X-linked, or a chromosomal abnormality; the cataract may arise secondarily to an intrauterine infection (e.g. rubella).
- Visual acuity testing
- Refraction
- Intraocular pressure
- *Undilated and dilated slit-lamp examination*: Other ocular congested toe anomalies may occur along with a congenital cataract, such as colobomata of the iris
- *Dilated fundus examination*: especially in infants and young children; other ocular congenital anomalies may occur along with a congenital cataract, such as colobomata of the choroid
- Appropriate evaluation of any underlying cores as indicated.

Differential Diagnosis

Cataracts in children can be secondary to:
- Tumor (e.g. retinoblastoma)
- Trauma (Fig. 1)
- Intraocular inflammation, e.g. rubella (Fig. 2)
- Metabolic (e.g. galactosemia) or systemic (e.g. diabetes mellitus) diseases.

Cause

- Congenital (accounts for approx. 50% of all childhood cataracts)
- Genetic without systemic abnormalities (e.g. autosomal dominant cataract)
- Genetic with systemic abnormalities (e.g. oculocerebral syndrome of Lowe, incontinentia pigmenti)
- Metabolic (e.g. galactosemia, diabetes mellitus)
- Chromosomal abnormalities [e.g. trisomies 13 (Patau syndrome) and 21 (Down syndrome)]
- Intrauterine (e.g. rubella), or postpartum intraocular infection
- Therapeutic drugs (e.g. steroids).

Epidemiology

Cataracts occur in approx. 0.3% of all children; most have no known cause or associated systemic conditions.

Classification

- Infantile cataracts occur from 0 to 10 years
- Juvenile cataracts occur from 11 to 20 years
- Presenile cataracts occur ≤ 45 year.

Associated Features

Approximately 50% of patients have no associated systemic features, but some may have other ocular abnormalities (e.g. amblyopia, strabismus, intraocular structural abnormalities).

In the other 50%, associated features depend on the underlying cause (e.g. chromosomal or metabolic disorders, systemic syndromes with ocular manifestations, trauma, infections).

Pathology

The pathology depends on the type of cataract, with degenerative changes found in the nucleus, cortex, and anterior or posterior subcapsular areas.

Diagnosis continued on p. 74

TREATMENT

Diet and Lifestyle

In the vast majority of patients, diet and lifestyle have no effect on the cataracts. However, in patients with metabolic cataracts (e.g. galactosemia), appropriate diet can have a dramatic effect on the cataract.

Galactosemia is an autosomal recessive disease resulting from a deficiency of the galactose-1-phosphate uridyl transferase. The cataract usually is noted a few days to a few months after birth.

Pharmacologic Treatment

In the vast majority of patients, pharmacologic treatment has no effect on the cataracts. However, in metabolic cataracts (e.g. diabetes mellitus), appropriate therapy can impede or even reverse the cataract.

Nonpharmacologic Treatment

If visual potential exists in the eye, surgical treatment is indicated. Extracapsular cataract extraction (ECCE), usually by the irrigation-and-aspiration (I&A) technique and patients $\leq$ 30 years of age and by I&A or phacoemulsification in older patients. Depending on the patient's age, intraocular lens implantation may or may not be indicated.

Special care must be taken if congenital ectopic cataracts are present, such as Marfan's syndrome (autosomal dominant; excessive hydroxyproline urinary excretion) and homocystinuria (autosomal recessive; deficiency of cystathionine synthetase). In these patients, the cataractous lens generally is subluxated (in posterior chamber but not in normal position) or dislocated (out of posterior chamber into the vitreous or anterior chamber).

Treatment Aims

- To improve vision
- To prevent or treat amblyopia and strabismus.

Prognosis

Prognosis depends on many factors, such as age at onset, other associated intraocular abnormalities, and presence of amblyopia. In young children approx. 10 years of age, special attention must be paid to visual rehabilitation and the prevention or treatment of amblyopia. Children approx. 10 years of age who have blurred vision in one eye (e.g. from unilateral congenital cataract) tend to rotate that eye internally or externally so that the image does not fall on the macula. Although these children are able to suppress the image in the deviating eye, thereby avoiding the debilitating symptom of double vision (diplopia), the deviating eye itself becomes "lazy", and amblyopia develops. After good vision is restored by cataract surgery, this type of amblyopia often can be treated successfully by patching the nonamblyopic eye. Once the amblyopic child passes the age of approx. 10–12 years, however, the amblyopia becomes so deep seated that it cannot be reversed by patching or any other means.

Follow-up and Management

Long-term follow-up is needed to ensure proper visual rehabilitation and treatment of such postoperative complications as glaucoma and retinal detachment.

Treatment continued on p. 75

Cataract, Infantile, Juvenile, and Presenile (366.0)

DIAGNOSIS—cont'd

Complications

- *Amblyopia*: if strabismus develops because of a unilateral cataract, the child will not use the macula properly. Thus, the image can become suppressed. The advantage is a lack of diplopia. The disadvantage is the resulting "lazy eye".
- *Phacolytic glaucoma*: a mature cataract can "leak" fluid through an intact capsule causing a secondary glaucoma. The lens proteins gain access to the anterior chamber, acting as a weak antigen. Macrophages engulf the proteins, swell, and block the angle.

Pearls and Considerations

Cataracts can be caused by ocular developmental dysgenesis, intrauterine infections, metabolic syndromes, gene mutation, or as a part of a systemic syndrome. Infantile cataract is of particular concern because of the potential for deprivation amblyopia and secondary glaucoma. Early detection and intervention are keys to a desirable visual outcome. Not all cataracts are visually significant. Cataracts not visually significant should be monitored regularly because of the potential for progression.

Commonly Associated Conditions

Microphthalmia is often associated with congenital cataracts. This is also found in the following conditions:
- *Intrauterine infection*: rubella, varicella, toxoplasmosis, herpes simplex, bacterial, or fungal endophthalmitis, cytomegalovirus
- *Metabolic disorders*: Galactosemia, hypocalcemia, hypoglycemia, diabetes mellitus, hyperferritinemia, Wilson syndrome, Fabry syndrome, Refsum syndrome, homocystinuria, myotonia dystrophy, pseudohypoparathyroidism
- *Chromosomal*: Trisomy 21, Turner syndrome, Trisomy 13, Trisomy 18, cri du chat syndrome
- *Renal disease*: Lowe syndrome, Alport syndrome, Hallermann-Streiff-Francois syndrome
- *Central nervous system diseases*: Marinesco-Sjögren syndrome, Sjögren syndrome
- *Mandibulofacial syndromes*: Pierre Robin syndrome, Treacher Collins syndrome
- *Dermal syndromes*: incontinentia pigmenti, congenital ectodermal dysplasia, Werner syndrome, Rothmund-Thomson syndrome
- *Others*: Norrie disease, aniridia, retinitis pigmentosa, persistent fetal vasculature, retinopathy of prematurity, endophthalmitis.

Referral Information

Cataract surgeon when visually significant or causing ocular complications.

TREATMENT—cont'd

The residual lens epithelium in children is quite reactive, and opacification of the posterior capsule after ECCE is almost inevitable. Most surgeons, therefore, will perform a posterior capsulotomy (opening) or capsulectomy (removal) at the time of ECCE.

Because the eye does not reach adult size until the middle to late teens, the decision whether or not to implant an intraocular lens at the time of cataract surgery in a child is controversial. Although some advocate postoperative contact lenses, posterior chamber lens implantation is generally desirable. The strength of the lens must be estimated because the eye is still growing.

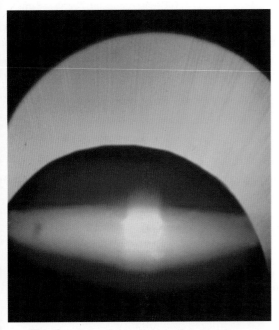

Fig. 1: Inferior dislocated lens following trauma.

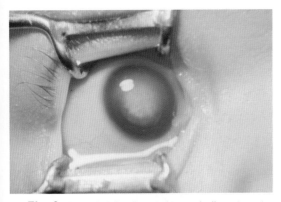

Fig. 2: Typical, infantile, nuclear, rubella cataract.

GENERAL REFERENCES

Bashour M, Menassa J, Gerontis CC. Congenital cataract. [online]. Available from www.emedicine.com

Bateman JB, Johannes M, Flodman P, et al. A new locus for autosomal dominant cataract on chromosome 12q13. Invest Ophthalmol Vis Sci. 2000;41(9): 2665-70.

Bateman JB, Johannes M, Flodman P, et al. A new locus for autosomal dominant cataract on chromosome 12q13. Invest Ophthalmol Vis Sci. 2000;41(9): 2665-70.

Conley YP, Erturk D, Keverline A, et al. A juvenile-onset, progressive cataract locus on chromosome 3q21-q22 is associated with a missense mutation in the beaded filament structural protein-2. Am J Hum Genet. 2000;66(4):1426-31. Epub 2000 Mar 22.

Haargaard B, Wohlfahrt J, Fiedelius HC, et al. A nationwide Danish study of 1027 cases of congenital/infantile cataract: etiological and clinical classifications. Ophthalmology. 2004;111: 2292-8.

Haargaard B, Wohlfahrt J, Fledelius HC, et al. A nationwide Danish study of 1027 cases of congenital/infantile cataracts: etiological and clinical classifications. Ophthalmology. 2004;111(12): 2292-8.

Junk AK, Stefani FH, Ludwig K. Bilateral anterior lenticonus: Scheimpflug imaging system documentation and ultrastructural confirmation of Alport syndrome in the lens capsule. Arch Ophthalmol. 2000;118(7):895-7.

Kramer PL, LaMorticella D, Schilling K, et al. A new locus for autosomal dominant congenital cataracts maps to chromosome 3. Invest Ophthalmol Vis Sci. 2000;41(1):36-9.

Kröger A, Bachli EB, Mumford A, et al. Hyperferritinemia without iron overload in patients with bilateral cataracts: a case series. J Med Case Reports. 2011;5:471.

Lambert SR, Drack AV. Infantile cataracts. Surv Ophthalmol. 1996;40(6): 427-58.

Lambert SR, Drack AV. Infantile cataracts. Surv Ophthalmol. 1996;40(6): 427-58.

Yanoff M, Sassani JW. Ocular Pathology, 6th edition. St Louis: Mosby; 2001. pp 361-5.

Cavernous Sinus Syndrome (Cavernositis 607.2)

DIAGNOSIS

Definition

Refers to a myriad of disease processes occurring within the cavernous sinus with resultant signs and symptoms of ophthalmoplegia, chemosis, proptosis, Horner's syndrome, or trigeminal sensory loss.

Synonyms

None

Symptoms

- Diplopia
- Ptosis
- Painful or painless.

Signs

- Ptosis
- Ophthalmoparesis
- Third-, fourth-, and sixth-nerve palsies
- Oculosympathetic paresis (Horner's syndrome: postganglionic third-order neuron affected)
- *Proptosis*: Up to 4 mm
- Loss of sensation along V1, V2.

Investigations (Figs 1A to G)

- *Anisocoria*: Check in bright and dim illumination
- *Cocaine ophthalmic solution (4–10%) or paredrine (hydroxyamphetamine; Pharmics, Salt Lake City, Utah) pupil testing*: No dilation to both in Horner's syndrome.
- Forced ductions
- Magnetic resonance imaging
- Lumbar puncture
- Indirect pharyngoscopy
- Biopsy of nasopharynx
- Laboratory studies (e.g. MMA-TP, RPR, ANA, ESR, CXR).

Pearls and Considerations

Varied and dependent on the etiology of the disease

Referral Information

A full medical workup and imaging are required to determine the nature of the disease.

Differential Diagnosis

- Myasthenia gravis
- Giant cell arteritis
- Ischemic ocular syndrome
- Chronic progressive external ophthalmoplegia (bilateral)
- Miller-Fisher variant of Guillain-Barré syndrome
- Botulism.

Cause

- Trauma
- Intracavernous carotid artery aneurysm
- Carotid cavernous fistula or thrombosis
- Neoplasm
- Metastases
- Inflammation/infection (e.g. herpes zoster, mucormycosis, *Treponema pallidum, Mycobacterium tuberculosis*)
- Sarcoidosis
- Wegener's granulomatous disease
- *Tolosa-Hunt syndrome (THS)*: Diagnosis of exclusion; inflammatory, painful idiopathic ophthalmoplegia.

Classification

- Retrocavernous sinus involvement is suggested by involvement of V1, V2 and V3.
- Inferior cavernous sinus involvement is indicated by parasympathetic paresis of the pupil and loss of sensation in V1.
- Involvement of the anterior cavernous sinus/superior orbital fissure is implied by proptosis and involvement of the optic nerve.

TREATMENT

Diet and Lifestyle

No special precautions are necessary.

Pharmacologic Treatment

- Treatment directed toward underlying cause
- *Tolosa-Hunt syndrome*: Oral prednisone, 1–1.5 mg/kg/day; possible initial IV steroids; exclude infection before initial steroid therapy.

Nonpharmacologic Treatment

No nonpharmacologic treatment is recommended.

Treatment Aims
Depends on cause.

Prognosis
Depends on cause.

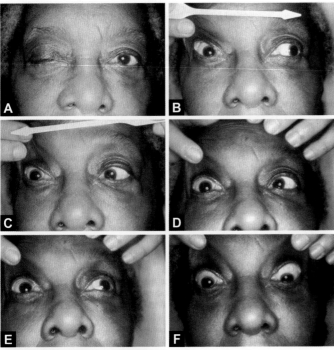

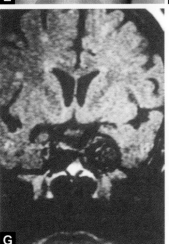

Figs 1A to G: (A) Woman aged 55 years has acute onset of right ophthalmoparesis; (B) While lifting her eyelid, she is unable to adduct her right eye; (C) She is also unable to abduct her right eye; (D) and cannot elevate it up and in (E) or up and out; (F) She is equally unable to depress her right eye, which is consistent with third-, fourth-, and sixth-nerve palsies. Furthermore, the right pupil is miotic and implicates the oculosympathetic fibers; and (G) This constellation of signs localized a lesion to the cavernous sinus. This coronal T1-weighted magnetic resonance image shows an aneurysm involving the right cavernous sinus.

GENERAL REFERENCES

Kattah J, Pula J (2006). Cavernous sinus syndromes. [online] Available from www.emedicine.com

Keane JR. Cavernous sinus syndrome: analysis of 151 cases. Arch Neurol. 1996; 53(10):967-71.

Levin A. Neuro-ophthalmology. New York: Thieme Medical Publishers; 2005.

Zarei M, Anderson JR, Higgins JN, et al. Cavernous sinus syndrome as the only manifestation of sarcoidosis. J Postgrad Med. 2002;48(2):119-21.

Chemical Burns (941.02)

DIAGNOSIS

Definition

Traumatic injury to the eye or adnexa resulting from contact with any chemical agent.

Synonyms

None

Symptoms

- Pain
- Photophobia
- Burning
- Foreign body sensation
- Decreased vision
- Epiphora.

Signs

Mild to Moderate Burns

- *Corneal epithelial defects*: from superficial punctate keratitis to focal epithelia loss to sloughing of the entire epithelium (Fig. 1)
- Conjunctival hyperemia/injection
- No signs of absent blood vessels, conjunctival chemosis, hyperemia, or hemorrhage.

Moderate to Severe Burns

- Corneal edema and opacification
- Significant chemosis and perilimbal blanching
- High intraocular pressure
- Poor fluorescein stain despite complete epithelial loss
- Conjunctival ischemia/absent blood vessels.

Investigations

- *History*: time of injury, type of chemical, duration of exposure, duration of irrigation
- Visual acuity test
- *Slit-lamp examination and eyelid eversion*: to look for foreign body
- Intraocular pressure
- Dilated fundus examination.

Differential Diagnosis

- Traumatic corneal abrasion
- Dry eyes
- Episcleritis
- Scleritis
- Stevens-Johnson syndrome
- Ocular cicatricial pemphigoid.

Cause

Alkali (lye, cements, plasters), acids, solvents, detergents, mace.

Classification

Alkali burns: Penetrate ocular surface easily.
Acid burns: Coagulate surface tissue.

Pathology

- Acids denature and precipitate proteins in tissue. Tissue damage is mainly at the surface, and the coagulated surface forms a barrier against penetration of the agent.
- Alkylating agents raise the pH of tissue and cause saponification of fatty acids in cell membranes, subsequently disrupting them. The agent is then able to penetrate the ocular tissue rapidly, entering the anterior chamber, where it causes intense inflammation.

Diagnosis continued on p. 80

TREATMENT

Diet and Lifestyle

Protective eyewear around chemicals.

Pharmacologic Treatment

Emergency treatment is mandatory. Copious irrigation of the eyes with saline or with nonsterile water if it is the only liquid available. This might take up to 4–6 L to neutralize the pH. Place a lid speculum and topical anesthesia in the eye before irrigation. Inspect the upper and lower fornices well, sweep with moistened cotton swab, and irrigate thoroughly. Use IV tubing connected to an irrigating solution to facilitate irrigation.

For Mild Burns

- After the eye is irrigated and the pH is neutral, instill cycloplegia
- *Standard dosage*: Homatropine 5%, two times daily
- Place topical antibiotic ointment
- *Standard dosage*: Erythromycin, four times daily
- Consider pressure patch for 24 hours.

For Moderate to Severe Burns

- Debride necrotic tissue, instill cycloplegia (see for mild burns), place topical antibiotic ointment up to eight times daily (see for mild burns), and apply topical steroid
- *Standard dosage*: Prednisolone acetate 1%, four to eight times daily for 1–2 weeks, then rapid taper
- *Special points*: Consider pressure patch between drops
- If the intraocular pressure is elevated, administer antiglaucoma medication. Destroy conjunctival adhesions using a glass rod with antibiotic ointment
- If corneal melt occurs, may use collagenase inhibitors (e.g. Mucomyst every 4 hours), and if melting progresses, consider cyanoacrylate adhesive
- Consider doxycycline (100 mg twice daily) for its collagenase inhibitor effect and vitamin C, 2 g daily (1 g twice daily or 500 mg four times daily), to promote collagen synthesis
- Frequent lubrication with preservative-free tears, every 1–2 hours, essential in promoting re-epithelialization
- Consider topical citrate 10%, four to eight times daily, for its anticollagenase effect and topical ascorbate 10%, four to eight times daily, to promote collagen synthesis.

Treatment Aims

To reduce and prevent further breakdown of tissue and to promote healing.

Prognosis

Poor for severe burns, especially those caused by alkylating agents.

Follow-up and Management

Mild burns

Recheck daily, consider patching, until corneal abrasion heals.

Moderate to Severe Burns

Daily follow-up with aggressive lubrication and antibiotic coverage; severely dry eyes may require a tarsorrhaphy; a conjunctival autograft may be performed if the injury is unilateral.

Treatment continued on p. 81

Chemical Burns (941.02)

DIAGNOSIS—cont'd

Complications

- Corneal ulceration and infection
- Corneal opacity and vascularization
- Corneal melt and perforation
- Symblepharon formation
- Anterior-segment ischemia
- Cataract
- Local necrotic retinopathy.

Pearls and Considerations

Treatment with copious irrigation should be instituted immediately, even before testing vision or undertaking any other testing, and should be continued until a neutral pH is achieved.

Referral Information

Depends on severity of disease; referral for hospitalization, palliative care, or corneal graft surgery may be required depending on the severity of the burn.

TREATMENT—cont'd

Nonpharmacologic Treatment

- Soft/bandage contact lenses, patching, tarsorrhaphy, and amniotic membrane transplantation may be required to promote re-epithelialization
- Corneal transplant may be performed either as an emergency procedure for corneal melt or perforation or later because of corneal scarring
- Limbal stem cell transplant may be necessary to replace damaged limbal stem cells, alone or before corneal transplantation.

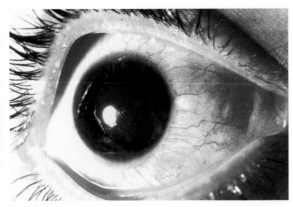

Fig. 1: Corneal and conjunctival abrasion after chemical burn caused by car battery explosion (HNO_3). There is no limbal ischemia.

GENERAL REFERENCES

Albert DM, Jakobiec FA (Eds). Principles and practice of ophthalmology, vol 1. Philadelphia: WB Saunders; 2000.

American Academy of Ophthalmology. Basic and Clinical Science. San Francisco: The Academy; 2006-2007.

Kunimoto DY, Kanitkar KD, Makar M. Chemical burns. In: Friedberg MA, Rapuano CJ (Eds). The Wills eye manual: office and emergency room diagnosis and treatment of eye disease, 4th edition. Philadelphia: Lippincott Williams & Wilkins; 2004. pp. 14-6.

Wright K. Textbook of ophthalmology. Baltimore: Lippincott Williams & Wilkins; 1997.

Chiasmal Syndrome (377.5)

DIAGNOSIS

Definition

Loss of vision and visual field from direct involvement of the optic chiasm, its blood supply, or the adjacent optic tract (Fig. 1).

Synonyms

None

Symptoms

- Painless, asymmetric visual loss
- *Hemifield slide phenomenon*: in a complete bitemporal hemianopia, the intact nasal visual fields of each eye may overlap or separate; this can cause a sensory diplopia, or an object may seem to disappear from central vision.
- *Postfixation blindness*: in a complete bitemporal hemianopia, when a patient converges to a point, the blind hemianopic visual fields align behind fixation; when the patient attempts to thread a needle, for example, the thread enters the eye of the needle but does not appear to exit on the other side.
- Cerebrospinal fluid rhinorrhea (sphenoid sinus eroded by pituitary adenoma)
- Headache
- Decreased libido, impotence
- Amenorrhea
- Galactorrhea, oligomenorrhea
- Infertility
- Asthenia.

Signs

- Visual field loss that respects the vertical meridian
- *Optic nerve dysfunction*: may include visual acuity loss, relative afferent pupillary defect, dyschromatopsia, pallor of the neuroretinal rim of the optic disk, and dropout of the nerve fiber layer.
- Acquired cupping (rare) and neuroretinal rim pallor
- Proptosis.

Investigations

Magnetic resonance imaging: sella optic chiasm, suprasellar cistern (Fig. 2).

Endocrinologic evaluation: may include cortisol measurement for adrenal axis, thyroid tests, sex hormone measurement for gonadal axis, prolactin test, growth hormone assay, plasma and urine osmolality measurement for postetior pituitary, insulin tolerance test, and releasing hormone tests.

Differential Diagnosis

- Pseudo-visual field defect (e.g. from ptosis)
- Bilateral cecocentral scotomas
- Enlarged blind spots
- Peripheral visual field contraction
- Retinitis pigmentosa.

Cause

- Pituitary adenoma, 50–55%
- Craniopharyngioma, 20–25%
- Meningioma, 10%
- Gliomas, 7%.

Classification

- The anterior chiasmal syndrome refers to a central scotoma in one eye with superior temporal visual field loss respecting the vertical hemianopic meridian in the fellow eye.
- The middle chiasmal syndrome describes the bitemporal (often asymmetric) visual field defect.
- The posterior chiasmal syndrome is characterized by a central bitemporal hemianopia respecting the vertical hemianopic meridian, a bitemporal hemianopia respecting the vertical hemianopic line (more dense below than above), or an incongruous homonymous hemianopia resulting from the lesion affecting the junction of the optic tract at the optic chiasm.

Diagnosis continued on p. 84

TREATMENT

Diet and Lifestyle

No special precautions are necessary.

Pharmacologic Treatment

- If the pituitary tumor is secreting prolactin, administration of bromocriptine is indicated
- *Replacement therapy*: depending on hormonal involvement.

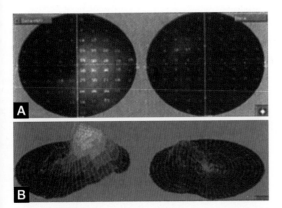

Figs 1A and B: (A) Visual field of a 41-year-old man who has progressively lost vision in his right eye. A temporal defect in his left eye respects the vertical hemianopic line. This is right anterior chiasmal syndrome; (B) This three-dimensional visual representation demonstrates loss in the hill of vision in the same patient.

Treatment Aims

- To decompress the optic chiasm to regain vision or at least prevent further visual loss
- To normalize pituitary function.

Prognosis

Depends on the sellar lesion and the degree of involvement of the optic nerves and optic chiasm.

Follow-up and Management

Because of the recurrence of pituitary adenomas, craniopharyngiomas, and meningiomas, the patient must undergo at least yearly serial visual field testing and magnetic resonance imaging.

Treatment continued on p. 85

DIAGNOSIS—cont'd

Complications

Pituitary adenoma can hemorrhage, become secondary, or undergo necrosis: this results in further visual loss as the optic nerve and chiasm are compressed. Ophthalmoparesis (usually third-nerve palsy) occurs as the enlarged tumor involves the cavernous sinus and subarachnoid space. There is a high mortality rate because of panhypopituitarism and subarachnoid hemorrhage. Immediate treatment is mandatory, with high-dose systemic corticosteroids and stabilization of electrolyte balance.

Pregnancy: Sheehan's syndrome refers to the postpartum infarction of a normal pituitary gland.

Pearls and Considerations

Varied and dependent on the etiology of the disease.

Referral Information

Patients with chiasmal syndrome should be referred for imaging, blood work, and subspecialist consultation (e.g. endocrinologist, oncologist) depending on the etiology of the disease.

TREATMENT—cont'd

Nonpharmacologic Treatment

- Trans-sphenoidal hypophysectomy
- Transfrontal craniotomy for large masses
- *Radiation therapy*: rarely used as a primary treatment.

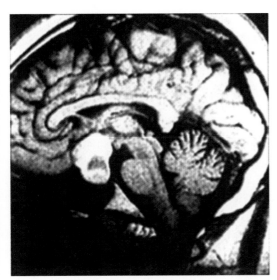

Fig. 2: T1-weighted sagittal magnetic resonance image revealing pituitary adenoma with hemorrhage (pituitary apoplexy) compressing the chiasm from below.

GENERAL REFERENCES

Foroozan R. Chiasmal syndromes. Curr Opin Ophthalmol. 2003;14(6):325-31.

Hedges TR. Optic chiasm field defects. In: Walsh TJ (Ed). Visual Fields: Examination and Interpretation. San Francisco: American Academy of Ophthalmology; 1990. pp. 151-77.

Ruben RM, Sadun AA, Pava A. Optic chiasm, parasellar region, and pituitary fossa. In: Yanoff M, Duker JS (Eds). Ophthalmology, 2nd edition. St. Louis: Elsevier; 2006.

Trevino R. Chiasmal syndrome. J Am Optometr Assoc. 1995;66(9):559-75.

Chorioretinitis (363.0)

DIAGNOSIS

Definition

Inflammation of the retina and choroid secondary to underlying infection or chronic granulomatous disease.

Synonyms

None; associated abbreviation: POHS (presumed ocular histoplasmosis syndrome).

Symptoms

Presumed Ocular Histoplasmosis

Patients are usually asymptomatic; secondary choroidal neovascularization (CNV) may cause distortion, decreased vision and scotomas.

Toxoplasmosis

Floaters, decreased vision, distortion of central vision.

Signs

Presumed Ocular Histoplasmosis

- Classic triad of clinical findings (*see* Fig. 1)
- Peripapillary pigment alteration
- Multiple punched-out atrophic lesions in the peripheral fundus
- Choroidal neovascularization in the macula.

Toxoplasmosis

- *Anterior-chamber inflammation*: may be seen
- Vitreous cells
- *Active retinitis*: with an adjacent chorioretinal scar with overlying vitreous cells ("headlight in the fog") (*see* Fig. 2)
- *Subretinal hemorrhage, subretinal scar formation*: from secondary CNV
- *Macular or peripheral chorioretinal scar*: implies a previous infection
- Congenital cases may have associated microphthalmia, vitritis, glaucoma and ocular palsies
- Immunocompromised patients have a more severe retinochoroiditis that tends to be bilateral and multifocal.

Investigations

Presumed Ocular Histoplasmosis

- *Careful history*: most patients with this disease have lived in the central and eastern river-valley regions of the United States
- Slit-lamp and dilated eye examination
- *Fluorescein angiography*: to determine the presence of active CNV
- *Histoplasmin skin test*: not helpful in making the diagnosis.

Differential Diagnosis

Presumed Ocular Histoplasmosis
- Idiopathic CNV
- Multifocal choroiditis.

Toxoplasmosis
- Sarcoidosis and multifocal choroiditis.

Cause

Presumed Ocular Histoplasmosis
- *Histoplasma capsulatum* is a dimorphic soil mold. Infection results from inhalation of spores and is usually asymptomatic.
- In immunocompromised individuals, disseminated disease (characterized by hepatosplenomegaly, lymphadenopathy and pancytopenia) can occur.

Toxoplasmosis
- *Toxoplasma gondii* is an obligate intracellular parasite of humans and animals. The tachyzoite form invades tissue during an acute infection, which usually follows ingestion of contaminated meat or cat feces.
- Tachyzoites spread hematogenously; they can cross the placental barrier, causing acute infection in the fetus.

Epidemiology

Toxoplasmosis
- Congenital chorioretinitis infection has a propensity for the macular region and is bilateral in 85% of cases.
- Four percent of seropositive individuals will show evidence of chorioretinal lesions on fundus examination.

Associated Features

Toxoplasmosis
Systemic features in acute infection include fever, headache, lymphadenopathy, fatigue, malaise, myalgias, urticaria and erythematous macular rashes. Mild secondary leukopenia and pancytopenia are common. Patients with severe disease have pneumonitis, splenomegaly, encephalitis and myocarditis.

Pathology

Presumed Ocular Histoplasmosis
Peripheral lesions: Clinically, they are 0.2–0.6 disk diameter in size, discrete, and often have pigmented borders; histologically, areas show varying degrees of inflammation with aggregates of lymphocytes in the choroid; eventually there is a loss of overlying retinal pigment epithelium and a degeneration of the rods and cones in this area.

Diagnosis continued on p. 88

TREATMENT

Diet and Lifestyle

Presumed Ocular Histoplasmosis

No special precautions are necessary.

Toxoplasmosis

Pregnant women need to avoid cat litter, undercooked meats, and foods made with raw eggs.

Pharmacologic Treatment

Presumed Ocular Histoplasmosis

A series of intravitreal injections with either Avastin or Lucentis often improves the visual acuity and induces regression of the choroidal neovascular vessels. Fewer injections are required than in patients with CNV due to macular degeneration.

Toxoplasmosis

Standard dosage: Prednisone 40–80 mg/day depending on weight, with taper over 1–2 months in addition to antibiotics.
Sulfadiazine, 4–6 g divided in 4 daily doses for 4–6 weeks.

Special points: If sulfadiazine is not available, clindamycin may be used (300 mg PO divided in 4 daily doses for 4–6 weeks).

Complications

Presumed Ocular Histoplasmosis

Secondary CNV

Toxoplasmosis

Permanent decreased vision: from macular scar formation from an active lesion or secondary CNV.

Cataracts, glaucoma, cystoid macular edema: caused by chronic active inflammation.

Pearls and Considerations

- Lesions from histoplasmosis typically present as peripapillary atrophy, punched-out lesions of the periphery, and CNV of the macula (or resultant disciform scar after resolution of CNV)
- Geographically, histoplasmosis is most common in the Ohio and Mississippi river valleys
- Systemic histoplasmosis and toxoplasmosis usually present as a mild to moderate respiratory infection
- Recurrence of toxoplasmosis infection is common because of the rupture of cysts, which form in any organ
- *Toxoplasma* infection can pass to infant (congenital toxoplasmosis) via transplacental transmission.

Referral Information

Refer to retinal specialist for intravitreal injections or laser photocoagulation.

Treatment Aims

Presumed Ocular Histoplasmosis
None
Toxoplasmosis
- To control reactivation
- To educate the patient on the possible secondary complications of glaucoma, cataract, macular edema and CNV.

Prognosis

Presumed Ocular Histoplasmosis
Good, unless macular CNV occurs.
Toxoplasmosis
- Prognosis is good in adult patients when the lesion is peripheral
- Macular reactivation can cause significant visual loss
- Immunocompromised patients have a worse prognosis
- Patients with congenital disease are often legally blind.

Follow-up and Management

Presumed Ocular Histoplasmosis
Amsler grid to detect early signs of secondary CNV; otherwise, annual dilated eye examinations.
Toxoplasmosis
- Active lesions are followed closely until they subside
- Chorioretinal scars can be followed on an annual basis.

Treatment continued on p. 89

Chorioretinitis (363.0)

DIAGNOSIS—cont'd

Toxoplasmosis

Careful history: previous exposure to cat feces, poorly cooked meats, raw eggs.

Careful slit-lamp and dilated fundus examination: necessary because the diagnosis is often clinical.

Immunoglobulin M and G titer: rising in acute infections; low or absent in chronic infections.

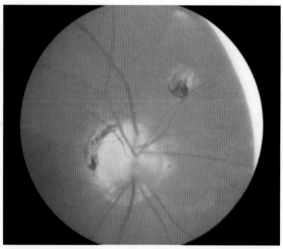

Fig. 1: Presumed ocular histoplasmosis. Two components of the classic triad can be seen here: peripapillary atrophy and a peripheral punched-out lesion.

TREATMENT—cont'd

Nonpharmacologic Treatment

Presumed Ocular Histoplasmosis

Thermal laser photocoagulation to CNV, if extrafoveal location. For subfoveal CNV use intravitreal Avastin or Lucentis. Photodynamic therapy is only used in selected cases of subfoveal CNV.

Toxoplasmosis

No nonpharmacologic treatment is recommended.

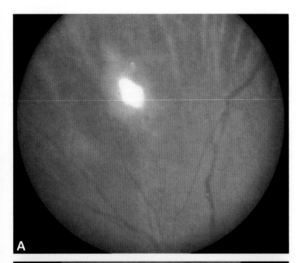

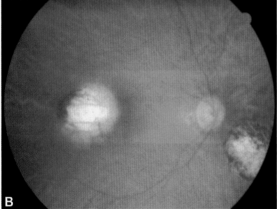

Figs 2A and B: Toxoplasmosis. (A) Active retinitis with an adjacent chorioretinal scar and overlying vitreous cells; (B) Macular and peripheral chorioretinal scars in a patient with congenital toxoplasmosis.

GENERAL REFERENCES

Adams WH, Kindermann WR, Walls KW, et al. Toxoplasmic antibodies and retinochoroiditis in the Marshall Islands and their association with exposure to radioactive fallout. Am J Trop Med Hyg. 1987;36:315-20.

Jabs DA, Nguyen QD. Ocular toxoplasmosis. Retina, 4th edition. St Louis: Elsevier; 2006.

Makley TA, Craig EL, Werling K. Histopathology of ocular histoplasmosis. Int Ophthalmol Clin. 1983;23:1-18.

Schadlu R, Blinder KJ, Shah GK, et al. Intravitreal bevacizumab for choroidal neovascularization in ocular histoplasmosis. Am J Ophthalmol. 2008;145(5): 875-8.

Chorioretinopathy, Central Serous (362.41)

DIAGNOSIS

Definition

A disease of the choroid and retina characterized by accumulation of clear fluid at the posterior pole of the fundus.

Synonyms

None; abbreviated CSC or CSR (central serous retinopathy).

Symptoms

- Gradual decrease in vision
- Metamorphopsia
- Alteration in color vision
- Micropsia.

Signs (Figs 1-3)

- Shallow, round accumulation of subretinal fluid
- Subretinal precipitates
- Subretinal fibrin
- *Changes in the retinal pigment epithelium (RPE)*: suggest a previous episode
- Extramacular RPE atrophic tracts
- Multiple bullous, serous, retinal and RPE detachments.

Investigations

Fluorescein angiography: demonstrates pinpoint leakage that increases in size as the angiogram continues; late phases of the angiogram show pooling of dye into the subretinal space; a "smokestack" leakage pattern (*see* Fig. 2), although less common, is characteristic. Indocyanine green angiography may be done if fluorescein angiography does not reveal the leak.

Complications

- *Permanently decreased vision*: can occur with repeated bouts of CSC
- Secondary choroidal neovascularization.

Differential Diagnosis

- Pigment epithelial detachment
- Choroidal neovascularization
- Optic nerve pit with subretinal leakage
- Choroidal tumors
- Choroidal inflammation
- Choroidal ischemia.

Cause

- Central serous retinopathy is thought to result from focal leakage caused by alterations of the RPE that allow fluid from the choroidal layer to seep through to the subretinal space. This is somehow hormonally induced, as steroids can cause recurrences while inhibition of steroids can result in resolution of the fluid.
- There may be a correlation to stress, as the condition is more common in patients with Type A personality.

Epidemiology

- More common in males aged 25–50 years
- Spontaneously resolves over 6 months
- Can recur
- Occurs bilaterally in 10% of cases
- Has been seen in pregnant females.

Associated Features

- Migraine headaches
- Type A personality traits
- Hypochondria and hysteria.

Pathology

Unknown, but believed to be multifactorial, in which one of the risk factors is stress; it is difficult to determine if CSC is a primary choroidal problem, a primary RPE problem, or combination of the two.

Diagnosis continued on p. 92

TREATMENT

Diet and Lifestyle

If related to stress, attempts to decrease stress may allow the disease to resolve more quickly.

Pharmacologic Treatment

- Oral steroids are contraindicated.
- Small studies suggest that glucocorticoid receptor antagonism with oral mifepristone is beneficial in refractory cases.

Nonpharmacologic Treatment

If the fluid does not resolve over 4 months or the patient's occupation requires clear binocular vision, thermal laser photocoagulation to the leakage spot may be applied. Photodynamic therapy may be used for subfoveal leakage not amenable to thermal laser; complications of this may include tears of the retinal pigment epithelium.

Treatment Aims

To resolve fluid

Prognosis

- Eighty to ninety percent of patients resolve spontaneously.
- Visual deterioration to less than 20/200 is uncommon.

Follow-up and Management

- Patients should be followed periodically until the fluid resolves.
- Patients need to be educated on the risk of recurrence and involvement of the second eye.

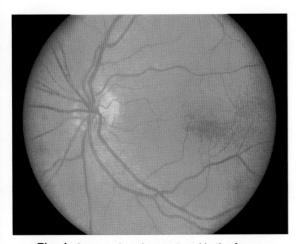

Fig. 1: Serous elevation centered in the fovea.

Treatment continued on p. 93

Chorioretinopathy, Central Serous (362.41)

DIAGNOSIS—cont'd

Pearls and Considerations

- Optical coherence tomography (OCT) can be useful in quantifying serous detachment and in tracking its resolution
- Central serous retinopathy has not been reported in patients under 20 years of age
- Use of oral or even inhaled steroids may cause exacerbation of the condition.

Referral Information

Refer for photocoagulation if fluid does not resolve on its own.

TREATMENT—cont'd

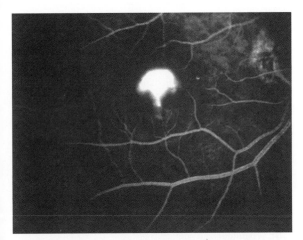

Fig. 2: Classic "smokestack" fluorescein pattern in a patient with central serous chorioretinopathy.

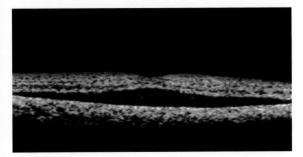

Fig. 3: Optical coherence tomography demonstrates subneurosensory fluid with no intraretinal fluid. Foveal contour is preserved.

GENERAL REFERENCES

Folk J, Oh K. (2005). Chorioretinopathy, central serous. [Online]. Available from www.emedicine.com/oph/topic 689.htm.

Guyer DR, Gragoudas ES. Central serous chorioretinopathy. In: Albert DM, Jakobiec FA (Eds). Principles and Practice of Ophthalmology. Philadelphia: Saunders; 1994. pp. 818-25.

Klais CM, Ober MD, Ciardella AP, et al. Central serous chorioretinopathy. Retina, 4th edition. St Louis: Elsevier; 2006.

Nielsen JS, Jampol LM. Oral mifepristone for chronic central serous chorioretinopathy. Retina. 2011;3(9): 1928-36.

Ober MD, Yannuzzi LA, Do DV, et al. Photodynamic therapy for focal retinal pigment epithelial leaks secondary to central serous chorioretinopathy. Ophthalmology. 2005;112(12): 2088-94.

Choroid Dystrophies (363.5)

DIAGNOSIS

Definition

Degeneration of the choriocapillaris caused by gene mutations affecting function of the retinal pigment epithelium (RPE), resulting in choroidal dystrophies (e.g. gyrate atrophy and choroideremia).

Symptoms

Gyrate Atrophy

- *Gradual decrease in vision to legal blindness*: by age 40–55 years
- Night blindness.

Choroideremia

Progressive visual loss, visual field constriction, and decreased night vision with advancing age: men more than 60 years of age rarely retain central vision.

Signs

Gyrate Atrophy

Multiple sharply defined, scalloped areas of chorioretinal atrophy: separated from each other by thin margins of pigment; these lesions begin in the midperiphery, eventually coalescing to involve the entire fundus (*see* Fig. 1).

Choroideremia

- *Diffuse, progressive atrophy of the choriocapillaris and RPE*: these changes start at the midperiphery and develop into scalloped edges that extend both anteriorly and posteriorly (*see* Fig. 2)
- Retinal arteriolar attenuation
- Clumped pigment dispersed in the periphery.

Investigations

Gyrate Atrophy

- *Detailed family history*: for decreased vision and blindness
- Slit-lamp and dilated fundus evaluation
- *Visual field test*: will show constriction
- *Electroretinogram*: shows reduced rod and cone responses with the rods affected worse in the early phases
- Abnormal dark adaptation shows elevated rod thresholds
- *Amino acid evaluation*: decreased lysine levels; elevated plasma ornithine levels in all body fluids.

Choroideremia

- Slit-lamp and dilated fundus examinations
- *Dark adaptation thresholds*: increase with age
- *Visual field thresholds*: demonstrate constriction over time
- *Electroretinogram*: will be greatly reduced.

Differential Diagnosis

Gyrate Atrophy
- Choroideremia
- Paving-stone degeneration
- High myopia
- Thioridazine (Mellaril) retinopathy.

Choroideremia
- Gyrate atrophy
- Retinitis pigmentosa
- Toxic retinopathy
- Albinism.

Cause

Gyrate Atrophy
- Autosomal recessive inheritance pattern

Choroideremia
- X-linked recessive trait found on the q21 band of the X chromosome.

Epidemiology

Choroideremia

Asymptomatic carriers have normal visual acuity; dark adaptation, and visual fields. Fundus examination may show clumping of RPE and depigmentation of the pigment layer.

Associated Features

Gyrate Atrophy
- Seizures have been reported in some patients despite normal neurologic evaluation
- Electron microscopy reveals morphologic changes in muscle fibers and hair shafts.

Pathology

Gyrate Atrophy

Swollen mitochondria in the retina lack ornithine ketoacid aminotransferase, the mitochondrial matrix that catalyzes the intraconversion of ornithine and a-ketoglutarate to pyrroline and glutamate; ornithine ketoacid aminotransferase is assigned to chromosome 10.

Choroideremia

Irregular pigmentation with a well-defined zone of midperipheral depigmentation of the RPE; optic nerve and arterioles appear normal; atrophy of the outer segments of the photoreceptors; choriocapillaris atrophy; thickening of Bruch's membrane.

Diagnosis continued on p. 96

TREATMENT

Diet and Lifestyle

Gyrate Atrophy

- Reduce dietary protein consumption
- Avoid arginine amino acid in food products.

Choroideremia

No precautions are necessary.

Pharmacologic Treatment

Gyrate Atrophy

Standard dosage: Supplemental vitamin B$_6$ (pyridoxine), 20 mg/day PO to start; increase up to 500 mg/day.

Special points: A 30–50% decrease in plasma ornithine levels will occur in 1 week.

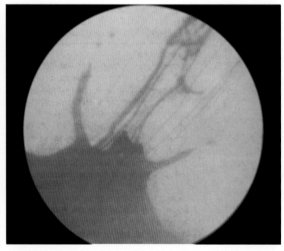

Fig. 1: Gyrate atrophy. Note the scalloped, well-defined areas of chorioretinal atrophy in the midperipheral retina.

Treatment Aims

Choroideremia
Unfortunately, there is no effective treatment. Low-vision aids may be of some benefit.
Gyrate Atrophy
To lower plasma levels of ornithine through diet control (early detection is therefore of utmost importance), although the long-term benefit to visual preservation is unknown.

Other Treatments

- Darkly tinted sunglasses
- Genetic counseling: Gyrate atrophy is an autosomal recessive disorder caused by mutations in the ornithine aminotransferase gene on chromosome 10. Choroideremia is an X-linked recessive disease caused by the deletion of the Rab escort protein 1.

Prognosis

Poor, because patients with either gyrate atrophy or choroideremia often lose vision to legal blindness.

Follow-up and Management

Gyrate Atrophy

- Ornithine levels need to be checked to determine the amount of vitamin B$_6$ needed to stabilize the ornithine levels.
- Serum ammonia levels are followed to monitor dietary arginine restriction.

Treatment continued on p. 97

Choroid Dystrophies (363.5)

DIAGNOSIS—cont'd

Complications

Gyrate Atrophy

Legal blindness

Choroideremia

Progressive, extensive visual loss

Referral Information

Refer to eye care physician to rule out conditions that may mimic gyrate atrophy and choroideremia (e.g. retinitis pigmentosa).

TREATMENT—cont'd

Choroideremia

No pharmacologic treatment is recommended.

Nonpharmacologic Treatment

No nonpharmacologic treatment is recommended.

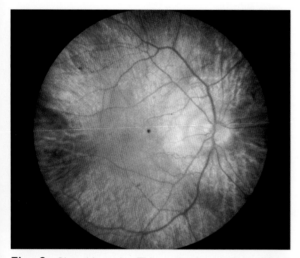

Fig. 2: Choroideremia. This patient's eye has diffuse progressive atrophy of the choriocapillaris and retinal pigment epithelium, retinal arteriolar attenuation, prominent large choroidal vessels, and clumped pigment dispersed in the periphery.

GENERAL REFERENCES

Berson EL. Retinitis pigmentosa and allied diseases. In: Albert DM, Jakobiec FA, (Eds). Principles and Practice of Ophthalmology. Philadelphia: Saunders;1994. pp. 1225-6.

Flannery JG, Bird AC, Farber DB, et al. A histopathologic study of a choroideremia carrier. Invest Ophthalmol Vis Sci. 1990;31:229-36.

Choroidal Detachment (after Filtration Surgery) (363.70)

DIAGNOSIS

Definition

Displacement of the choroid from the sclera caused by accumulation of fluid in the virtual space between them.

Synonyms

None

Symptoms

Decreased vision: Visual acuity is typically decreased after filtration surgery for a few days to several weeks; however, choroidal detachment is associated with a loss of vision that becomes more profound than expected or a worsening of vision over time during the postoperative period; in the presence of a large choroidal detachment, patients may be aware of a black area in the field of vision corresponding to the location of the choroidal detachment.

Pain: Pain associated with postoperative choroidal detachment is variable; many patients report no discomfort at all; some patients report mild to moderate pain with the onset of the choroidal detachment: if the detachment is hemorrhagic, pain may be quite severe.

Signs

Hypotony: Choroidal detachments are generally associated with a very low intraocular pressure (IOP) postoperatively, usually caused by decreased ciliary body function due to the fluid collection in the suprachoroidal and supraciliary space; also, overfiltration may be associated with an abnormally large filtering bleb; a wound leak from the filtration site can be detected with the Seidel test; with a hemorrhagic choroidal detachment, the IOP may be elevated.

Shallowing of the anterior chamber: Because of the fluid collection between the choroid and sclera and the associated anterior displacement of the ciliary body, and because of the hypotony, the anterior chamber will be abnormally shallow; there may be peripheral iris-cornea touch (Grade 1), central iris-cornea touch (Grade 2), or lens, implant or vitreous-cornea touch (Grade 3). Lens, implant or vitreous-cornea touch will result in injury to the corneal endothelium, permanent corneal edema and opacification if not corrected promptly.

Elevation of the choroid and retina: The choroid and overlying retina will be elevated; if the fundus can be seen, this will appear as a smooth, bullous, orange-brown elevation, usually arising from the inferior fundus; if the fundus cannot be seen, B-scan ultrasonography will usually reveal the detachment.

Differential Diagnosis

The diagnosis of choroidal detachment following filtration surgery is usually fairly obvious. It is important to distinguish serous from hemorrhagic choroidal detachment. Differential diagnosis would include:
- Retinal detachment
- Choroidal melanoma or metastatic tumor.

Etiology

It is thought that the sudden decrease in IOP after filtration surgery causes the choroidal vessels to leak fluid into the suprachoroidal space. This sets up a vicious cycle because the resulting ciliochoroidal detachment prevents the ciliary body from producing aqueous. The resulting hypotony then tends to worsen the choroidal effusion, which in turn prolongs the hypotony.

Classification

Choroidal detachments are classified as either *serous* (363.71) or *hemorrhagic* (363.72) depending on the nature of the fluid found in the suprachoroidal space.

Complications

Permanent loss of vision: Choroidal detachment, especially if hemorrhagic, is often associated with injury to the photoreceptor cells of the retina and with varying degrees of permanent loss of vision.

Corneal edema and cataract: In severe cases of anterior-chamber shallowing, the corneal endothelium and lens epithelium may be damaged, leading to irreversible corneal edema and cataract formation.

Failure of filtration: If ciliary body shutdown caused by choroidal detachment is prolonged, the filtering bleb will flatten and become adherent to the sclera with scar formation, leading to failure of the filtration surgery.

Hypotonous maculopathy: Prolonged hypotony may result in injury to the macula.

Diagnosis continued on p. 100

TREATMENT

Diet and Lifestyle

No precautions are necessary.

Pharmacologic Treatment

Topical corticosteroids and atropine: These agents are useful in reducing inflammation and decreasing vascular permeability; the atropine also causes relaxation and posterior movement of the ciliary muscle, resulting in deepening of the anterior chamber.

Analgesics: Systemic analgesics, including narcotics, may be necessary for severe pain.

Nonpharmacologic Treatment

Overfiltration: In cases of choroidal detachment associated with overfiltration, pressure patching, or the use of special contact lenses (e.g. the Simmons Compression Shell) may help reduce overfiltration, restore a normal IOP, and resolve the choroidal detachment; if this fails, surgery to resuture the sclerostomy may be necessary.

Pearls and Considerations

On B-scan ultrasonography, *choroidal* detachments appear as stable, fluid-filled, dome-shaped pockets and can be differentiated from *retinal* detachments, which are mobile and highly reflective. Serous detachments are hypoechoic (i.e. black due to lack of reflectivity) while hemorrhagic detachments are hyperechoic (i.e. white due to hyper-reflectivity).

Treatment Aims

To bring about a rapid resolution of the choroidal detachment while preserving the function of the retina, lens, cornea, and filtering bleb.

Prognosis

The prognosis is guarded. Serous choroidal detachments that are not associated with marked degrees of anterior-chamber shallowing will usually resolve without surgical treatment, but there is often some loss of central visual acuity. Hemorrhagic choroidal detachments are often associated with severe vision loss unless they are very small. Choroidal detachments that require surgery are often associated with loss of retinal function, corneal edema, cataract, and failure of filtration. Patients with choroidal detachment in the immediate postoperative period are at higher risk for developing late-onset choroidal detachment months or even years after glaucoma filtering surgery.

Follow-up and Management

Patients should be followed frequently and carefully after filtration surgery. If the choroidal detachment resolves without complication, follow-up may be the same as for any postoperative glaucoma patient, but the patient must be monitored in case the choroidal detachment worsens or other complications develop that may require additional surgery.

Treatment continued on p. 101

DIAGNOSIS—cont'd

Investigations

Visual acuity testing: The visual acuity should be determined at each visit to monitor the effect of the choroidal detachment on vision.

Slit-lamp examination: The depth of the anterior chamber should be assessed and recorded at each visit using a recognized grading system; the size and appearance of the filtering bleb should be noted.

Seidel test: Using a fluorescein strip to paint the bleb and conjunctival wound area, a Seidel test should be performed to look for aqueous leakage.

Intraocular pressure: The IOP should be measured at each postoperative visit.

Ultrasonography: B-scan ultrasonography is useful in the diagnosis of choroidal detachment (*see* Fig. 1) and the differentiation of choroidal from retinal detachment; B-scan ultrasonography can also be used to distinguish between hemorrhagic and serous choroidal detachments; ultrasonography will also help in monitoring the progress or resolution of the choroidal detachment as well as help plan the incision site for choroidal drainage surgery, if necessary.

Blood coagulation studies: In patients with hemorrhagic choroidal detachment, especially if there are recurrent episodes of hemorrhage, evaluation of clotting factors may reveal a cause for the hemorrhage.

TREATMENT—cont'd

Referral Information

If detachment persists beyond 7 days, consider referral for drainage of the suprachoroidal fluid.

Wound leak: In cases of choroidal detachment associated with a wound leak, a variety of treatments have been tried, including pressure patching, contact lenses, tissue glue, and injection of autologous blood into the bleb; if the wound leak persists, surgical repair is usually necessary.

Choroidal drainage and anterior chamber reformation: In cases of persistent choroidal detachment or where the anterior-chamber shallowing has resulted in lens-cornea touch, surgical drainage of the suprachoroidal space and reformation of the anterior chamber with a viscoelastic substance are usually required.

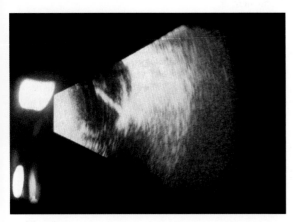

Fig. 1: B-scan ultrasound demonstrating choroidal detachment after glaucoma filtering surgery.

GENERAL REFERENCES

Bellows AR, Chylack LT, Hutchinson BT. Choroidal detachment: clinical manifestation, therapy and mechanism of formation. Ophthalmology. 1981;88:1107-13.

Fourman S. Management of cornea-lens touch after filtering surgery for glaucoma. Ophthalmology. 1990;97:424-8.

Liebmann JM, Sokol J, Ritch R. Management of chronic hypotony after glaucoma filtration surgery. J Glaucoma. 1996;5:210-20.

Shields MB. Filtering surgery. Textbook of glaucoma, 4th edition. Baltimore: Williams & Wilkins; 1998. pp. 518-27.

Traverso CE. (2005). Choroidal detachment [online]. Available from www.emedicine.com.

Choroidal Rupture (363.63)

DIAGNOSIS

Definition

Breaks in the choroid, Bruch's membrane and retinal pigment epithelium (RPE) usually in the posterior pole; generally associated with blunt ocular trauma.

Synonyms

None

Symptoms

- Decreased vision after trauma
- *Acute decreased vision*: may be permanent if fovea is involved
- Central or paracentral scotoma.

Signs

- *Yellow-white curvilinear streak(s)*: located concentric to the optic nerve or in the papillomacular bundle (Figs 1 A and B)
- *Subretinal hemorrhage*: may obscure the rupture initially
- Hemorrhagic detachment of the macula
- *Commotio retinae*: white appearance to the retina due to edema
- *Decreased intraocular pressure*: if the rupture is large
- Subretinal fibrosis
- Subretinal neovascularization.

Investigations

- *Detailed history*: for previous eye trauma or history of angioid streaks
- Slit-lamp and dilated fundus evaluation
- *Fluorescence angiography (FA)*: will show early hypofluorescence because of damage to the choriocapillaris; late hyperfluorescent staining seen in the area of the break
- *Fundus autofluorescence (FAF)*: choroidal ruptures typically appear as hypo-autofluorescent crescent-shaped lesions on FAF images due to the underlying RPE defect. The full extent of the rupture can often be seen on FAF with a clarity not seen on FA or fundus photography.

Complications

Patients may experience permanent visual loss from the rupture itself if it involves the fovea or if the following complications occur:

- Subretinal fibrosis
- Subretinal neovascularization
- Choroidal anastomosis.

Pearls and Considerations

- Initially, the choroidal rupture may be obscured by overlying hemorrhage
- Deep choroidal vessels are usually spared
- Neovascularization is an expected part of the healing process and will usually resolve spontaneously [anti-vascular endothelial growth factor (VEGF) treatment may hasten this process].

Referral Information

Refer for laser photocoagulation or anti-VEGF injections if central vision is threatened.

Differential Diagnosis

Angioid streaks: often emanate from the disk.
Lacquer cracks: associated with high myopia; appear as small, linear streaks in the macula.

Cause

Trauma

Associated Features

The clinician should look for other signs of ocular trauma, such as:

- *Sclopetaria*: pigment disruption in the peripheral retina from trauma
- Retinal detachment or retinal dialysis
- Cataract
- Iris sphincter tears
- Pigment on the surface of the lens.

Pathology

Splitting of the Bruch's membrane and choriocapillaris, or entire choroid

- The overlying RPE and neurosensory retina may be normal, atrophic or ruptured (rarely)
- When the globe is compressed in an anterior-posterior direction in blunt trauma, the sclera and retina are usually elastic enough to resist tearing. Bruch's membrane, although relatively inelastic, makes it vulnerable to rupture, along with the choriocapillaris and RPE.

TREATMENT

Diet and Lifestyle

Safety glasses during future sports activities

Pharmacologic Treatment

The mainstay of pharmacologic treatment options lies in the anti-VEGF class of agents. Options include intravitreal bevacizumab (Avastin, Genentech), ranibizumab (Lucentis, Genentech).

Nonpharmacologic Treatment

- *Laser photocoagulation to secondary choroidal neovascularization (CNV)*: may be necessary if it threatens the fovea
- If CNV is juxtafoveal or subfoveal, can consider pars plana vitrectomy with membrane extraction.

Treatment Aims

To stabilize vision

Prognosis

Good if fovea is not involved
- In 15–30% of patients, CNV may occur and lead to hemorrhagic or serous macular detachment, with concurrent central vision loss
- Most secondary subretinal neovascular membranes resolve spontaneously and do not require treatment.

Follow-up and Management

- Amsler grid testing daily to detect early distortion or visual loss from subretinal neovascularization
- Fundus examination every 3–6 months until findings are stable.

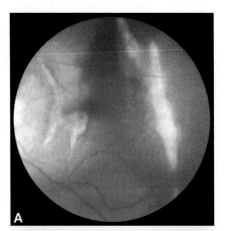

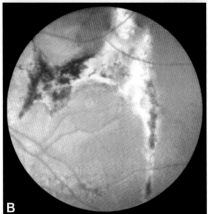

Figs 1A and B: Choroidal rupture. (A) The patient sustained a blunt trauma that resulted in choroidal ruptures in the posterior pole and subneural retinal hemorrhages. The optic nerve head is on the left in this eye; (B) One year later, considerable scarring has taken place. These patients must be watched closely for the occurrence of subneural retinal neovascularization that may occur at the edge of the healed rupture.

GENERAL REFERENCES

Aguilar JP, Green RG. Choroidal rupture. A histopathologic study of 47 cases. Retina. 1984;4:269-75.

Dugel PU, Win PH, Ober RR. Posterior segment manifestations of closed-globe contusion injury. In: Ryan SJ (Ed). Retina, 4th edition. St. Louis: Elsevier; 2006.

Federman JL, Gouras P, Schubert RT, et al. Trauma. In: Podos SM, Yanoff M (Eds). Textbook of Ophthalmology. London: Mosby; 1994. pp. 15.2-15.6.

Gass JDM. Stereoscopic Atlas of Macular Diseases, 3rd edition. St. Louis: Mosby; 1987. p. 170.

Wu L. (2012). Choroidal rupture. [online] Available from http://emedicine.medscape.com/article/1190735-overview [Accessed April, 2013].

Commotio Retinae (Berlin's Edema) (921.3)

DIAGNOSIS

Definition

A complication of blunt ocular trauma characterized by a milky opacification of the macular retina.

Synonyms

None

Symptoms

Acute visual loss after trauma

Signs

White discoloration to the outer retina: located in the posterior pole or peripheral retina (*see* Fig. 1)

Signs of trauma: hemorrhage, retinal detachment, sclopetaria.

Investigations

- *Careful history*: to determine if the preceding trauma was blunt or from a penetrating injury; visual acuity
- *Pupil examination*: to look for an afferent pupillary defect indicating optic nerve or widespread retinal injury
- Slit-lamp and dilated retinal examination
- *Fluorescence angiography*: may show abnormal vascular permeability or blockage of choroidal fluorescence.

Complications

Loss of vision

Pearls and Considerations

- If only the outer segments of the photoreceptors are damaged, they will regenerate, and retinal and visual function will recover
- Optical coherence tomography (OCT) evaluation will demonstrate increased reflectivity at the level of the photoreceptors.

Referral Information

None; patients should be observed for resolution.

Differential Diagnosis
- Myelinated nerve fibers
- Central retinal artery occlusion.

Cause
Trauma to the eye

Associated Features
Other ocular findings seen with trauma (e.g. vitreous hemorrhage, retinal detachment, choroidal rupture)

Pathology
- Disruption of the outer segments of the retina
- No evidence of actual retinal edema.

TREATMENT

Diet and Lifestyle

Safety glasses during sports-related activities

Pharmacologic Treatment

No pharmacologic treatment is recommended

Nonpharmacologic Treatment

Observation

Treatment Aims

To observe patient

Prognosis

Depends on whether the macula is involved; there may be permanent damage to the retina and late pigmentary changes that lead to loss of vision.

Follow-up and Management

Depends on the extent of ocular damage from the trauma; once stable, a yearly dilated eye examination is indicated.

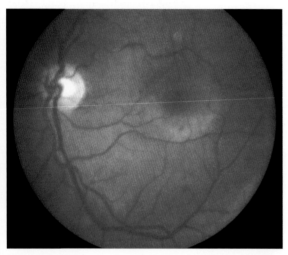

Fig. 1: Patient who sustained blunt trauma to the left eye exhibits retinal whitening of the macula on fundus examination.

GENERAL REFERENCES

Balles M. Traumatic retinopathy. In: Albert DM, Jakobiec FA (Eds). Principles and Practice of Ophthalmology. Philadelphia: Saunders; 1994. pp. 1027-8.

Dugel PU, Win PH, Ober RR. Posterior segment manifestations of closed-globe contusion injury. Retina, 4th edition. St Louis: Elsevier; 2006.

Sony P, Venkatesh P, Gadaginomath S, et al. Optical coherence tomography findings in commotio retinae. Clin Exp Ophthalmol. 2006;34:621-3.

Conjunctival Degenerations: Pinguecula (372.51) and Pterygium (372.40)

DIAGNOSIS

Definition

Pinguecula: area of thickening of the bulbar conjunctiva adjacent to the limbus and within the palpebral fissure

Pterygium: a growth of fibrovascular tissue onto the cornea from the conjunctiva.

Synonyms

None

Symptoms

- Patients are usually asymptomatic
- *Cosmetic concerns*: common
- *Photophobia, tearing, foreign body sensation*: less common
- *Decreased vision*: if pterygium is close to visual axis or causing astigmatic changes *(usually* irregular astigmatism).

Signs

- *Pingueculae are usually seen on the conjunctiva adjacent to nasal limbus*: they have the appearance of yellow-white, amorphous, subepithelial deposits (Fig. 1).
- Pterygium is a triangular-shaped fold of conjunctival and fibrovascular tissue that has advanced to the corneal surface (Fig. 2).

Investigations

- History
- *Visual acuity testing*: may be decreased from centralization of the pterygium, or irregular astigmatism
- Refraction: may have astigmatism from pterygium
- *Intraocular pressure*: usually normal
- *Slit-lamp examination*: may note an iron line (Stocker's line) in front of the pterygium, which usually indicates growth stabilization
- *Dilated fundus examination*: usually normal.

Differential Diagnosis

- *Conjunctival intraepithelial neoplasia*: unilateral jelly like or white mass, often elevated, vascularized; not in a wing shape
- Limbal dermoid
- Pannus.

Cause

Related to sun exposure, dust, and wind (chronic irritation)

Epidemiology

Common in the 30–50 age group and in tropical climate.

Pathology

- The subepithelial tissue shows senile elastosis and dense subepithelial concretions not sensitive to elastase.
- Common ocular surface lesions thought to originate from limbal stem cells altered by chronic UV exposure. Traditionally regarded as a degenerative condition, pterygia also display tumor-like features, such as a propensity to invade normal tissue and high recurrence rates following resection, and may coexist with secondary premalignant lesions.

Diagnosis continued on p. 108

TREATMENT

Diet and Lifestyle

- Protect the eye from sun, dust, and wind (e.g. wear sunglasses or goggles)
- In one large study, there was an age-related increase in prevalence and severity of pinguecula in contact lenses over noncontact lens wearers. Wearing time and contact lens fit should be optimized in these patients.

Pharmacologic Treatment

- Artificial tears or mild topical vasoconstrictor
- Mild topical steroid (if severe).

Nonpharmacologic Treatment

- Surgical removal may be considered if: (1) the lesion interferes with contact lens wear; (2) patient experiences extreme irritation not relieved by the above treatments; (3) pterygium involves the visual axis or progresses; (4) patient has cosmetic concerns; or (5) if the lesion induces progressive refractive aberrations such as astigmatism not well corrected with spectacles or contact lenses.
- Surgery should not be performed casually because recurrent pterygia are often worse than primary ones. An estimated 40% recur; however, with conjunctival transplantation, the rate drops to 5%.
- The current recommended practice is not to leave the sclera exposed but to cover the region with a graft such as cryopreserved amniotic membrane transplantation or conjunctival autograft. In conjunctival autograft techniques, ipsilateral bulbar conjunctiva (usually from the superior region) is excised and grafted over the excised pterygium bed. Antiobiotic/steroid combination ointment is placed on the eye, and the eye is then patched until the next day. The patient is followed until epithelium heals over the cornea.
- Consider maintaining patients with large or recurrent pterygium on topical steroids for 3–6 months to prevent recurrence. Any patient receiving topical steroids should be monitored regularly.

Treatment Aims

To relieve symptoms and prevent worsening of visual acuity

Other Treatments

- Apply mitomycin-C (0.2 mg/cm^3) to bare sclera after excision (only in severe pterygium). Concentration and time of exposure are important (outside the scope of this book).
- Other adjuvant therapies include thiotepa, intralesional bevacizumab (Avastin, Genentech), and beta radiation, all of which have associated ocular complications.
- Complications include scleral necrosis, cataract, persistent epithelial defects, and visual loss.

Prognosis

Aggressive recurrence may occur after excision (the rate of recurrence with bare sclera removal technique is 20–89%, minimized by conjunctival autograft and antifibrotic agents).

Follow-up and Management

- Asymptomatic patients may be checked every 1–2 years
- If treating with topical vasoconstrictor or topical steroid, check every 1–2 weeks to monitor inflammation and intraocular pressure. Taper steroid dose over several days once the inflammation has abated.

Treatment continued on p. 109

DIAGNOSIS—cont'd

Complications

- Dellen formation adjacent to pingueculae
- *Corneal scarring*: with pterygium
- *Recurrence of pterygium*: after excision
- *Inflammation of the pinguecula*: pingueculitis.

Pearls and Considerations

- Pingueculae should be observed and noted at each exam as they may have the potential for progressing to pterygia.
- Protective eyewear against ultraviolet (UV) radiation should be recommended to patients with either pinguecula or pterygia, which may impede further growth.

Referral Information

Refer for surgical excision as appropriate.

TREATMENT—cont'd

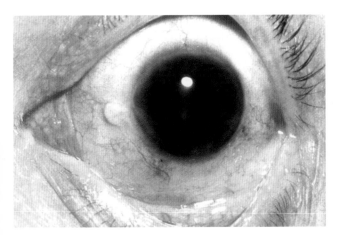

Fig. 1: Nasal pinguecula.

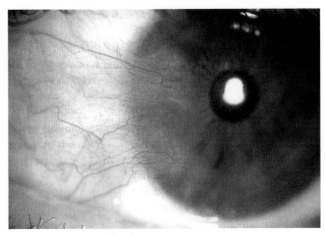

Fig. 2: Nasal pterygium.

GENERAL REFERENCES

American Academy of Ophthalmology. Basic and Clinical Science. San Francisco: The Academy; 2006-2007.

Farjo QA, Sugar A. Conjunctival and corneal degenerations. In: Yanoff M, Duker JS (Eds). Ophthalmology. St Louis: Elsevier; 2006.

Murube J. Pterygium: evolution of medical and surgical treatments. The Ocular Surface. 2008;6(4):155-61.

Mimura T, Usui T, Mori M, et al. Pinguecula and contact lenses. Eye. 2010;24:1685-91.

Smolin G, Thoft RA. The cornea. Scientific Foundation and Clinical Practice. Boston: Little, Brown; 2004.

Wright K. Textbook of ophthalmology. Baltimore: Williams & Wilkins; 1997.

Conjunctivitis, Acute (372.0)

DIAGNOSIS

Definition
Inflammation of the conjunctiva of less than 4 weeks' duration secondary to infection, allergen, toxin, or chemical insult.

Synonyms
"Pinkeye"

Symptoms
- Discharge
- Eyelid sticking
- Red eye
- Foreign body sensation: of less than 4 weeks' duration.

Signs
- Severe purulent discharge, marked chemosis, conjunctival papillae, preauricular adenopathy: in gonococcal conjunctivitis
- Purulent discharge of moderate degree, conjunctival papillae: other bacterial conjunctivitis (Fig. 1)
- Mucus discharge, conjunctival follicles, preauricular adenopathy, subconjunctival hemorrhage, conjunctival pseudomembranes, subepithelial infiltrates (may be late sign): in viral conjunctivitis
- Thick ropy discharge, large conjunctival papillae under the upper lid or along the limbus, superior corneal-shield ulcer, limbal or palpebral raised white dots (Horner-Trantas dots): vernal/atopic conjunctivitis
- Chemosis, conjunctival papillae, scant mucus discharge, mild edema and erythema of eyelids: allergic conjunctivitis.

Investigations
- *History*: severe purulent discharge within 12 hours (gonococcal), recent upper respiratory tract infection or contact with someone who has red eye (adenoviral), seasonal recurrences (vernal), history of allergies (atopic or allergic)
- Visual acuity test
- Slit-lamp examination
- Conjunctival swab for culture and sensitivities: e.g. blood agar, chocolate agar, Thayer- Martin plate, stat Gram stain if severe.

Differential Diagnosis
- Episcleritis
- Scleritis
- Uveitis
- Acute angle-closure glaucoma
- Corneal ulcer
- Dural-cavernous fistulae
- Kawasaki syndrome.

Cause and Classification
Infectious
- *Bacterial*: Staphylococcus aureus, Streptococcus pneumoniae, Haemophilus influenzae, Neisseria gonorrhoeae
- *Viral*: adenovirus, herpes simplex.

Noninfectious
- Allergic
- Vernal/atopic.

Diagnosis continued on p. 112

TREATMENT

Diet and Lifestyle

- In *adenoviral* conjunctivitis, wash hands frequently and avoid hand contacts
- In *allergic* conjunctivitis, avoid allergen or eliminate the inciting agent.

Pharmacologic Treatment

For Adenoviral Conjunctivitis

- Administer artificial tears four to eight times daily; apply cool compresses several times daily
- Vasoconstrictor/antihistamines help itching.

Standard dosage: fluorometholone or prednisolone acetate 0.125%, four times daily

Special points: used for pseudomembranes or corneal subepithelial infiltrate or if vision is reduced. Taper steroid slowly once resolved. Gently peel off membrane if present.

For Herpes Simplex Conjunctivitis

Apply cool compresses several times daily.

Standard dosage: trifluorothymidine (trifluridine) 1% (Viroptic) drops, five times daily.

For Bacterial Conjunctivitis (General)

Standard dosage: ciprofloxacin drops or erythromycin ointment, four times daily for 7 days.

For Haemophilus influenzae Conjunctivitis

Standard dosage: amoxicillin/clavulanate, 20–40 mglkg/day PO in three divided doses.

Special points: Oral dose because of nonocular involvement (e.g. otitis media, pneumonia, meningitis).

For Gonococcal Conjunctivitis

Treatment is initiated if the Gram stain shows Gram-negative intracellular diplococci or if there is a high suspicion of gonococcal conjunctivitis clinically.

Standard dosage: ceftriaxone, 1 g IM in single dose, or ceftriaxone 1 g IV every 12–24 hours if severe with lid swelling and corneal involvement; patient should be hospitalized; duration based on clinical response.

Topical bacitracin or erythromycin ointment four times daily, or ciprofloxacin drops every 2 hours.

Tetracycline or erythromycin, 250–500 mg PO four times daily for 2–3 weeks.

Special points: irrigate the eye with saline four times daily until the discharge is eliminated.

Treatment Aims

- To relieve symptoms of adenoviral and atopic/vernal conjunctivitis
- To prevent corneal involvement in herpes simplex, gonococcal conjunctivitis
- To minimize symblepharon formation.

Prognosis

- Acute conjunctivitis has a duration of ~4 weeks and usually is self-limited except in gonococcal conjunctivitis
- Recurrence of vernal/atopic conjunctivitis is common.

Follow-up and Management

- *Adenovirus*: every 1–3 weeks
- *Herpes simplex*: every 2–3 days initially to monitor corneal involvement, then every 1–2 weeks
- *Bacterial*: every 1–2 days initially, then every 2–5 days until resolved (gonococcal conjunctivitis needs to be followed daily until improvement noted, then every 2–3 days)
- *Vernal/atopic*: every 1–3 days in the presence of a shield ulcer, otherwise every few weeks. Cromolyn sodium is maintained for the duration of the season
- *Allergic*: 1–3 weeks to determine response to treatment. Continue to follow frequently if using topical steroids, until tapered.

Treatment continued on p. 113

Conjunctivitis, Acute (372.0)

DIAGNOSIS—cont'd

Complications

- Corneal ulcer, scarring, perforation: gonococcal conjunctivitis
- Phlyctenules and marginal infiltrates
- Recurrence: herpes simplex infection.

Pearls and Considerations

- If herpetic infection is suspected, steroid treatment is contraindicated due to the potential for worsening the disease
- *Epidemic keratoconjunctivitis* (EKC) is highly contagious and easily spread to other patients through improperly disinfected slit lamps, tonometers and other instruments. Careful disinfection of all instrumentation is critical in avoiding nosocomial infection of other patients.
- Gonococcal conjunctivitis is an emergency, given possible rapid progression and risk of corneal perforation, that requires systemic treatment.

Referral Information

None

TREATMENT—cont'd

For Vernal/Atopic or Allergic Conjunctivitis

- Mild Infection:
  - Administer artificial tears.
- Moderate infection:
  - *Standard dosage*: Levocabastine (Livostin) or olopatadine HCl 0.1% (antihistamines), four times daily
  - Ketorolac, four times daily.
- Severe infection:
  - *Standard dosage*: fluorometholone, four times daily for 1–2 weeks
  - *Special points*: add topical cromolyn sodium 4% or lodoxamide (Alomide) for vernal/atopic disease. If shield ulcer is present, add topical steroid and topical antibiotic (e.g. erythromycin ointment or Polytrim drops four times daily).

For Allergic Conjunctivitis

- Eliminate inciting factor if possible
- Apply cool compresses five times daily
- Mild cases:
  - Administer artificial tears four times daily.
- Moderate:
  - *Standard dosage:* olopatadine 0.1%, lodoxamide 0.1%, nedocromil 2%, or ketotifen 0.025%, twice daily.
- Severe:
  - *Standard dosage*: multitopical steroid (loteprednol or fluorometholone) four times daily with taper
  - *Special points*: Consider oral antihistamine if concomitant hay fever or systemic allergy symptoms for moderate or severe cases.

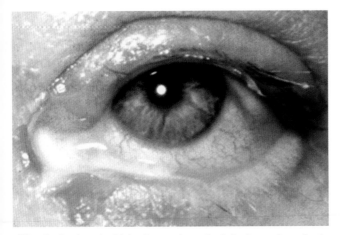

Fig. 1: Conjunctival injection and purulent discharge in patient with bacterial conjunctivitis.

GENERAL REFERENCES

Albert OM, Jakobiec FA (Eds). Principles and Practice of Ophthalmology. Philadelphia: Saunders; 2000.

American Academy of Ophthalmology. Basic and Clinical Science. San Francisco: The Academy; 2006-2007.

Stefkovicovaa M, Vicianova V, Sokolik J, et al. Causes and control measures in hospital outbreaks of epidemic keratoconjunctivitis. Indoor Built Environ. 2006;15:111-4.

Wright K. Textbook of ophthalmology. Baltimore: Williams & Wilkins; 1997.

Conjunctivitis, Chronic (372.1)

DIAGNOSIS

Definition
Inflammation of the conjunctiva of greater than 4 weeks' duration secondary to toxin or infection.

Synonyms
"Pinkeye"

Symptoms
- Discharge or eyelid "sticking," typically worse in the morning
- *Red eye and ocular irritation*: of longer than 4 weeks' duration.

Signs
Chlamydial inclusion conjunctivitis: inferior tarsal conjunctival follicles, superior corneal pannus, palpable preauricular node (PAN), gray-white subepithelial infiltrates (SEI), and stringy mucus discharge.

Trachoma stage 1: superior tarsal follicles, mild superficial punctate keratitis, and pannus (often preceded by purulent discharge and tender PAN).

Trachoma stage 2: significant superior tarsal follicular reaction and papillary hypertrophy associated with pannus, SEI, and limbal follicles.

Trachoma stage 3: follicles and scarring of superior tarsal conjunctiva.

Trachoma stage 4: extensive conjunctival scarring.

Molluscum contagiosum: dome-shaped, umbilicated (usually multiple) nodules on the eyelid or eyelid margin; follicular conjunctival response from toxic viral products (Fig. 1).

Toxic conjunctivitis/medicamentosa: inferior papillary reaction, especially with aminoglycosides, antivirals and preservatives; follicular response may be seen with atropine, miotics, epinephrine agents, topical glaucoma agents, and antiviral medications.

Investigations
- *History of exposure to sexually transmitted diseases (STDs)*: vaginitis, cervicitis, or urethritis may be present in chlamydial inclusion conjunctivitis
- *History of exposure to areas with high incidence of trachoma*: North Africa, Middle East, India, Southeast Asia
- *History of eyedrop use*: especially for glaucoma
- Visual acuity test
- Slit-lamp examination
- Dilated fundus examination
- *Conjunctival scraping for Giemsa stain (basophilic and intracytoplasmic inclusion bodies in epithelial cell)*: found in chlamydial inclusion conjunctivitis and trachoma.

Diagnosis continued on p. 116

Differential Diagnosis
- Herpes simplex conjunctivitis
- Adenoviral keratoconjunctivitis
- Ocular rosacea.

Cause
As described in Signs section; also allergic reactions (atropine, brimonidine, miotics, epinephrine, antivirals) and Reiter's syndrome.

Epidemiology
Trachoma is endemic in North Africa, Middle East, South and Southeast Asia, and rarely the United States.

TREATMENT

Diet and Lifestyle

- Promote sanitary living conditions and good facial hygiene in trachoma-endemic areas
- Patients with chlamydial inclusion conjunctivitis and their sexual partners should be evaluated by their medical physicians for other STDs.

Pharmacologic Treatment

For Chlamydial Inclusion Conjunctivitis

Standard dosage: Tetracycline, 250–500 mg PO four times daily x 1 week (avoid in pregnancy or children <8 years); or
Doxycycline, 100 mg PO BID x 1 week; or
Erythromycin, 500 mg PO four times daily; for 1 week.
Erythromycin ointment, two to three times daily for 2–3 weeks.
Azithromycin, 1 g PO for one dose.

Special points: These drugs should be given to patients and their sexual partners.

For Trachoma

Treatment is same as for chlamydial inclusion conjunctivitis but for 3–4 weeks' duration, unless surgical intervention required in severe disease.

For Toxic Conjunctivitis

- Discontinue the offending agent, if possible
- Artificial tears without preservatives should be administered four to eight times daily; can also administer mast-cell stabilizers such as olapatadine 0.1% (Patanol, Alcon) BID for comfort and to blunt the allergic response.

Treatment Aims

Treatment is usually curative.

Prognosis

Trachoma must be treated in early stages to prevent significant corneal scarring.

Follow-up and Management

Every 1–3 weeks, depending on the severity. Occasionally, a 6-week course of doxycycline is warranted.

Treatment continued on p. 117

Conjunctivitis, Chronic (372.1)

DIAGNOSIS—cont'd

Complications

- *Corneal scarring and pannus*: mild to severe
- *Late complications of trachoma*: severely dry eyes, trichiasis, entropion, keratitis, corneal scarring, superficial fibrovascular pannus, Herbert's pits (scarred limbal follicles), corneal bacterial superinfection, and ulceration.

Pearls and Considerations

Chronic follicular conjunctivitis may represent *Parinaud 's oculoglandular syndrome,* an ocular manifestation of cat-scratch disease (CSD). A full dilated examination should be performed to rule out additional, more serious complications of CSD, including neuroretinitis (optic nerve swelling and macular star) and focal chorioretinitis.

Referral Information

Dependent on etiology and extent of ocular involvement.

TREATMENT—cont'd

Nonpharmacologic Treatment

For Molluscum Contagiosum

Remove lesions by simple excision and curettage or by cryosurgery.

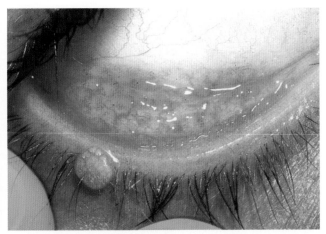

Fig. 1: Eyelid nodule with follicular conjunctivitis in patient with molluscum contagiosum.

GENERAL REFERENCES

Albert DM, Jakobiec FA (Eds). Principles and Practice of Ophthalmology. Philadelphia: Saunders; 2000.

American Academy of Ophthalmology. Basic and Clinical Science. San Francisco: The Academy; 2006-2007.

Cunningham ET, Keohler JE. Ocular bartonellosis. Am J Ophthalmol. 2000; 130:340-9.

Wright K. Textbook of ophthalmology. Baltimore: Lippincott Williams & Wilkins; 1997.

Katusic D, Petricek I, Mandic Z, et al. Azithromycin vs. doxycycline in the treatment of inclusion conjunctivitis. Am J Ophthalmol. 2003;135:447-51.

Thanathanee O, O'Brien TP. Conjunctivitis: systematic approach to diagnosis and therapy. Current Infectious Disease Reports. 2011;13(2):141-8.

Wright HR, Turner A, Taylor HR. Trachoma. The Lancet. 2008;371(9628):1945-54.

Chen YM, Hu FR, Hou YC. Effect of oral azithromycin in the treatment of chlamydial conjunctivitis. Eye. 2010;24: 985-9. doi: 10.1038/eye.2009. 264.

Corneal Abrasions (918.1) and Foreign Body (930.0)

DIAGNOSIS

Definition

A defect of the corneal epithelium with or without an associated foreign body.

Synonyms

None

Symptoms

- Pain
- Photophobia
- Foreign body sensation
- Tearing
- Blurred vision (secondary to tearing, ciliary body spasm, and/or if abrasion lies in visual axis).

Signs

- Epithelial staining defect with fluorescein: conjunctival injection and swollen eyelid may have mild anterior-chamber reaction (Fig. 1)
- Corneal foreign body, rust ring or both
- Conjunctival injection.

Investigations

History: often a history of scratching the eye, contact lens use/abuse (particularly overnight wear), objects blown into the eye (e.g. sand or debris), or foreign body from metal striking metal. Unconscious or sedated patients are particularly prone to iatrogenic abrasion.

Visual acuity test: may require topical anesthesia to complete.

Slit-lamp examination: with the use of fluorescein and eversion of the eyelids to evaluate for foreign body; if there is corneal whitening, rule out infection. Check for inflammation; there may be mild anterior-chamber reaction present, but if severe, rule out endophthalmitis.

Dilated fundus examination: rule out intraocular foreign body, especially with a history of striking metal against metal.

Imaging: particularly with high-velocity injuries (e.g. metal-on-metal, lawn mower), orbital computed tomography (metallic) and/or magnetic resonance imaging (nonmetallic) may be indicated. B-scan may also be useful in case of poor view on dilated examination. Optical coherence tomography has also proven useful in several cases in the literature in diagnosing otherwise missed intraocular foreign bodies.

Differential Diagnosis

- Corneal laceration
- Corneal ulcer or ulcerative keratitis
- Corneal melt
- Acute angle closure glaucoma
- Corneal dystrophy
- Herpes simplex dendritic keratitis
- Herpes zoster ophthalmicus
- Iritis, iridocyclitis, uveitis
- Blepharitis
- Trigeminal neuralgia.

Etiology

Scratching the eye: fingernail, contact lens, rubbing, paper cut, tree branch, toxic chemicals (e.g. inappropriate drops)
Iron shavings: most common foreign body.

Associated Features

Sterile corneal infiltrate: need to rule out infection.

Pathology

- Superficial epithelial defect or full epithelial defect: by definition, corneal abrasions only involve epithelial defects, and do not cross Bowman's membrane
- Corneal foreign body may or may not penetrate Bowman's membrane
- The cornea normally swells 2–4% during sleep. With a contact lens, overnight swelling increases to an average of 15%, and gross stromal edema can be present on awakening. In some patients, induced corneal swelling can be sufficient to cause bullae; these can rupture leading to epithelial defects.
- Corneal abrasion and inflammation, paracentesis, intraocular infection, and uveal inflammation all cause a breakdown of the blood-aqueous barrier so that plasma proteins and inflammatory cells pour into the anterior chamber. As a result, inflamed aqueous humor has increased levels of serum proteins, including immunoglobulins and complement components C1-C7.
- Hemidesmosomes anchor the epithelium to its basement membrane. The number of hemidesmosomes in people with diabetes is markedly reduced, impairing healing and predisposing patients to recurrent erosion.

Diagnosis continued on p. 120

TREATMENT

Diet and Lifestyle

- Safety goggles for prevention when striking metal on metal, or in other high-risk occupations or activities
- Ultraviolet (UV) protective goggles or sunglasses for those with a high likelihood of increased UV light exposure
- Advise patients to avoid bright light or to wear sunglasses for comfort if they have notable photophobia
- Lid closure (e.g. taping of lids) for unconscious or sedated patients, or in Bell's palsy
- Ensure proper fit, hygiene and wearing time for contact lenses.

Pharmacologic Treatment

Corneal Abrasion

Cycloplegia for aching pain/photophobia: e.g. homatropine 5% TID or cyclopentolate 1% TID (Cyclogyl, Alcon). Ensure patient does not have narrow angles given resultant mydriasis.

Topical antibiotics: routine use of antibiotics for corneal abrasions is somewhat controversial; many emergency physicians no longer use topical antibiotics for minor, clean abrasions. However, given that de-epithelialized cornea is more susceptible than intact cornea to infection (whether from the traumatic source or simply the normal conjunctival flora), ophthalmologists generally do prescribe antibiotics in corneal abrasion treatment, whether felt to be "clean" or otherwise.

- Noncontact lens wearers: erythromycin ointment 0.5% QID for 3–5 days (particularly useful in small children); or sulfacetamide 10% QID ointment or solution; or polymixin-trimethoprim (Polytrim, Allergan) QID for 3–5 days; ciprofloxacin 0.3% (Ciloxan, Alcon) QID for 3–5 days; or ofloxacin 0.3% (Ocuflox, Allergan) QID for 3–5 days
- Contact lens wearers (much more vigilance required, and no contact lens use until cornea healed completely): moxifloxacin 0.5% (Vigamox, Alcon) q2h while awake for 2 days, then q4–8h for 5 days; or levofloxacin 0.5% (Quixin, Vistakon) q2h while awake for 2 days, then q4–8h for 5 days; or ofloxacin 0.3% (Ocuflox, Allergan) QID for 3–5 days; or entamicin 0.3% (Garamycin, Fera); or tobramycin 0.3% (Tobrex, Alcon)
- Large or dirty abrasions: use broad-spectrum antibiotic drops, such as polytrim, sulfacetamide, an aminoglycoside or fluoroquinolone (most commonly used)
- Antibiotic formulations containing neomycin should be generally avoided given the high incidence of allergy in the general population to this agent.

Topical analgesics: diclofenac 0.1% QID (Voltaren, Novartis) for less than 2 weeks; or ketorolac 0.4% QID (Acular, Allergan)

- Multiple randomized trials have found significant pain relief with topical diclofenac
- Alternatively, oral analgesia may be used in the initial period of healing.

Lubrication: artificial tears (preservative-free formulations may be less irritating) Q1h–QID while awake, depending on the size and severity of injury

Treatment Aims

Quick healing of the corneal defect, pain relief during healing, prevention of corneal infection or other complications

Prognosis

- Corneal abrasions usually heal with no scarring
- Removal of the foreign body usually leaves minimal scarring, depending upon the size and depth of penetration.

Follow-up and Management

- Follow daily for large or dirty abrasions and contact lens-related abrasions. Avoid pressure patching in patients who wear contact lenses.
- If superficial punctate keratitis remains, treat with topical antibiotic for up to 4 days
- If a corneal infiltrate is observed, appropriate smears and cultures should be obtained; treat as a corneal ulcer. In contact lens users or if vegetable matter involvement, consider *Pseudomonas*, amebic, and fungal involvement.
- Advise eye rest (i.e. no reading or work that requires substantial eye movement and blinking that might interfere with re-epithelialization)
- Minor abrasions should heal within 24–48 hours and may not require follow-up if the patient is completely asymptomatic at 48 hours.
- Nonhealing or recurrent corneal abrasions that do not resolve with the use of routine prophylactic antibiotics must be evaluated for conditions that impede healing, e.g. infection, neurotrophic keratopathy and topical anesthetic abuse.

Treatment continued on p. 121

Corneal Abrasions (918.1) and Foreign Body (930.0)

DIAGNOSIS—cont'd

Complications

Infectious corneal infiltrate: with or without significant anterior-chamber reaction.

Decreased vision: secondary to central corneal scar.

Recurrent corneal erosions: days to years following re-epithelialization. In cases secondary to trauma, occur more often with a history of paper cut or fingernail abrasion; however, can also occur spontaneously secondary to a predisposing factor such as diabetes, neurotrophic conditions (check corneal sensitivity), history of limbal stem cell damage, or underlying corneal dystrophy (e.g. Fuchs'). Patients often report sharp pain and characteristic symptoms upon awakening from sleep.

Epidemiology

- The most common eye injuries especially prevalent among people who wear contact lenses
- Corneal abrasions account for about 10% of eye-related emergency visits.

Pearls and Considerations

- The Seidel test can be used to rule out penetration and open-globe injury. Apply sodium fluorescein to the suspected site of penetration and observe under a slit lamp for sign of streaming (diluted fluorescein running from the wound site). A positive Seidel sign indicates penetrating injury and open globe.
- If corneal ulcer is suspected (e.g. corneal edema which may represent infectious infiltrate) or feared to be impending (e.g. dirty trauma or extended contact lens wear), consider obtaining bacterial cultures prior to instilling antibiotics.
- The pattern of staining may offer valuable clues as to the mechanism of injury; for instance, multiple vertical, linear abrasions suggest a hidden foreign body under the upper eyelid (evert the eyelid to check).
- Never allow a patient to use topical anesthetics (e.g. proparacaine) outside of monitored clinical setting aside from topical NSAIDs.

Referral Information

Refer for surgical evaluation if penetrating injury is suspected. Recurrent cases may warrant referral to a cornea subspecialist.

TREATMENT—cont'd

Corneal Foreign Body

- Cycloplegia: e.g. homatropine or cyclopentolate as above
- Antibiotic: e.g. fluoroquinolone (see above) after removing the foreign body; consider pressure patching for 24 hour (controversial)
- Apply topical anesthetic (e.g. proparacaine) and remove the foreign body in one piece if possible with 25-gauge needle using the slit lamp. Rust ring can be removed with an Alger brush. If the rust ring is too deep for safe one-step removal at the slit lamp, leave it and allow time for the rust to migrate to the corneal surface.
- Full dilated fundoscopic examination and lid eversion should be performed to locate all foreign body fragments and ensure no intraocular penetration. Special care and follow-up should be taken with dirty foreign bodies, contact lens wearers, and vegetable matter, carefully monitoring for signs of fungal or amebic keratitis. Many metal foreign bodies elicit an intense inflammatory response, which should be monitored for, and the entirety of the metal removed from the eye expediently.

Nonpharmacologic Treatment

- Pressure patching for 24 hours for clean corneal abrasions or recurrent erosions is a traditional treatment. However, multiple randomized controlled trials, as well as a systematic review and meta-analysis have demonstrated no evidence for this intervention, with higher rates of healing and pain relief in fact found in patients with topical antibiotics and cycloplegia. Patching should never be applied in cases of "dirty" trauma (such as fingernail or tree-branch scratch) or in a patient who wears contact lenses.
- Therapeutic lenses such as self-dissolving porcine collagen bandage contact lenses are sometimes used, particularly in uncomplicated corneal abrasions in which a collagen lens could be an alternative to a pressure dressing. However, one study showed that with common corneal abrasions, collagen lenses resulted in unexpected discomfort rather than decreased symptoms. Another showed no benefit in healing persistent epithelial defects after penetrating keratoplasty. Additionally, many patients have difficulty in handling the lenses, which can fall out prior to follow-up examination.
- Cold compresses/ice packs can be used for 24–48 hours to reduce edema. Warm compresses can be used thereafter.

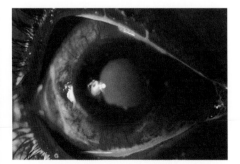

Fig. 1: Central corneal abrasion staining with fluorescein.

GENERAL REFERENCES

Albert DM, Jakobiec FA, (Eds). Principles and Practice of Ophthalmology, Vol. 1. Philadelphia: Saunders; 2000.

Basic and Clinical Science Course (BCSC): External Disease and Cornea Section 8. San Francisco: American Academy of Ophthalmology; 2006–2007.

Calder LA, Balasubramanian S, Fergusson D. Topical nonsteroidal anti-inflammatory drugs for corneal abrasions: meta-analysis of randomized trials. Acad Emerg Med. 2005;12:467-73.

Dua HS, Gomes JA, Singh A. Corneal epithelial wound healing. Br J Ophthalmol. 1994;78(5):401-8.

Fraser S. Corneal abrasion. Clin Ophthalmol. 2010;4:387-90.

Groden LR, White W. Porcine collagen corneal shield treatment of persistent epithelial defects following penetrating keratoplasty. CLAO J. 1990;16(2):95-7.

Jayamanne DG, Fitt AW, Dayan M, et al. The effectiveness of topical diclofenac in relieving discomfort following traumatic corneal abrasions. Eye. 1997;11(Pt 1): 79-83.

Turner A, Rabiu M. Patching for corneal abrasion. Cochrane Database Syst Rev. 2006;(2):CD004764.

Verma A. (2011). Corneal abrasion. [online] Available from http://emedicine.medscape.com/article/1195402-overview [Accessed April, 2013].

Wright K. Textbook of Ophthalmology. Baltimore: Lippincott Williams & Wilkins; 1997.

Wylegala E, Dobrowolski D, Nowińska A, et al. Anterior segment optical coherence tomography in eye injuries. Graefes Arch Clin Exp Ophthalmol. 2009;247(4):451-5.

Corneal Edema (371.24)

DIAGNOSIS

Definition

Swelling of the cornea. Though the term is often used loosely by clinicians, corneal edema technically refers to a cornea hydrated beyond its normal 78% water content.

Synonyms

None

Symptoms

- Blurry vision
- Haloes
- Pain: if corneal epithelial defects or bullae are present.

Signs

- Stromal edema
- Epithelial edema
- Bullous epithelial changes
- Endothelial corneal (Fuchs') dystrophy (cornea guttata) (Fig. 1)
- Abrasion
- Intraocular pressure (IOP): may be elevated.

Investigations

- *History*: note any history of ocular surgery (e.g. cataract surgery, LASIK) or trauma. Check for history of amantadine use (for influenza or Parkinson's treatment), which has been implicated in inducing bilateral corneal edema in some patients.
- *Visual acuity test*: usually decreased relative to severity of edema
- *Slit-lamp examination*: pigmented guttata often visible in Fuchs' endothelial dystrophy and microcystic epithelial edema; bullous changes on the corneal surface are a sign of marked endothelial dysfunction. Carefully assess other eye for signs of Fuchs' dystrophy.
- *Intraocular pressure*: may be low as in patients with ocular ischemia and corneal edema as well as uveitis with ciliary body shutdown; may also be elevated as in phakic patients with angle closure caused by corneal edema and trauma.
- *Pachymetry and/or specular/confocal microscopy*: to confirm that corneal edema is present, and to what degree
- Dilated fundus examination.

Complications

- Corneal abrasion/ruptured bullae
- Infectious corneal ulcer
- Angle-closure glaucoma.

Differential Diagnosis

- Interstitial keratitis
- Infectious keratitis
- Corneal dystrophy
- Corneal scar (inert).

Cause

Endothelial dysfunction or elevated IOP

Endothelial Cell Dysfunction

- Pseudophakic/aphakic bullous keratopathy (cataract surgery)
- Fuchs' endothelial dystrophy (common) and other endothelial dystrophies (rare)
- Trauma (e.g. Descemet's rupture/detachment)
- Slowly healing corneal abrasion
- Corneal infiltrate, ulcers, endophthalmitis
- Herpetic disciform keratitis: associated with mild anterior uveitis
- Corneal hydrops secondary to keratoconus: usually with severe thickening of the cornea
- Toxic anterior segment syndrome (toxic substances in anterior chamber)
- Ocular ischemia: associated with hypotony, conjunctival injection and anterior uveitis.

High Intraocular Pressure

- Acute angle-closure or other uncontrolled glaucoma (e.g. neovascular glaucoma)
- Postoperative pressure spikes, retained viscoelastic material
- Medications (e.g. topical steroids).

Pathology

The cornea is normally 78% water; corneal edema (with resultant scattering of light and decreased transparency) occurs when this level of hydration is increased to more than 5% above baseline.

With corneal edema secondary to endothelial cell dysfunction, it is typically only around a central endothelial cell density of 500 cells/mm^2 (down from normal lifetime averages of 5,000 cells/mm^2 to 2,500 cells/mm^2) that corneal edema manifests clinically.

Diagnosis continued on p. 124

TREATMENT

Varies by underlying cause

Diet and Lifestyle

A hair drier may be cautiously used to blow air on the cornea (not at high heat levels!) to increase evaporation.

Pharmacologic Treatment

For Mild Cases (Nonglaucomatous)

Sodium chloride (NaCl) 5% solution or ointment (e.g. Muro 128, Bausch and Lomb) four times daily; decrease IOP if elevated or in high teens with antiglaucoma medication.

For Acute Glaucoma

Decrease IOP with antiglaucoma medication and topical as well as oral carbonic anhydrase inhibitors and hyperosmotic agents.

Treatment Aims

- To improve visual acuity
- To relieve pain.

Other Treatments

Gundersen conjunctival flap (superior conjunctiva transposed over cornea): mainly performed to promote nonhealing abrasion and to relieve pain in eyes with poor visual potential.

Prognosis

- After corneal transplantation, recent research has linked viability with being highly dependent upon donor age, and possibly final endothelial cell densities and viability of the graft
- A recent large study found that for primary adult penetrating keratoplasty, the 5-year probability of graft survival was 96.2% for keratoconus, 39.4% for corneal edema, 71.1% for stromal scarring, and 85.2% for stromal dystrophy, with surprisingly low graft survival rates found in patients treated for corneal edema, far below rates for other indications.

Follow-up and Management

Fuchs' endothelial dystrophy: every 1–3 months
Pseudophakic/aphakic bullous keratopathy: 1–3 months
Traumatic: weekly
Nonhealing epithelial defect: every 3–5 days
Acute angle-closure glaucoma: weekly after successful laser iridectomy or trabeculectomy
Corneal hydrops: every 1–2 weeks

Treatment continued on p. 125

Corneal Edema (371.24)

DIAGNOSIS—cont'd

Pearls and Considerations

- Corneal edema may also be associated with contact lens over wear. A thorough history of the patient's lens-wearing habits should be obtained
- Patients should be advised beforehand that Muro 128 normally stings/burns, and that this is generally not a reason to discontinue use
- With mild to moderate intraoperative corneal edema (e.g. in vitreoretinal surgery), performing an anterior chamber paracentesis to fill the anterior chamber with the viscoelastic agent Viscoat (Alcon Laboratories, Ft. Worth, TX) has been found to clear corneal edema and provide significant improvement in the surgical view within 15–20 minutes.

Referral Information

Varied and dependent on etiology. In difficult to manage cases, or in cases that may require surgical intervention, referral to a cornea subspecialist may be warranted.

- Epithelial edema
  - Microcystic appearance (reduces vision and increases glare)
  - Bullae (with severe edema; sometimes very painful and leads to epithelial erosions)
- Stromal edema
  - Cloudy thickening (reduces vision and increases glare)
  - Descemet's membrane folds (reduces vision)
- *Fuchs' endothelial dystrophy*: Descemet's membrane with nodular excrescences (guttata) and decrease in endothelial cell numbers
- *Trauma*: discontinuation of Descemet's membrane with rolling of the edges
- *Bullous keratopathy*: fluid accumulating under epithelial tissue, elevating it to form a bullous appearance.

TREATMENT—cont'd

Nonpharmacologic Treatment

- Bandage contact lens: for severe cases
- Penetrating keratoplasty, Descemet's membrane-stripping endothelial keratoplasty: ultimately may be needed for visual rehabilitation and comfort
- Laser peripheral iridectomy and trabeculectomy (if necessary): for corneal edema secondary to acute glaucoma
- For painful bullous keratopathy in eye with poor visual potential, consider anterior stromal puncture or amniotic membrane transplantation.

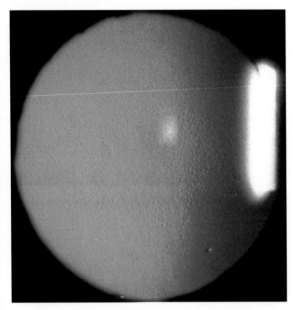

Fig. 1: Corneal guttata seen in retroillumination.

GENERAL REFERENCES

Albert DM, Jakobiec FA (Eds). Principles and Practice of Ophthalmology, Vol. 1. Philadelphia: Saunders; 2000.

Basic and Clinical Science Course (BCSC): External Disease and Cornea Section 8. San Francisco: American Academy of Ophthalmology; 2006–2007.

Ghaffariyeh A, Honarpisheh N. Amantadine-associated corneal edema. Parkinsonism Relat Disorders. 2010;16(6):427.

Levin LA, Albert DM. Ocular Disease: Mechanisms and Management. Philadelphia: Saunders; 2010. pp. 64-73.

McCannel CA. Improved intraoperative fundus visualization in corneal edema: the Viscoat trick. Retina. 2012;32(1):189-90.

Wagoner MD, Gonnah ES, Al-Towerki AE. Outcome of primary adult optical penetrating keratoplasty with imported donor corneas. Int Ophthalmol. 2010;30 (2):127-36.

Wright K. Textbook of Ophthalmology. Baltimore: Lippincott Williams & Wilkins; 1997.

Cyclodeviations (378.33)

DIAGNOSIS

Definition
Rotational deviation of the eye

Synonyms
Torsional deviation, cyclotropias, cyclophorias

Symptoms
• Diplopia and visual confusion in patients who cannot suppress
• Asthenopia.
Note: Cyclodeviations do not cause head tilts

Signs (Figs 1A to D)
• *Objective*: Fundus torsion
• *Subjective*: Torsional results on sensory testing
• *Visual field testing*: Cyclodisplacement of blind spot.

Investigations
• *Objective*: Typically (in fundus photography), fovea is located 1/3 distance up from the bottom of optic nerve. If it is located higher, it indicates incyclotorsion; if lower, it indicates excyclotorsion. The reverse is true using indirect ophthalmoscopy.
• *Subjective*: Maddox rod shows line 90° from strong cylinders in rod. For both eyes, use differing colors
• *Visual field test*: shows torsional displacement of blind spot from usual position
• *Cover testing*: no torsional correction for either cyclotropia or cyclophoria
• *Lancaster red-green test*: allows diagnosis but not quantification of torsion.

Complications
Longstanding cyclodeviations may not elicit target torsion, but will have fundus torsion.

Commonly Associated Conditions
• Oblique muscle dysfunction
• Cyclovertical muscle palsies.

Referral Information
To ophthalmologist for surgical correction when affecting primary gaze or cosmetic appearance.

Differential Diagnosis
• Patients with dissociated vertical deviation will not have torsion in primary position
• Patients with oblique muscle dysfunction will have objective torsion in primary position, and possibly subjective torsional findings as well.

Causes
• Primary and secondary oblique muscle dysfunctions
• Cyclovertical muscle palsies
• Occasionally, fibrotic muscle syndromes
• After strabismus surgery (especially oblique muscle surgery and rectus muscle translations for alphabet patterns).

Associated Features
• Oblique muscle dysfunctions
• Cyclovertical muscle palsies.

TREATMENT

Diet and Lifestyle

No special precautions are necessary.

Pharmacologic Treatment

No pharmacologic treatment is recommended.

Nonpharmacologic Treatment

- Many patients have vertical deviations as well. Prism treatment may permit these patients to fuse
- Some require strabismus surgery on oblique or rectus muscles for intorsion/extorsion
- *Intorsion*: recession of lengthening of superior oblique tendon, nasal translation of superior rectus muscle, temporal translation of inferior rectus muscle; disinsertion of anterior half of superior oblique tendon
- *Extorsion*: Harada-Ito procedure, temporal translation of superior rectus muscle, nasal translation of inferior rectus muscle; weakening procedure on inferior oblique muscle; recession, disinsertion, myectomy, and advancement to inferior rectus insertion.

Treatment Aims

Achieving comfortable single binocular vision in all gaze positions

Prognosis

- Medical and surgical treatment is typically effective
- Patients should be warned of possible postoperative torsional spatial distortion.

Follow-up and Management

Individualized according to patient needs

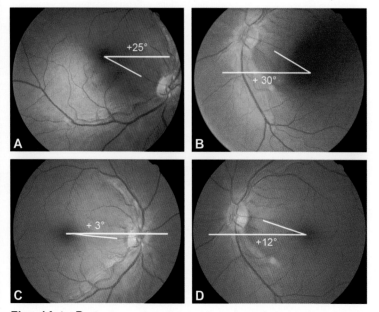

Figs 1A to D: Ocular cyclotorsion measured at admission (see A for the right eye and B for the left eye) and after 3 days in the right eye (C) and in the left eye(D).
(*Source*: http://www.neurology.org/content/77/24/2137/F1.expansion.html).

GENERAL REFERENCES

Bixenmann W, von Noorden GK. Apparent foveal displacement in normal subjects and in cyclotropia. Ophthalmology. 1982; 89:58-63.

Brazis PW, Lee AG. Binocular vertical diplopia. Mayo Clin Proc. 1998;73(1): 55-66.

Guyton DI, von Noorden GK. Sensory adaptations to cyclodeviations. In: Reinecke RD (Ed). Strabismus. New York: Grune & Stratton; 1978. pp. 399-412.

Guyton DL. Clinical assessment of ocular torsion. Am Orthop J. 1983;33: 7-12.

Locke JC. Heterotopia of the blind spot in ocular vertical muscle imbalance. Trans Am Ophthalmol Soc. 1967;65: 306-16.

Schworm HD, Eithoff S, Schaumberger M, et al. Investigations on subjective and objective cyclorotatory changes after inferior oblique muscle recession. Invest Ophthalmol Vis Sci. 1997;38(2): 405-12.

Dacryoadenitis (375.0)

DIAGNOSIS

Definition

An inflammatory enlargement of the lacrimal gland

Synonyms

None

Symptoms

- Pain (more commonly with acute presentation; often painless if chronic)
- Double vision: occasionally.

Signs

- Swelling of the lateral third of the upper eyelid with "S-shaped" appearance
- Nut-size mass (not connected to orbit or lid margin)
- Conjunctival injection and chemosis
- Palpable preauricular or submandibular lymph nodes
- Enlarged parotid gland (e.g. in acute pediatric dacryoadenitis secondary to mumps)
- Ptosis
- Restriction of ocular motility: uncommon
- Proptosis: occasionally
- Globe displacement inferiorly and medially
- Increased severity of signs and symptoms if orbital lobe involvement.

Investigations

- Medical history
- Presence of other skin lesions
- Lymph node enlargement
- Orbital computed tomography (CT) scan with contrast or magnetic resonance imaging (MRI) with gadolinium contrast. Can show marked enhancement if acute, whereas no marked enhancement in chronic disease. May show concomitant orbital myositis in some cases, typically with tendon involvement.
- No compressive changes in contiguous bone/globe should be seen
- If such compressive changes seen, consider lacrimal gland tumors
- B-scan ultrasonography: may be useful in diagnosis. Using high-resolution mode, dacryoadenitis is echographically characterized by enlargement of the lacrimal gland with smooth, clear contours, irregular structure, and reduced echogenicity of the parenchyma.
- Smear and cultures: if discharge
- Blood cultures: if infectious etiology suspected
- Lacrimal gland biopsy: must be excisional if benign mixed tumor is suspected
- Blood count: to rule out elevated white blood cell counts or abnormal lymphoproliferative disorders.

Differential Diagnosis

- Chalazion
- Hordeolum
- Orbital/preseptal cellulitis
- Prolapsed lacrimal gland
- Lymphoma
- Malignant or benign lacrimal tumors
  - Inflammation occurs in a 3:1 ratio to neoplastic swelling of the lacrimal gland.

Cause

- Infectious disease (viral or bacterial)
- Lymphoproliferative disease (e.g. mumps, infectious mononucleosis, influenza virus, herpes zoster)
- Granulomatous disease (e.g. sarcoidosis)
- Sjögren's syndrome, Graves' disease, Wegener's disease, lupus.

Classification

Acute: rare; symptoms occurring over hours or days. Typically presents as unilateral swelling with pain and pressure.
- Children: usually a complication of viral infection including mumps, Epstein-Barr virus, measles or influenza, but sometimes due to bacterial or fungal infection
- Adults: *Neisseria gonorrhoeae* may be responsible.

Chronic: Typically presents as a painless, nontender bilateral swelling present for more than 1 month.
- Frequently associated with systemic diseases such as sarcoidosis, Graves' disease, Sjögren's syndrome, amyloidosis, Wegener's granulomatosis, IgG4-positive systemic disease (previously known as autoimmune pancreatitis), and lymphoma.
- Called Mikulicz's syndrome when combined with parotid gland swelling
- Infectious causes are rare, but include syphilis, tuberculosis, leprosy and trachoma.

Pathology

May result in lymphocytic infiltration of the gland with foci of granulomatous or nongranulomatous inflammation; underlying pathology depends on the systemic process (if present), with resultant blockage between the lacrimal ductules and conjunctiva.

Diagnosis continued on p. 130

TREATMENT

Diet and Lifestyle

Chronic swelling can result from nutritional deficiencies, alcohol, diabetes or drug use.

Pharmacologic Treatment

- Treat underlying disease process; may require systemic steroids
- If bacterial etiology suspected in acute cases, can initiate first-generation cephalosporins (e.g. Keflex 500 mg qid) until culture results available.

Treatment Aims

To resolve symptoms of inflammation and decrease swelling

Other Treatments

Treatment of possible underlying disease entities

Prognosis

Dependent on underlying cause; if associated with systemic disease, prognosis may vary widely.

Follow-up and Management

Dependent on the underlying cause of glandular swelling; necessary for ancillary treatment of systemic illness.

- Refer patient to rheumatologist if collagen vascular or other autoimmune disease is suspected. Good coordination with the patient's internist is important if considering sarcoidosis, tuberculosis (TB), Sjögren's syndrome, or Graves' disease.

Treatment continued on p. 131

Dacryoadenitis (375.0)

DIAGNOSIS—cont'd

Pearls and Considerations

- Dacryoadenitis is usually representative of underlying systemic disease. A thorough history may shed light on its etiology
- The swelling is usually unilateral and localized over the lateral one-third of the upper eyelid, imparting an "S-shaped" curve to the lid margin
- In children, acute dacryoadenitis is most often seen as a complication of mumps with accompanying bilateral parotid swelling
- Approximately half of the lacrimal gland masses are inflammatory; the other halves are neoplastic.

Referral Information

- Patients should be referred for biopsy, blood work and imaging as appropriate
- Patients should be referred to the appropriate subspecialist (e.g. rheumatology) for treatment of underlying systemic disease once identified.

TREATMENT—cont'd

Nonpharmacologic Treatment

- Supportive local treatment with heat (warm compresses); possible surgical incision and drainage
- Evaluation and treatment of underlying disease processes.

GENERAL REFERENCES

Fraunfelder F, Roy F (Eds). Current Ocular Therapy. Philadelphia: Saunders; 2000.

Kim UR, Khazaei H, Stewart WB, et al. Spectrum of orbital disease in South India: an aravind study of 6328 consecutive patients. Ophthal Plast Reconstr Surg. 2010;26(5):315-22.

Plaza JA, Garrity JA, Dogan A, et al. Orbital inflammation with IgG4-positive plasma cells: manifestation of IgG4 systemic disease. Arch Ophthalmol. 2011;129(4): 421-8.

Privalova E, Vyklyuk M. High-resolution ultrasonography as diagnostics of dacryocystitis and dacryoadenitis. Ultrasound Med Biol. 2011;37(8):S129.

Singh GJ. (2011). Dacryoadenitis. [online] Available from http://emedicine.medscape.com/article/1210342-overview [Accessed April, 2013].

Tasman W, Jaeger E (Eds). Duane's Clinical Ophthalmology, Vol. 4. Philadelphia: Lippincott-Raven; 2005.

Vagefi M, Sullivan JH, Corrêa ZM, et al. Lids and Lacrimal Apparatus. In: Riordan-Eva P, Cunningham Jr. ET (Eds). Vaughan & Asbury's General Ophthalmology, 18th edition. New York: McGraw-Hill; 2011.

Dacryocystitis [375.30 or 375.32 (Acute)]

DIAGNOSIS

Definition

Infection or inflammation of the lacrimal sac

Synonym

Lacrimal drainage inflammation (375.3)

Symptoms

- Tearing
- Mucous discharge
- Pain
- Lump in medial canthal area
- Episodes develop suddenly.

Signs

Mass in medial canthal area: with erythema extending along the inferior orbital area (Fig. 1).

Mucus reflux through the canaliculi: resulting from pressure on the sac.

Investigations

- External ocular examination
- *Evaluation of extent of erythema and tenderness*: for possible cellulitis
- *Local pressure on sac*: to see if reflux can be elicited
- *Puncture and aspiration*: in the case of abscess formation
- *Examination of nasal passages*: for possible rhinitis, septal deviation, or mass
- *General eye examination evaluating vision, motility, etc.*: to rule out evidence of orbital cellulitis
- *Sinus radiographs, computed tomography (CT) scan*: to rule out an underlying cause
- *Blood cultures and complete blood count (CBC)*: in severe disease, particularly in children
- Schirmer testing
- Dacryocystography
- *B-scan ultrasonography*: may be useful in diagnosis. Using high-resolution mode, dacryocystitis is echographically characterized by increased lacrimal sac size and diffusely thickened or distorted sac walls, with lacrimal sac contents visualized as homogeneous liquid with echogenic point inclusions.

Differential Diagnosis

- Sinusitis
- Preseptal/orbital cellulitis
- Canaliculitis.

Cause

- Cause is believed to be an anatomic abnormality that results in stasis of tear flow. The restriction of flow results in inflammation of the lacrimal passages, caused by an increase in the number of normal bacterial tear flora that accumulate in the blocked lacrimal sac. Causes of the anatomic abnormality include impatency, stone, trauma, sinus inflammation or infection, and stenosis of ostium.
- Rarely, systemic diseases have been associated, including sarcoidosis, tuberculosis, and collagen vascular disease.

Epidemiology

- Common incidence is in two age groups: less than 2 years and more than 40 years
- In adult forms, there is a female predominance.

Classification

Acute dacryocystitis: sudden onset, increased symptoms.
Chronic dacryocystitis: indolent chronic course.
Congenital dacryocystitis: usually caused by incomplete canalization at the valve of Hasner.

Immunology

- Although no immunologic factors are involved in the causes of lacrimal tract infections, the potency of the immune protection system may explain the relative rarity of the condition.
- High quantities of immunoglobulin A (IgA) are found in tears; also, IgA, IgD, and IgE are found in the conjunctivae that line the lacrimal system.

Pathology

Most believe that the agents responsible are *Staphylococcus aureus, Streptococcus pneumoniae, S. epidermidis, Streptococcus sp.*, and *Haemophilus* sp. (in young children), though Gram-negative isolates including *Pseudomonas aeruginosa* have been found responsible as well in patients with acute dacryocystitis.

Diagnosis continued on p. 134

TREATMENT

Diet and Lifestyle

No special precautions are necessary.

Pharmacologic Treatment

Systemic antibiotics: either intravenous (IV) or PO, depending on extent of infection

- Empiric treatment with oral antibiotics [e.g. amoxicillin/clavulanate (Augmentin, Dr. Reddy's) 875/125 mg PO q8h] and topical ciprofloxacin drops (Ciloxan, Alcon) QID x 7–10 days is appropriate first-line treatment in acute dacryocystitis in adults.
- Acute dacryocystitis with orbital cellulitis necessitates hospitalization with IV antibiotics
  - Appropriate neuroimaging studies should be obtained as above, and surgical exploration and drainage should be performed for focal collections of pus.
  - Intravenous empiric antimicrobial therapy for penicillin-resistant *Staphylococcus* (nafcillin or cloxacillin) should be initiated immediately.
  - Blood cultures and cultures of the lacrimal secretions should be obtained prior to antibiotic therapy.
  - Treatment with warm compresses may aid in resolution of the disease.
  - Impending perforation should be treated with a stab incision of the skin.
- Analgesics: for pain control
- Avoid antipyretics in order to assess whether patient becomes febrile.

Treatment Aims

To resolve pain and the infectious process through prevention of complications (e.g. cellulitis, fistula formation, chronic tearing)

Prognosis

- Congenital obstructions meet with good success if treated before 1 year of age with probing. Many will open spontaneously over the first several months of life.
- Acute and chronic obstructions may require surgical manipulation, but such surgeries reach high levels of success for ultimate patency and relief of symptoms.

Follow-up and Management

As needed to ensure adequate control of infection and subsequent restoration of system patency to prevent persistent epiphora (tearing).

133

Treatment continued on p. 135

Dacryocystitis [375.30 or 375.32 (Acute)]

DIAGNOSIS—cont'd

Complications

- If left untreated, can lead to *chronic obstructive problems* with marked tearing
- May result in *fistula formation* to skin if drainage occurs externally
- Can act as a potent reservoir of pyogenic infection, with further complications including *mucocele* formation, conjunctivitis, corneal ulceration, endophthalmitis, and *orbital cellulitis*.

Pearls and Considerations

- May be acute, subacute, or chronic
- Sixty percent of cases are recurrent
- Often characterized by a palpable, painful mass at the inner canthus
- The presence of a lacrimal sac mucocele in adults mandates treatment even if asymptomatic.

Referral Information

Consider referral to ENT specialist for co-management if obstruction felt secondary to sinus disease or similar anatomic obstruction; depending on the severity of disease, infectious disease and neurosurgery consultations may also be appropriate. Consider oculoplastics referral for DCR or other surgical management.

TREATMENT—cont'd

Nonpharmacologic Treatment

Acute dacryocystitis: digital decompression, if possible.

Chronic dacryocystitis: digital decompression of sac, but definitive treatment requires surgical intervention with probing and intubation or dacryocystorhinostomy (DCR). DCR has been shown to have a higher rate of success in management of nasolacrimal duct obstruction in patients with history of dacryocystitis, over probing and intubation.

Congenital dacryocystitis: massage of sac with digital decompression. If resolution fails to occur over a short treatment period, lacrimal system should be probed (because success rates of probing fall dramatically more than 1 year of age).

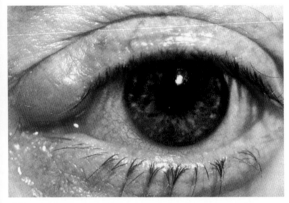

Fig. 1: Focal edema and erythema in area of left upper medial canthus in patient with *Leptothrix* canaliculitis.

GENERAL REFERENCES

Gilliland GD. (2012). Dacryocystitis. [Online] Available from www.emedicine.com.

Hill RH III, Norton SW, Bersani TA. Prevalence of canaliculitis requiring removal of SmartPlugs. Ophthalmic Plastic & Reconstructive Surgery. 2009; 25(6):437-9.

Hornblass A (Ed). Oculoplastic, Orbital, and Reconstructive Surgery, vol 2. Baltimore: Lippincott Williams & Wilkins; 1990.

Meyer D, Linberg J. Acute dacryocystitis. Oculoplastic and Orbital Emergencies. Norwalk, Conn: Appleton & Lange; 1990. pp. 29-43.

Privalova E, Vyklyuk M. High-resolution ultrasonography as diagnostics of dacryocystitis and dacryoadenitis. Ultrasound Med Biol. 2011;37(8):S129.

Pinar-Sueiro S, Sota M, Lerchundi TX, et al. Dacryocystitis: systematic approach to diagnosis and therapy. Curr Infect Dis Rep. 2012;14(2):137-46.

Shinder R. Nasolacrimal probing and intubation for children with nasolacrimal duct obstruction and history of dacryocystitis. J AAPOS. 2012;16(5):492.

Shah CP, Santani D. Bacteriology of dacryocystitis. Nepal J Ophthalmol. 2011;3(6): 134-9.

Tse D. Lacrimal system. In: Roy F (Ed). Ocular Differential Diagnosis. Baltimore: Lippincott Williams & Wilkins; 1997. pp. 127-45.

Tasman W, Jaeger E (Eds). Duane's Clinical Ophthalmology, vol 4. Philadelphia: Lippincott-Raven; 2005.

Delayed Visual-System Maturation (369.20)

DIAGNOSIS

Definition

A developmental delay in visual perception during the first year of life

Synonyms

None

Symptoms

Decreased visual acuity in a child younger than 1 year of age

Signs

- Decreased visual attentiveness
- No fixational ability until 6 or 12 months of age
- Normal or sluggish pupils; no afferent papillary defect
- No nystagmus
- Structurally normal eyes.

Investigations

- *Electroretinogram (ERG)*: Normal
- *Visual-evoked response (VER)*: Normal, reduced, or absent. Compared to age-matched, most kids with delayed visual maturation will have VERs normal for their age. Variations may represent resolution of the disorder.

Pearls and Considerations

- It usually corrects itself with time and further development
- Education and reassurance for parents is the aim of treatment
- Diagnosis of exclusion.

Commonly Associated Conditions

- More frequent in premature infants
- Apart from history of developmental delay and possible soft signs of cerebral palsy, no systemic associations are noted.

Referral Information

None

Differential Diagnosis

- *Cortical blindness*: Pupils are usually normal and patients don't develop nystagmus
- *Occurs in same population (premature and developmentally delayed)*: VER is absent typically; may need MRI; visual acuity does not improve with time.

Cause

Delay in synaptic development with normal myelination

Epidemiology

Most common in settings of prematurity and developmental delay; no racial or familial pattern.

Associated Features

Except for history of developmental delay and possible soft signs of cerebral palsy, no systemic associations are noted; more frequent in very premature infants.

TREATMENT

Diet and Lifestyle

It is reasonable to provide visual stimulation, but there is no proven benefit.

Pharmacologic Treatment

No pharmacologic treatment has been proven effective.

Nonpharmacologic Treatment

No nonpharmacologic treatment is recommended.

Treatment Aims

No specific treatment indicated.

Prognosis

Spontaneous recovery without treatment is typical.

Follow-up and Management

Reassurance to parents and 3-month follow-up is recommended.

GENERAL REFERENCES

Cole GF, Hungerford J, Jones RB. Delayed visual maturation. Arch Dis Child. 1984; 59(2):107-10.

Cole GF, Hungerford J, Jones RB. Delayed visual maturation in infancy. Arch Dis Child. 1984;59:107-110.

Harel S, Holtzman M, Feinsod M. Delayed visual maturation. Arch Dis Child. 1983; 58(4):298-9.

Hoyt CS, Jastrzebski G, Marg E. Delayed visual maturation in infancy. Br J Ophthalmol. 1983;67:127-30.

Illingworth RS. Delayed visual maturation. Arch Dis Child. 1961;36:407-9.

Lambert SR, Kriss A, Taylor D. Delayed visual maturation: a longitudinal clinical and electro-physiological assessment. Ophthalmology. 1989;96:524-9.

Skarf B, Panton C. VEP testing in neurologically impaired and developmentally delayed infants and young children: ARVO Abstracts. Invest Ophthalmol Vis Sci. 1987;28(suppl):302.

Dermatochalasis (374.87)

DIAGNOSIS

Definition
Redundant, lax skin of the upper eyelid, typically as a result of age-related degenerative changes.

Synonyms
None

Symptoms
Drooping of the eyelids: caused by aging, redundant eyelid skin (Fig. 1).

Signs
Redundant skin: usually located on the outer two-thirds of the lid; the excess skin may be so extensive that it can droop over the visual axis, obscuring vision.

Investigations
- *History*: evaluate for symptoms of discomfort or eye strain due to droopy lids, and patient's self-reported functional impairment
- Visual acuity test
- Margin reflex distance 1 (MRD$_1$) measurement: preoperative indicators of improvement include MRD$_1$ of 2 mm or less
- Brow position
- *Head position*: Evaluate for a chin-up backward head tilt due to visual axis obscuration
- Levator function
- Visual field test, with/without eyelids elevated/taped
  - May be required to be performed for insurance reimbursement to objectively document noncosmetic impact of dermatochalasis
  - Superior visual field loss of at least 12° or 24% is a preoperative indicator of success.
- Slit-lamp examination: to rule out anterior segment abnormality.

Complications
- Obscuration of the visual field
- Chin-up backward head tilt due to visual axis obscuration
- Symptoms of discomfort or eye strain due to droopy lids.

Differential Diagnosis
Blepharochalasis: a true swelling of the eyelid itself, typically resulting from recurrent inflammation.

Cause
- Generalized change of aging
- Thyroid eye disease
- Amyloidosis
- Floppy eyelid syndrome
- Ehlers-Danlos syndrome
- Blepharochalasis syndrome
- Trauma
- Medication (antiglaucoma prostaglandin analogs, e.g. latanoprost).

Pathology
- Involutional: stretching of skin
- In true dermatochalasis, the orbital septum is intact as opposed to *steatoblepharon*, in which fat extrudes through orbital septum.

Diagnosis continued on p. 140

TREATMENT

Diet and Lifestyle

No special precautions are necessary.

Pharmacologic Treatment

Some benefit (e.g. for patients who cannot undergo surgery) has been shown with a single dose of botulinum toxin type A (Botox, Allergan), 6U/brow.

Nonpharmacologic Treatment

Surgical removal of the redundant skin and underlying fat: The American Academy of Ophthalmology (AAO) evidence-based indications for surgical treatment of upper eyelid dermatochalasis and blepharoptosis include MRD_1 of 2 mm or less, superior visual field loss of at least 12° or 24%, down-gaze ptosis impairing reading and other close-work activities, a chin-up backward head tilt due to visual axis obscuration, symptoms of discomfort or eye strain due to droopy lids, central visual interference due to upper eyelid position, and patient self-reported functional impairment.

Nonsurgical management: Depending upon the pattern of aging changes in the individual patients, nonsurgical treatment options include neuromodulators (e.g. Botox), soft tissue fillers, laser and light energy-based devices, and adjunctive treatments, including chemical peels and topical therapies.

Treatment Aims

To remove redundant skin to restore full visual (i.e. field) and aesthetic potential.

Prognosis

After surgical removal, taking into account all relevant contributing conditions, prognosis is good.

Follow-up and Management

Surgical removal of skin is generally curative unless further laxity occurs with increased age.

Treatment continued on p. 141

Dermatochalasis (374.87)

DIAGNOSIS—cont'd

Pearls and Considerations

- Carbon dioxide (CO_2) laser resurfacing has been investigated for the treatment of dermatochalasis and may be considered a safe, effective and less invasive treatment for patients uncomfortable with traditional treatment methods
- Dermatochalasis-related excess skin may lead to "masquerade" visual field changes complicating diagnosis of other ophthalmic pathologic conditions if the lids are not taped during visual field testing
- Multiple conditions, such as steatoblepharon, blepharoptosis and brow ptosis, may coexist influencing the overall management and surgical approach of the dermatochalasis to be treated
- The aging face and in particular the aging eyelid is increasingly thought of as a process of both laxity and excess skin, and coexisting volume loss from multiple tissue planes (bone, muscle, subcutaneous fat and skin). The increasing use of filler products and changing surgical approaches in aesthetic surgery beyond simply "trimming the excess tissue" reflects this change in understanding.

Referral Information

Refer as appropriate (e.g. to an oculoplastic subspecialist) for excisional blepharoplasty with patients who either experience limited superior visual field or who have related cosmetic concerns.

TREATMENT—cont'd

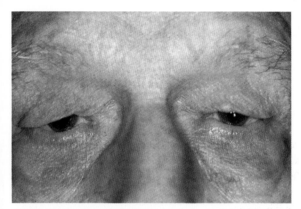

Fig. 1: Redundant skin of the upper eyelids is present diffusely but most marked on the outer two-thirds of the lids.

GENERAL REFERENCES

Alster TS, Bellew SG. Improvement of dermatochalasis and periorbital rhytides with a high-energy pulsed CO_2 laser: a retrospective study. Dermatol Surg. 2004; 30:483-7.

Cahill KV, Bradley EA, Meyer DR, et al. Functional indications for upper eyelid ptosis and blepharoplasty surgery: a report by the American Academy of Ophthalmology. Ophthalmology. 2011; 118(12):2510-7.

Cohen JL, Dayan SH. Botulinum toxin type A in the treatment of dermatochalasis: an open-label, randomized, dose-comparison study. J Drugs Dermatol. 2006;5(7): 596-601.

Fitzgerald R. Contemporary concepts in brow and eyelid aging. Clin Plastic Surg. 2013;40:21-42.

Fraunfelder F, Roy F (Eds). Current Ocular Therapy. Philadelphia: Saunders; 2000.

Gilliland GG. (2012). Dermatochalasis. [online] Available from http://emedicine. medscape.com/article/1212294-overview [Accessed April, 2013].

Hornblass A. Oculoplastic, Orbital and Reconstructive Surgery, vol. 2. Baltimore: Lippincott Williams & Wilkins; 1990.

Stewart W (Ed). Ophthalmic plastic and reconstructive surgery. San Francisco: American Academy of Ophthalmology; 1984.

Sundaram H, Kiripolsky M. Nonsurgical rejuvenation of the upper eyelid and brow. Clin Plastic Surg. 2013;40:55-76.

Ung T, Currie Z. Periocular changes following long-term administration of latanoprost 0.005%. Ophthal Plas Reconstr Surg. 2012;28(2):e42-3.

Diabetic Retinopathy (362.0)

DIAGNOSIS

Definition

Retinal vascular disease and visual loss associated with diabetes mellitus

Synonym

Proliferative diabetic retinopathy (PDR) and nonproliferative diabetic retinopathy (NPDR)

Symptoms

- Gradual decreased vision
- Floaters
- Acute loss of vision.

Signs

- Intraretinal hemorrhages (*see* Fig. 1)
- Retinal edema
- Intraretinal microvascular abnormalities
- Cotton-wool spots (*see* Fig. 1)
- Microaneurysms (*see* Fig. 1)
- Neovascularization of the disk and elsewhere (*see* Fig. 2)
- Venous beading
- Venous omega loops
- Vitreous hemorrhage
- Tractional retinal detachment
- Iris neovascularization.

Differential Diagnosis

- Ocular ischemic syndrome
- Hypertension
- Vasculitis
- Central, hemiretinal or branch retinal vein occlusion.

Cause

Diabetes mellitus

Epidemiology

- Diabetes accounts for 10% of new cases of legal blindness each year
- Incidence of diabetic retinopathy depends on the age of patients, duration of the disease, and insulin-dependent versus noninsulin-dependent diabetes mellitus.
- Twenty-five to fifty percent of insulin-dependent patients of 10–15-year duration will have signs of retinopathy.
- Twenty-three percent of noninsulin-dependent patients of 11–13-year duration will have signs of retinopathy.

Classification

Nonproliferative diabetic retinopathy: includes microaneurysms, cotton-wool spots, retinal edema, intraretinal lipid, intraretinal microvascular abnormalities, venous beading and venous omega loops.
Proliferative diabetic retinopathy: includes all the findings of nonproliferative disease plus neovascularization of the disk or elsewhere.

Pathology

- Decrease in pericytes in the retinal vascular endothelium
- Progressive thickening of the retinal capillary basement membrane
- Vascular occlusion
- Microaneurysms form in the superficial retinal capillaries
- Dot and blot hemorrhages in the outer plexiform and inner nuclear layer of the retina
- Breakdown of the blood retinal barrier
- Intraretinal lipid exudates.

Diagnosis continued on p. 144

TREATMENT

Diet and Lifestyle

- Maintain a normal blood glucose level
- Exercise.

Pharmacologic Treatment

For Neovascular Glaucoma

Standard dosage: Nonselective β-blockers, one drop twice daily

Selective β-blocker, one drop twice daily

Topical carbonic anhydrase inhibitor, one drop three times daily

Oral carbonic anhydrase inhibitor, 250 mg four times daily, or 500 mg twice daily

- If there is evidence of iris neovascularization, administer atropine sulfate 1%. One drop twice daily is recommended to maintain long-term pupil dilation
- Intravitreal Avastin or Lucentis can result in prompt regression of the iris vessels, but panretinal laser photocoagulation is necessary to prevent them from regrowing.

Nonpharmacologic Treatment

Focal thermal laser therapy: for macular edema if it is within 500 μm of the fovea with or without intraretinal lipid, or if there is an area of macular edema that is equal or greater in size than one disk area within 1 disk diameter of the fovea.

Panretinal laser photocoagulation: for PDR if there is neovascularization of the disk or moderate to severe neovascularization elsewhere.

Pars plana vitrectomy: for nonclearing vitreous hemorrhage or tractional diabetic detachment that threatens the fovea.

Intravitreal triamcinolone injection: for macular edema involving the fovea that is affecting visual acuity and has not responded to macular laser.

Intravitreal Avastin or Lucentis for both macular edema and proliferative disease (especially with vitreous hemorrhage) may be indicated.

Treatment Aims

- To stabilize vision or decrease the rate of visual loss
- To decrease macular edema
- To achieve regression of proliferative retinopathy
- To release traction if macula is threatened
- To clear vitreous hemorrhage if present greater than or equal to 2 months.

Prognosis

- Depends on the severity of the disease

Follow-up and Management

- Yearly screening dilated fundus examinations should be performed on all diabetic patients.
- If diabetic retinopathy is detected, follow-up examinations may be as frequent as every 2–3 months to observe the rate of progression.

Complications

- Cataracts
- Neovascular glaucoma secondary to ischemia with iris or angle neovascularization (*see* Pharmacologic Treatment)
- Tractional retinal detachment
- Vitreous hemorrhage
- Preretinal hemorrhage
- Macular edema
- Optic nerve damage.

Treatment continued on p. 145

Diabetic Retinopathy (362.0)

DIAGNOSIS—cont'd

Investigations

- *Careful slit-lamp examination*: to rule out neovascularization of the iris
- *Gonioscopy*: if there is a suspicion for neovascular glaucoma
- Dilated fundus examination
- Fluorescein angiography (*see* Fig. 3).

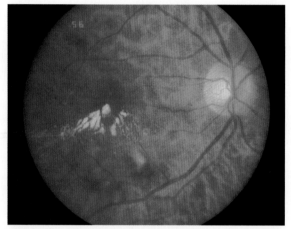

Fig. 1: Background diabetic retinopathy. Note intraretinal lipid, microaneurysms, intraretinal hemorrhages and cotton-wool spot.

TREATMENT—cont'd

Pearls and Considerations

Even asymptomatic patients may need to be treated to prevent future visual loss from macular edema or neovascularization.

Referral Information

Patients need an annual dilated fundus examination, with or without symptoms.

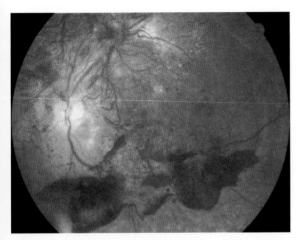

Fig. 2: Proliferative diabetic retinopathy. Note neovascularization of the disk, preretinal fibrosis superiorly and preretinal hemorrhage inferiorly.

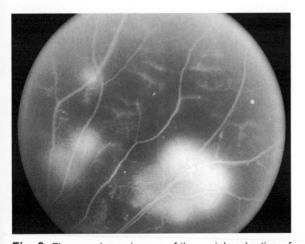

Fig. 3: Fluorescein angiogram of the peripheral retina of a patient with proliferative diabetic retinopathy, showing hyperfluorescent leakage secondary to neovascularization elsewhere (white areas with poorly defined borders) and capillary loss (dark areas between the blood vessels).

GENERAL REFERENCES

Aiello LM. Diagnosis, management, and treatment of nonproliferative diabetic retinopathy and macular edema. Prin Pract Ophthal. 1994;2: 747-60.

Avery RL, Pearlman J, Pieramici DJ, et al. Intravitreal bevacizumab (Avastin) in the treatment of proliferative diabetic retinopathy. Ophthalmology. 2006;113 (10):1695. e1-15.

Klein R, Klein BE, Moss SE, et al. The Wisconsin Epidemiologic Study of Diabetic Retinopathy. IX. Four-year incidence and progression of diabetic retinopathy when age of diagnosis is less than 30 years. Arch Ophthalmol. 1989; 107:237-43.

Klein R, Klein BE, Moss SE, et al. The Wisconsin Epidemiologic Study of Diabetic Retinopathy. X. Four-year incidence and progression of diabetic retinopathy when age of diagnosis is 30 years or more. Arch Ophthalmol. 1989;107:244-9.

Martidis A, Duker JS, Greenberg PB, et al. Intravitreal triamcinolone for refractory diabetic macular edema. Ophthalmology. 2002;109:920-7.

Miller JW, D'Amico DJ. Proliferative diabetic retinopathy. Prin Pract Ophthal. 1994;2:760-82.

Duane Syndrome (378.71)

DIAGNOSIS

Definition
A congenital miswiring of the medial and lateral rectus muscles, such that globe retraction on attempted adduction occurs, as well as limitation of adduction, abduction, or both.

Synonyms
Duane's retraction syndrome, retraction syndrome

Symptoms
Cosmetic deformity on lateral gaze

Signs (Figs 1A to E)
* Retraction of involved globe on adduction, attempted adduction; ptosis on adduction, or attempted adduction
* *Duane I*: absent abduction
* *Duane II*: absent adduction
* *Duane III*: limited abduction and adduction.

Investigations
* Magnetic resonance imaging to characterize upshoot and downshoot movements
* Hearing deficiency.

Complications
* *Duane I*: esotropia in 40% with head turn toward involved eye (≤30 prism diopters)
* *Duane II*: exotropia in 20% with head turn away from involved eye
* *Duane III*: either esotropia or exotropia, usually small in magnitude
* Amblyopia may develop in patients with strabismus and no head turn.

Pearls and Considerations
Usually do not experience diplopia

Commonly Associated Conditions
* *Klippel-Feil anomaly*: cervical vertebral fusion, platybasia, spina bifida, scapular elevation
* *Wildervanck syndrome*: Klippel-Feil anomaly, congenital labyrinthine deafness
* *Goldenhar syndrome*: epibulbar dermoids, auricular appendages, microtia, mandibular and vertebral anomalies
* *Vertical-retraction syndrome*: monocular retraction of globe with narrowing of lid fissure on attempted up- or downgaze: limitation of elevation or depression
* *Synergistic divergence*: "ocular splits"—simultaneous abduction of both eyes on gaze away from involved eye
* *Speculated miswiring of horizontal recti*: lateral rectus muscle innervated by both cranial nerve (CN6) and branch of inferior division of CN3.

Referral Information
Surgical referral for extraocular muscle surgery to limit retraction may be considered.

Differential Diagnosis
* Sixth nerve palsy
* Congenital esotropia
* Exotropia
* Orbital fracture, tumor, or restrictive infiltrative process
* *Mobius syndrome*: bilateral, no globe retraction or ptosis on adduction, associated CN7 and 12 palsies.

Cause
* Genes DURS1 and DURS2
* *Duane I*: depleted CN6 nucleus and absent CN6: lateral rectus innervated by branch of inferior division of CN3
* *Duane II*: lateral rectus innervated by both CN6 and branch of inferior division of CN3
* *Duane III*: both medial and lateral rectus muscles innervated by CN6 and brand of inferior division of CN3.

Epidemiology
* Accounts for 1% of all strabismus
* Type 1 is most common variant (85%) presents most in the left eye (60%)
  - Female predilection, with severely limited or absent abduction
* Type 2 represents 14% of patients
* Type 3 represents 1% of patients
* Autosomal dominant form exists.

Pathology
Duane I: depleted CN6 nucleus of absent nerve; lateral rectus partially or totally replaced with fibrous tissue

TREATMENT

Diet and Lifestyle

Patients may learn to turn the head to avoid a cosmetic blemish in side gaze.

Pharmacologic Treatment

No pharmacologic treatment is recommended.

Nonpharmacologic Treatment

Surgery indicated when strabismus is present in primary position.

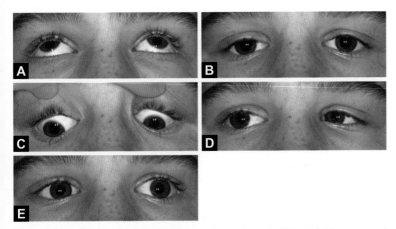

Figs 1A to E: Versions in Duane syndrome type I. This child has normal versions in her right eye and no abduction of the left eye beyond the midline. The lid fissure narrows on adduction of the left eye and widens on attempted abduction. The exotropia in upgaze is common in patients with Duane syndrome.

GENERAL REFERENCES

Barbe ME, Scott WE, Kutschke PJ. A simplified approach to the treatment of Duane's syndrome. Br J Ophthalmol. 2004;88(1):131-8.

Fells P, Lee JP. Strabismus. In: Spalton DJ, Hitchings RA, Hunter PA (Eds). Atlas of Clinical Ophthalmology. London, New York: Gower Medical Publishing; 1984.p.6.7.

Hotchkiss MG, Miller NR, Clark AW, et al. Bilateral Duane's retraction syndrome: a clinico-pathologic report. Arch Ophthalmol. 1980;98:870-6.

Huber A. Electrophysiology of the retraction syndrome. Br J Ophthalmol. 1974; 58:293-5.

Miller MT. Association of Duane retraction syndrome with craniofacial malformations. J Craniofac Genet Dev Biol Suppl. 1985;1:273-8.

Moster ML. Paresis of isolated and multiple cranial nerves and painful ophthalmoplegia. In: Yanoff M, Duker JS (Eds). Ophthalmology. St Louis: Elsevier; 2006.

Pressman SH, Scott WE. Surgical treatment of Duane's syndrome. Ophthalmology. 1986;93:29-83.

Yüksel D, Optican LM, Lefèvre P. Properties of saccades in Duane retraction syndrome. Invest Ophthalmol Vis Sci. 2005;46(9):3144-51.

Esotropia (378.0)

DIAGNOSIS

Definition
Inward deviation of the visual axis

Synonyms
- "Cross-eye"
- Convergent strabismus
- Internal strabismus.

Symptoms
- Asthenopia
- Likely loss of stereopsis
- Possibly cosmetic deformity.

Signs (Figs 1 and 2)
- Intermittent or constant inward deviation of the visual axes, especially when tired or ill
- Squinting or rubbing of one or both eyes.

Investigations (Figs 3A to C)
- General medical and neurological examination
- Family history, trauma, recent immunizations
- Age of onset, change in frequency and amplitude of deviation
- Measurement of alignment at near, distance, and all gaze positions
- Evaluation of ductions and versions.

Complications
- Amblyopia
- Surgery can result in under- or overcorrections
- Surgery also associated with rare complications including infection, hemorrhage, loss of vision, slipped or lost muscles
- Decreased horizontal visual field.

Pearls and Considerations
- Must evaluate alignment and motility in all gaze positions to assess commitance
- Full cycloplegic refraction is essential
- Continuous monitoring for diplopia.

Differential Diagnosis
- Pseudoesotropia, myasthenia, thyroid eye disease
- Nystagmus blockage (compensation) syndrome
- Mobius syndrome
- Duane syndrome
- Cyclic esotropia
- Congenital sixth-nerve palsy
- Neurologic impairment.

Cause
- *Early-onset esotropia*: either congenital lack of binocular vision with resultant esotropia or mismatch between sensory input and motor response systems with resultant esotropia.
- *Accommodative esotropia*: either high hyperopia or increased ratio of accommodative convergence to accommodation (or both).
- *Duane syndrome*: esotropia found in 40% of Type I, with absence of sixth cranial nerve and miswiring of lateral rectus muscle by a branch of the lower division of the third cranial nerve; autosomal dominant form exists.
- *Cyclic esotropia*: presumed inherent biologic clock
- *Sixth-nerve palsy*: increased intracranial pressure, mass, infection, or inflammation of cavernous sinus or Dorello canal; occlusion of vessel to nerve; pontine infarct or mass.
- *Sensory esotropia*: poor acuity in one eye; often caused by congenital cataract, corneal opacity, strabismic or anisometropic amblyopia.
- *Möbius syndrome*: unknown
- *Strabismus fixus*: presumably caused by congenital fibrosis of the medial recti.

Epidemiology
- Congenital esotropia occurs in roughly 1% of the population, typically more in children who have neurological disorders.
- Accommodative esotropia occurs between 6 months and 7 years of age typically toward the end of the day or when the child is very tired, ill, or daydreaming.

Pathology
Most cases have no known pathophysiology attributed to ocular muscles, orbit, or cranial nerves.

Diagnosis continued on p. 150

TREATMENT

Diet and Lifestyle

No special precautions are necessary.

Pharmacologic Treatment

- Infants and myopic patients can be treated for accommodative esotropia with phospholine iodide drops (0.125% in both eyes before each bedtime) to lower ratio of accommodative convergence to accommodation
- Botulinum toxin injection into medial recti of affected patients usually requires general anesthesia in children; found to be less successful than surgery in most published series.

Nonpharmacologic Treatment

- *Glasses and contact lenses:* foundation of initial treatment for accommodative esotropia; the full hyperopic correction with bifocals, if necessary, is prescribed for young children
- *Base-out prisms:* may be helpful in some patients with intermittent esotropia.
- *Strabismus surgery:* necessary for eye alignment in most patients in whom glasses are not effective; procedures include symmetric medial rectus recessions, monocular recession of medial rectus and resection of lateral rectus, and symmetric lateral rectus resections.
- Many patients with esotropia are amblyopic and should be treated in the usual manner.

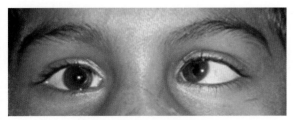

Fig. 1: Congenital esotropia.

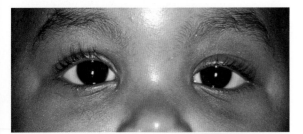

Fig. 2: Pseudostrabismus: This results from a flat nasal bridge, wide epicanthal folds, and small interpupillary distance.

Treatment continued on p. 151

Esotropia (378.0)

DIAGNOSIS—cont'd

Commonly Associated Conditions

- Amblyopia
- *All forms*: alphabet-pattern strabismus with greater esotropia in upgaze (A pattern) or downgaze (V pattern)
- *Early-onset esotropia*: inferior oblique overaction (75%), superior oblique overaction (5%), dissociated vertical deviation (75%), latent nystagmus (50%), rotary nystagmus (20%), amblyopia (40%); deviation is the same at distance and at near fixations.
- *Accommodative esotropia*: inferior oblique overaction (50%); deviation initially greater at near than at distance fixation.
- *Duane syndrome*: esotropia (40% in type I); overelevation or overdepression in adduction; retraction of globe into orbit with adduction; pseudoptosis with adduction; may be associated with Klippel-Feil anomaly, Goldenhar syndrome, Wildervanck syndrome (Klippel-Feil anomalad, Duane syndrome, congenital labyrinthine deafness).
- *Möbius syndrome*: upper-motor-neuron seventh-nerve palsies, lower-motor-neuron twelfth-nerve palsies, mental retardation, polydactyly, syndactyly, brachydactyly, clubbed feet, peculiar gait, peroneal muscle atrophy.

Referral Information

- Consider neurology or neurosurgery for cases of suspected intracranial pathology or myasthenia
- Orbital specialist for thyroid eye disease.

TREATMENT—cont'd

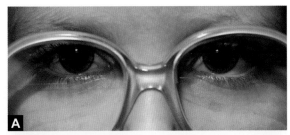

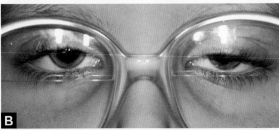

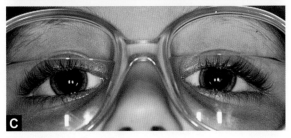

Figs 3A to C: Hyperopic child with right esotropia. (A) Esotropia controlled at distance fixation through distance (top) segment of bifocals; (B) Esotropia near fixation through distance segment of bifocals; (C) Aligned eyes at near fixation through near (bottom) segment of bifocals.

GENERAL REFERENCES

Baker JD, Parks MM. Early-onset accommodative esotropia. Am J Ophthalmol. 1980;90:11-8.

Birch EE, Wang J. Stereoacuity outcomes after treatment of infantile and accommodative esotropia. Optom Vis Sci. 2009; 86(6):647-52.

Cheng KP, Biglan AW, Hiles DA. Pediatric ophthalmology. In: Zitelli BJ, Davis HW (Eds). Atlas of pediatric physical diagnosis, 2nd edition. New York: Gower Medical Publishing; 1992. p.19.1.

Henderson JC. The congenital facial diplegia syndrome: clinical feature, pathology, and etiology: a review of 61 cases. Brain. 1939;62:381-4.

Hitchkiss MG, Miller NR, Clark AW, et al. Bilateral Duane's retraction syndrome: a clinical-pathologic report. Arch Ophthalmol. 1980;98:870-90.

Ing MR. Early surgical alignment for congenital esotropia. Trans Am Ophthalmol Soc. 1981;79:625-33.

Louwagie CR, Diehl NN, Greenberg AE, et al. Long-term follow-up of congenital esotropia in a population-based cohort. J AAPOS. 2009;13(1):8-12. Epub 2008.

Pediatric Eye Disease Investigator Group. Interobserver reliability of the prism and alternate cover test in children with esotropia. Arch Ophthalmol. 2009;127(1):59-65.

Exophthalmos, Noninfectious and Nonendocrine (376.3)

DIAGNOSIS

Definition

Abnormal protrusion of the globe from the bony orbit

Synonym

Bulging eye

Symptoms

- Swelling/pressure
- *Red, painful eye*: if exophthalmos is excessive, exposure keratitis may cause redness and pain in the eye
- Tearing
- Blurred vision
- Strabismus and diplopia (double vision).

Signs

- *Exophthalmos (ocular proptosis)*: a lesion within the muscle cone causes more exophthalmos than a similar-sized lesion outside the muscle cone; paresis of the extraocular muscles as a result of inflammation (ophthalmoplegia) can cause 2.0 mm of ocular proptosis.
- *Chemosis of conjunctiva*: may be so severe that the chemotic conjunctiva protrudes through the semiclosed eyelids
- Lid swelling
- *Redness*: neoplasms (e.g. rhabdomyosarcomas) may present initially with redness and swelling of the lids, causing a misdiagnosis of orbital cellulitis
- Strabismus and diplopia (double vision).

Investigations

History

- Especially presence of breast or lung cancer, lymphoma, or leukemia
- Duration: Benign neoplasms [e.g. orbital cavernous hemangioma (the most common primary orbital neoplasm that causes exophthalmos and benign mixed tumor; see Figs 1 and 2)] tend to have a long history of slow growth, whereas malignant neoplasms [e.g. adenoid cystic carcinoma of lacrimal gland or rhabdomyosarcoma (the most frequent primary mesenchymal malignant neoplasm of the orbit)] tend to have a rapid, short course.
- Age at onset: Congenital orbital tumors (e.g. dermoids) usually are diagnosed at a very early age. Cavernous hemangioma, although congenital, is not usually diagnosed until the fourth or fifth decade. The vast majority of orbital rhabdomyosarcomas occur before age 20 years. Other malignant tumors, such as fibrosarcoma and adenoid cystic carcinoma, tend to occur in middle-aged to elderly individuals.
- Orbital metastasis from lung cancer usually occurs early in the course of the disease. Conversely, orbital metastasis from breast cancer tends to occur late in the disease.

Differential Diagnosis

Benign Neoplasms

Cavernous hemangioma (most common), lymphangioma, orbital varix, dermoid, hemangiopericytoma, reactive fibrous proliferations, fibrous dysplasia, neurofibroma, neurilemmoma, meningioma, optic nerve glioma, benign mixed tumor of lacrimal gland, Langerhans granulomatoses, sinus histiocytosis.

Malignant Neoplasms

Kaposi's sarcoma, fibrous histiocytoma, rhabdomyosarcoma, adenoid cystic carcinoma and malignant mixed tumors of lacrimal gland, lymphoma, leukemia.

Cause

Unknown in most cases

Epidemiology

- All orbital neoplasms, benign and malignant, are extremely rare.
- Cavernous hemangioma is the most common benign tumor, followed by orbital dermoid.
- Rhabdomyosarcoma is the most common primary mesenchymal orbital malignant tumor, followed by lymphoma and leukemia.
- Lung, breast, and neuroblastoma are the most common metastatic tumors in men, women, and children, respectively.

Classification

- Orbital tumors can be classified as primary or secondary or according to tissue of origin.
- Hamartomas (e.g. cavernous hemangiomas) are congenital tumors of tissue normally present in the orbit.
- Choristomas (e.g. dermoids) are congenital tumors of tissue not normally present in the orbit.

Associated Features

Depend on the cause [e.g. metastatic orbital tumors have systemic findings; Kaposi's sarcoma usually is associated with acquired immune deficiency syndrome (AIDS)].

Pathology

Depends on the type of lesion present in the orbit; basically, soft tissue tumor pathology is involved.

Diagnosis continued on p. 154

TREATMENT

Diet and Lifestyle

No special precautions are necessary.

Pharmacologic Treatment

In general, pharmacologic treatment is ineffective, except in special cases of chemotherapy (e.g. for rhabdomyosarcoma).

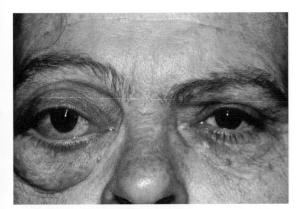

Fig. 1A: Right eye exophthalmos caused by orbital cavernous hemangioma.

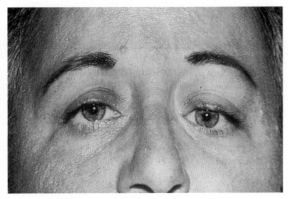

Fig. 1B: Another patient with right eye exophthalmos caused by orbital cavernous hemangioma.

Treatment Aims

- To preserve vision
- To eradicate the tumor.

Other Treatments

If the tumor is part of a systemic process (e.g. metastatic tumor, neurofibromatosis, Langerhans granulomatoses), further study is indicated.

Prognosis

Prognosis depends on the type of tumor and whether it is benign or malignant.

Follow-up and Management

- Close initial follow-up is essential to monitor effectiveness of therapy
- Long-term follow-up is necessary to recognize any early recurrence.

Treatment continued on p. 155

Exophthalmos, Noninfectious and Nonendocrine (376.3)

DIAGNOSIS—cont'd

Ocular Examination

Visual acuity, ocular motility, complete external examination, exophthalmometry (measurement of exophthalmos by an exophthalmometer), intraocular pressure, undilated and dilated slit-lamp examination and dilated fundus examination.

General Examination

Physical examination and any indicated laboratory test

Special Examination

Orbital imaging by computed tomography, magnetic resonance imaging, and orbital ultrasound is the benchmark of orbital tumor diagnosis; this type of imaging often is diagnostic of the process and allows for anatomic delineation of the tumor from a surgical point of view.

Complications

- Visual loss
- Exposure keratitis
- Cosmetic appearance permanent (exophthalmos)
- Strabismus and diplopia.

Morbidity and Mortality

If caused by malignant neoplasm

Pearls and Considerations

- Orbital metastasis from lung usually occurs early in the disease, whereas from breast usually occurs late
- Generally, a difference of greater than 2 mm proptosis between the two eyes is considered abnormal
- An average exophthalmometry reading is 21 mm, although this figure is somewhat variable by race and gender.

Referral Information

Refer to appropriate subspecialist (e.g. oncologist, endocrinologist) for management of underlying systemic pathology.

TREATMENT—cont'd

Nonpharmacologic Treatment

- Orbital biopsy usually is necessary for diagnosis, especially of malignant tumors
- Local excision is adequate for most benign tumors, whereas exenteration may be necessary for malignant tumors
- Radiation therapy may be appropriate for certain malignant neoplasms (e.g. malignant lymphomas).

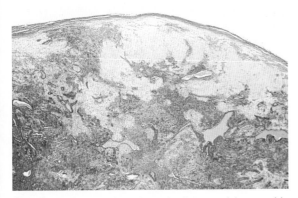

Fig. 2: Histology of benign mixed tumor (pleomorphic adenoma) shows diphasic pattern: pale background, myxomatous stroma, and relatively amorphous; and contiguous cellular areas that contain mainly epithelial cells.

GENERAL REFERENCES

Demirici H, Shields CL, Shields JA, et al. Orbital tumors in the older population. Ophthalmology. 2002;109(2): 243-8.

Feurman JM, Flint A, Elner VM. Cystic solitary fibrous tumor of the orbit. Arch Ophthalmol. 2010;128:385.

Kodsi SR, Shetlar DJ, Campbell RJ, et al. A review of 340 orbital tumors in children during a 60-year period. Am J Ophthalmol. 1994;117:177-82.

McNab AA, Satchi K. Recurrent lacrimal gland pleomorphic adenoma: clinical and computed tomography features. Ophthalmology. 2011;118:2088.

Sharara N, Holden JT, Woho TH, et al. Ocular adnexal lymphoid proliferations: clinical, histologic, flow cytometric, and molecular analysis of forty-three cases. Ophthalmology. 2003;110(6):1245-54.

Shields CL, Shields JA. Rhabdomyosarcoma: review for the ophthalmologist. Surv Ophthalmol. 2003;48 (1):39-57.

Yanoff M, Sassani JW. Ocular Pathology, 6th edition. Philadelphia: Mosby; 2009. pp. 529-32,540-85.

Exotropia (378.1)

DIAGNOSIS

Definition

Strabismus in which manifest deviation of the visual axis of one eye occurs away from that of the other eye, resulting in diplopia.

Synonyms

Divergent strabismus, external strabismus, "walleye" (Fig. 1).

Symptoms

- Asthenopia (headaches, irritability, visual discomfort): with onset of strabismus
- *Probable loss of stereoscopic ability*: when strabismic
- Possible cosmetic deformity
- Children less than 7–9 years of age who are binocular will develop sensory adaptations of suppression and anomalous retinal correspondence. They will also be asymptomatic.
- Children less than 7–9 years of age who are binocular will develop diplopia and visual confusion.

Signs

- *Intermittent or constant outward deviation of the visual axes*: especially when tired or ill
- *Squinting or rubbing of one or both eyes*: especially in bright sunlight.

Investigations

- *General medical and neurologic examinations*: as appropriate to exclude intracranial masses, myasthenia gravis, vascular disease, etc. as cause of exotropia
- History of other affected family members, trauma
- Age of onset, previous treatment, change in frequency and amplitude of deviation
- Sensory testing
- Measurement of alignment near, at distance, and in all gaze positions
- Evaluation of ductions and versions.

Complications

- *Amblyopia*: if exotropia is not alternating and age of onset is less than 5 years
- Probable loss of stereoptic ability while eyes are strabismic
- Cosmetic deformity.

Differential Diagnosis

- *Early-onset exotropia*: large angle; age of onset is approximately 6 weeks; no binocular vision unless eyes aligned less than 2 years of age
- *Intermittent exotropia*: typical age of onset is approximately 18 months; exotropia greater at distance than at near fixation in most patients
- Third-nerve palsy
- *Consecutive exotropia*: after treatment (usually surgical) for esotropia
- *Exotropia associated with osteologic, cranial and facial disorders*: Crouzon, Apert, Pfeiffer and Carpenter syndromes
- *Duane syndrome*: type II associated with exotropia in 20%.

Cause

- *Early-onset exotropia*: either congenital lack of binocular vision with resultant exotropia or mismatch between sensory input and motor response systems with resultant exotropia
- *Intermittent exotropia*: deficient fusional convergence amplitudes
- *Third-nerve palsy*: midbrain masses or infarcts, infection or inflammation of cavernous sinus, occlusion of vessels to third cranial nerve
- *Consecutive exotropia*: after surgery for exotropia
- *Duane syndrome*: type II postulated to occur because of combined innervation of lateral rectus muscle by sixth cranial nerve and branch of lower division of third nerve.

Epidemiology

- *Early-onset exotropia*: 10% as frequent as early-onset esotropia; no gender or race predilection
- *Intermittent exotropia*: 1% of children; no race or gender predilection
- *Duane syndrome*: type II uncommon; no race, gender or eye predilection.

Diagnosis continued on p. 158

TREATMENT

Diet and Lifestyle

No special precautions are necessary.

Pharmacologic Treatment

No pharmacologic treatment is recommended.

Nonpharmacologic Treatment

Glasses or contact lenses: may be effective in myopic exotropic patients by stimulating accommodative convergence.

Base-in prisms: may be helpful in some patients with intermittent exotropia.

Fusional training exercises: may be helpful in some patients with intermittent exotropia, especially those who have convergence insufficiency (greater exotropia at near than distance fixation).

Alternate-eye occlusion: has been helpful in some patients with intermittent exotropia.

Treatment Aims

- To achieve excellent visual acuity in each eye
- To achieve straight eyes with comfortable single binocular vision and stereopsis
- To remove cosmetic deformity.

Prognosis

- *Early-onset exotropia*: about one-third of cases will spontaneously resolve before 1 year of age; strabismus surgery is approximately 70% successful after one operation, 90% after two.
- *Intermittent exotropia*: approximately one-third of patients will respond to medical treatment; two-thirds will require strabismus surgery; surgery is approximately 85% successful.
- *Third-nerve palsy*: depends on cause and severity of involvement; total palsy is difficult to treat.
- *Consecutive exotropia*: usually responds to medical or surgical treatment.
- *Duane syndrome*: surgery for type II will result in straight eyes in primary position in almost all patients, but adduction beyond primary position will rarely be obtained.

Follow-up and Management

Care is individualized depending on cause and type of exotropia.

Treatment continued on p. 159

Exotropia (378.1)

DIAGNOSIS—cont'd

Associated Features

Early-onset exotropia: risk of amblyopia 40%; overaction of inferior oblique muscles (50%), but dissociated vertical deviation is rare; often spontaneously resolves by 1 year of age.

Intermittent exotropia: overaction of inferior oblique muscles (35%), overaction of superior oblique muscles (15%), amblyopia (25%); alphabet-pattern strabismus with greater exotropia in upgaze (V pattern) or downgaze (A pattern).

Third-nerve palsy: pupillary dilation and paralysis of accommodation, simultaneous fourth-, fifth-, and sixth-nerve palsies; involved eye exotropic, hypotropic with ptosis; limitation of elevation, depression, adduction.

Consecutive exotropia: consider slipped or lost medial rectus muscle if postoperative patient and if adduction is limited.

Exotropia associated with osteologic or facial abnormalities: overelevation in adduction caused by horizontal rectus muscle displacement from horizontal meridians; absent superior rectus or superior oblique muscles or tendons.

Duane syndrome: type II associated with limitation of adduction, full abduction, retraction of globe on attempted adduction, overelevation or depression of globe on attempted adduction.

TREATMENT—cont'd

Strabismus surgery: will be necessary for those patients in whom the previous treatments are unsuccessful; procedures include symmetric lateral rectus muscle recessions, monocular lateral rectus recession combined with medial rectus resection, and symmetric medial rectus resections; occasionally, patients will require a single lateral rectus recession.

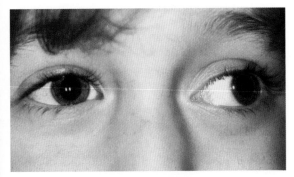

Fig. 1: Constant exotropia at distance fixation.

GENERAL REFERENCES

Gregeeson E. The polymorphous exo patient: analysis of 231 consecutive cases. Acta Ophthalmol. 1969;47:579-83.

Hardesty HH, Boynton JR, Kennan JP. Treatment of intermittent exotropia. Arch Ophthalmol. 1978;96:268-80.

Hoyt WF, Nachtigaller H. Anomalies of the ocular motor nerves: neuroanatomic correlates of paradoxical innervation in Duane's syndrome and related congenital oculomotor disorders. Am J Ophthalmol. 1965;60:443-51.

Moore S, Cohen RL. Congenital exotropia. Am Orthop J. 1985;35:68-74.

Raab EL, Parks MM. Recession of the lateral recti: early and late postoperative alignments. Arch Ophthalmol. 1969; 82:203-11.

Eyelid Ectropion (374.1)

DIAGNOSIS

Definition

An outward turn (eversion) of the eyelid margin and lashes

Synonyms

None

Symptoms

- Corneal irritation
- Foreign body sensation
- Blurred vision
- Tearing.

Signs

- Conjunctival chemosis
- Conjunctivitis (chronic)
- Corneal exposure
- Corneal drying/keratitis.

Investigations

- Visual acuity test
- Evaluation of lid/lash position
- *Slit-lamp examination*: to evaluate cornea for ulceration
- *Fluorescein staining of cornea*: for exposure.

Complications

- *Corneal scarring*: from chronic irritation
- *Corneal ulcerations*: in severe cases, can lead to corneal melt and even perforation
- Thickening of the lid margin
- Keratinization of conjunctival surface (Fig. 1).

Pearls and Considerations

- Patients with ectropion may be constantly wiping their eyes, which will exacerbate lid laxity and ectropion
- Interim bandage contact lens treatment is often helpful in maintaining patient comfort and minimizing corneal desiccation.

Referral Information

Consider oculoplastics referral for surgical repair.

Differential Diagnosis

Flaccid types: involutional, paralytic
Cicatricial: traumatic, spastic
Mechanical: tumor, swelling

Cause

Involutional: most common type; relaxation of the orbicularis muscle
Cicatricial: history of burns, use of periocular medications (e.g. topical dorzolamide, brimonidine, timolol and 5-fluorouracil), scars from lacerations, complications of blepharoplasty result in shortening of the anterior lid lamella.
Mechanical: caused by weight of lid tumors
Paralytic: such as in cases of Bell's palsy or seventh nerve palsy.

Classification

- Congenital (rare)
- Cicatricial
- Involutional.

Pathology

See Cause section.

TREATMENT

Diet and Lifestyle

No special precautions are necessary.

Pharmacologic Treatment

- *Adequate lubrication*: artificial tears (preservative-free formulations may be less irritating), lubricating ointment (e.g. Lacrilube or erythromycin ointment if coexisting blepharitis)
- Cicatricial ectropion felt secondary to topical drug administration may require topical steroid use after stopping the offending agent.

Nonpharmacologic Treatment

- Interim taping of the eyelids when sleeping, if significant corneal exposure noted
- Surgical repair depending on the type and cause; possible surgery includes diathermy, lazy-T resection, V-Y plasty or Z-plasty, horizontal shortening, and canthal tendon surgery
- Interestingly, certain ectropion repair lid tightening procedures (e.g. the Kuhnt-Szymanowski-Smith method) have been used successfully to treat entropion. Based upon the successful use of this procedure to correct both involutional entropion and ectropion, the difference between the two conditions is felt to strongly depend upon on how strong the contraction of the orbicularis muscle is in the patient.

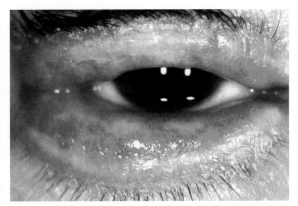

Fig. 1: Ectropion of lower lid with keratinization of palpebral conjunctiva in child with ichthyosis congenita.

Treatment Aims

To restore the lid tension and position to allow proper apposition of the lid relative to the globe and redirection of tear flow.

Prognosis

The variety of procedures shows that no single repair will work at all times. Care must be taken to tailor an appropriate functional and anatomic result for the individual patient.

Follow-up and Management

As needed

GENERAL REFERENCES

Asamura S, Chichikawa K, Nishiwaki H, et al. Why does the corrective procedure of the ectropion work for repairing the entropion? J Craniofac Surg. 2012;23(4):1133-6.

Damasceno RW, Osaki MH, Dantas PE, et al. Involutional entropion and ectropion of the lower eyelid: prevalence and associated risk factors in the elderly population. Ophthal Plast Reconstr Surg. 2011;27(5):317-20.

Fraunfelder F, Roy F (Eds). Current Ocular Therapy. Philadelphia: Saunders; 2000.

Hegde V, Robinson R, Dean F, et al. Drug-induced ectropion: what is best practice? Ophthalmology. 2007;114(2):362-6.

Hornblass A. Oculoplastic, Orbital, and Reconstructive Surgery, vol. 2. Baltimore: Lippincott Williams & Wilkins; 1990.

Ing E. (2005). Ectropion. [online] Available from http://emedicine.medscape.com/article/1212398-overview [Accessed April, 2013].

Tasman W, Jaeger E (Eds). Duane's Clinical Ophthalmology, vol. 5. Philadelphia: Lippincott-Raven; 1995.

Eyelid Entropion (374.0)

DIAGNOSIS

Definition

An inward turn (inversion) of the eyelid margin.

Synonyms

None

Symptoms

- Corneal irritation
- Foreign body sensation
- Blurred vision
- Tearing.

Signs

- Conjunctival chemosis: caused by irritation from internal turning of lid margin against the eye (Fig. 1)
- Conjunctivitis (chronic)
- Corneal ulcerations. In severe cases, can lead to corneal melt and even perforation
- Abnormal eyelash position (Fig. 2)
- Epiphora on examination.

Investigations

- Visual acuity test
- Evaluation of lid/lash position
- Evaluation of tarsal and palpebral conjunctiva. This may point to a cicatricial etiology for instance
- *Slit-lamp examination*: to evaluate cornea for ulceration
- *Fluorescein staining*: of cornea for abrasion
- *Snap test*: the eyelid margin is pulled away from the globe, with poor resultant snap back to the globe surface found in involutional entropion.

Complications

- Corneal scarring: from chronic irritation
- Corneal ulcerations.

Pearls and Considerations

- Small amounts of injected botulinum toxin A (Botox, Allergan) may be useful in managing spastic entropion
- It is important to identify and aggressively treat any blepharitis to reduce risk of corneal infection
- If entropion is suspected but not elicited when the patient is in an upright position, lay the patient in a supine position and have him or her squeeze the eyelids closed. This may manifest the entropion by allowing the orbital soft tissues to settle posteriorly, and the eyelid to turn inward.

Referral Information

Consider oculoplastics consult for surgical repair.

Differential Diagnosis

- Epiblepharon (extra fold of skin)
- Trichiasis (abnormal or misdirected lashes; may be coexistent or secondary to primary entropion)
- Distichiasis (extra row of lashes).

Cause

Congenital: rare.
- Dysgenesis of the lower eyelid retractors may lead to lid instability with consequent entropion, or a paucity of tissue vertically in the posterior lamella of the eyelid
- Structural defects in the tarsal plate may also result in tarsal kink syndrome, with entropion in the upper eyelid.

Cicatricial: history of ocular inflammation (e.g. Stevens-Johnson syndrome, trachoma, chemical or heat burns) resulting in shortening of the posterior lid surface.

Spastic: found with recent intraocular surgery or inflammation. Spastic closure of the eyelids allows the orbicularis oculi muscle to overwhelm the oppositional action of the lower eyelid retractors, resulting in inversion of the eyelid margin.

Involutional (senile): most common; considered to have multiple causative factors, including horizontal eyelid laxity with weakness of the inferior preseptal muscle, vertical eyelid laxity with attenuation or disinsertion of the lower eyelid retractors, or preseptal orbicularis overriding the pretarsal muscle.

Classification

- Congenital
- Cicatricial
- Spastic
- Involutional.

Pathology

See Cause section.

TREATMENT

Diet and Lifestyle

No special precautions are necessary.

Pharmacologic Treatment

Adequate lubrication: artificial tears (preservative-free formulations may be less irritating), lubricating ointment (e.g. Lacrilube or erythromycin ointment if coexisting blepharitis).

Nonpharmacologic Treatment

- Taping of the lid to evert the margin (often unsuccessful due to lubricating ointment causing tape to slip off the eyelids)
- Surgical repair.

Treatment Aims

To restore the lid anatomy to allow proper positioning of the lids and lashes relative to the globe, and the resolution of resultant trichiasis and corneal damage.

Prognosis

The abundance of surgical repair procedures shows that no single treatment is always sufficient to re-establish the lid contours. Care must be taken, therefore, to evaluate the cause and to tailor the procedure to the patient's functional and anatomic needs.

Follow-up and Management

As needed

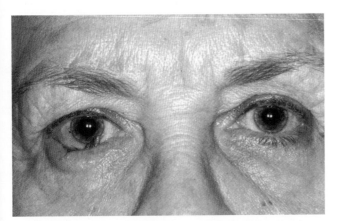

Fig. 1: The margin of the right lower lid is turned inward.

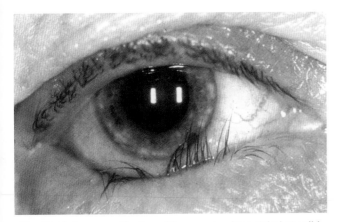

Fig. 2: Higher magnification of the margin of the right lower lid. Note the eyelashes rubbing against the cornea.

GENERAL REFERENCES

Asamura S, Chichikawa K, Nishiwaki H, et al. Why does the corrective procedure of the ectropion work for repairing the entropion? J Craniofac Surg. 2012; 23(4):1133-6.

DeBacker C. (2011). Entropion. [online] Available from http://emedicine.medscape.com/article/1212456-overview [Accessed April, 2013].

Fraunfelder F, Roy F (Eds). Current Ocular Therapy. Philadelphia: Saunders; 2000.

Hornblass A. Oculoplastic, Orbital, and Reconstructive Surgery, vol. 2. Baltimore: Lippincott Williams & Wilkins; 1990.

Tasman W, Jaeger E (Eds). Duane's Clinical Ophthalmology, vol. 5. Philadelphia: Lippincott-Raven; 1995.

Eyelid Hemorrhage (374.81)

DIAGNOSIS

Definition

Subepidermal bleeding of the skin around the eye

Synonyms

Ecchymosis, "black eye"

Symptoms

- Swelling
- Periorbital pressure
- Pain
- Lid discoloration
- Itching.

Signs

- Lid edema, lid ecchymosis (Fig. 1)
- Ptosis
- Double or blurred vision.

Investigations

- *Inspection of lids*: to rule out traumatic injury
- *Palpation of lids*: to rule out occult malignancy
- *History*: drug use, recent endoscopic or periorbital surgery (e.g. blepharoplasty), trauma, Valsalva (e.g. straining to void/defecate), medications with anticoagulant and cardiovascular effects (e.g. aspirin, nonsteroidal anti-inflammatory agents, platelet inhibitors (Plavix, Bristol-Meyers Squibb), low molecular weight heparin products (Lovenox, Aventis Pharmaceuticals), factor Xa inhibitors (Artixtra, Organon Sanofi-Sunthelablo), warfarin (Coumadin, Bristol-Meyers Squibb), large doses of vitamin E, gingko biloba extract, garlic, ginseng, kava, ephedra, and red wine (contains resveratrol, which may promote bleeding).
- *Visual acuity test*: may require speculum examination if lids are very edematous
- *Pupillary testing*: evaluating for the presence of relative afferent pupillary defect (RAPD)
- *Tonometry*: assess for high intraocular pressure (IOP)
- Ocular motility
- Slit-lamp examination
- Dilated fundus examination
- *Computed tomography (CT) scan*: of head and orbits evaluating for retrobulbar hemorrhage, optic nerve involvement, tenting of the posterior globe angle, globe involvement, periorbital fractures, extraocular muscle entrapment, proptosis/subluxation and periorbital foreign body.
- *B-scan ultrasonography*: may occasionally be helpful if retrobulbar hemorrhage suspected and a poor view available, although management of retrobulbar hemorrhage should not be delayed for such testing.

Differential Diagnosis

- Retrobulbar hemorrhage/orbital compartment syndrome
- Preseptal/periorbital cellulitis
- Penetrating trauma
- Henoch-Schonlein purpura
- Vascular malformation
- Rosacea
- Blepharochalasis
- Autoimmune orbital inflammation
- Thyroid ophthalmopathy
- Ruptured dermoid cyst
- Progressively enlarging masses; with unknown cause, occult tumor should be ruled out.

Cause

- Most common cause is trauma
- Rule out drug-induced side effect. Multiple drugs have been associated with spontaneous lid bleeding.
- Hutchinson's syndrome (adrenal cortex neuroblastoma with orbital metastasis) is rare.

Immunology

No immunologic factors have been associated with eyelid bleeding.

Diagnosis continued on p. 166

TREATMENT

Diet and Lifestyle

- Head elevation
- Avoidance of intense activity, bending, lifting or straining.

Pharmacologic Treatment

- Cessation/modification (if possible, in consultation with their primary care physician) of any medications that may worsen eyelid bleeding
- With planned surgery, some plastic surgeons will administer intraoperative IV dexamethasone along with cold saline compresses, which have been shown to reduce postoperative ecchymosis and edema.

Treatment Aims

To relieve lid swelling and discomfort

Other Treatments

Cessation of any drugs (e.g. aspirin) if possible given the patient's comorbidities that may promote hemorrhage with minimal trauma

Prognosis

In simple cases of isolated trauma-related ecchymosis, resolution should result in no permanent disfigurement or ocular dysfunction.

Follow-up and Management

- As needed to ensure that complete resolution occurs without residual ptosis from disruption of the levator muscle complex
- Management of other conditions if found, particularly if penetrating trauma or orbital compartment syndrome suspected.

Treatment continued on p. 167

Eyelid Hemorrhage (374.81)

DIAGNOSIS—cont'd

- In acute retrobulbar hemorrhage with severe IOP elevation, a "guitar pick" sign can be seen with tenting of the posterior globe and tethered optic nerve
- *Coagulation studies*: e.g. complete blood count (CBC), prothrombin time/partial thromboplastin time/international normalized ratio (PT/PTT/INR), sickle cell panel, D-dimer, liver function tests (LFTs), anti-Xa. Further testing for underlying blood dyscrasias (severe anemia, von Willebrand disease, hemophilia, leukemia, sickle cell disease, hepatitis) may be warranted based upon the patient presentation.

Complications

- Secondary ptosis: as a result of inflammation
- Associated orbital fractures
- Associated orbital hemorrhage/orbital compartment syndrome: with compressive neuropathy and potentially devastating vision loss.

Pearls and Considerations

- Evaluation of traumatic ecchymosis should include full dilated examination to rule out further ocular trauma and ocular motility testing to evaluate for orbital blow-out fracture or muscle entrapment
- Anticoagulation therapy is a common pharmacologic cause of ecchymosis, and occurs in up to 25% of patients receiving this therapy either spontaneously or secondary to trauma
- In cases of bilateral ecchymosis, consider CT imaging to evaluate for basilar skull fracture
- There is a significantly greater risk of lid hematoma developing in patients undergoing cataract surgery with retrobulbar block than peribulbar block (7.3% versus 2.7% in one study).

Referral Information

None unless further trauma or other complications require care

TREATMENT—cont'd

Nonpharmacologic Treatment

- Supportive treatment with use of continuous cool compresses (10 minutes on, and then 10 minutes off) to decrease swelling and for increased comfort over 3 days (except when eating or sleeping); warm compresses can be considered after this time.
- Care should be taken particularly in postoperative (e.g. post-blepharoplasty) cool compresses, not to use too heavy an ice pack, which may lead to wound dehiscence, or ice application directly to the skin, which may lead to necrosis.

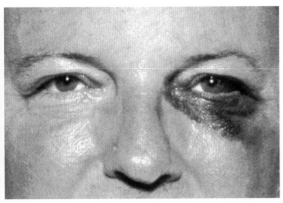

Fig. 1: Ecchymosis of the left eye. Trauma to the left eye causes hemorrhage mainly into left lower lid. Note also that the same trauma caused a conjunctival hemorrhage temporarily in the left eye.

GENERAL REFERENCES

Kaiser RS, Williams GA. Ocular manifestations of hematologic diseases. In: Tasman W, Jaeger EA (Eds). Duane's Clinical Ophthalmology (CD-ROM). Baltimore: Lippincott Williams & Wilkins; 2004.

Klapper SR, Patrinely JR. Management of cosmetic eyelid surgery complications. Semin Plast Surg. 2007;21:80-93.

Lima V, Burt B, Leibovitch I, et al. Orbital compartment syndrome: the ophthalmic surgical emergency. Surv Ophthalmol. 2009;54:441-9.

Patel B. Lids. In: Roy FH (Ed). Ocular Differential Diagnosis. Baltimore: Lippincott Williams & Wilkins; 1997.

Taskin U, Yigit O, Bilici S, et al. Efficacy of the combination of intraoperative cold saline-soaked gauze compression and corticosteroids on rhinoplasty morbidity. Otolaryngol Head Neck Surg. 2011;144:698-702.

Tasman W, Jaeger E (Eds). Duane's Clinical Ophthalmology, vol. 5. Philadelphia: Lippincott-Raven; 1995.

Theoret J, Sanz GE, Matero D, et al. The "guitar pick" sign: a novel sign of retrobulbar hemorrhage. CJEM. 2011; 13(3): 162-4.

Eyelid Noninfectious Dermatoses (373.3)

DIAGNOSIS

Definition

Inflammation of the eyelid skin by other than an infectious agent

Synonyms

Includes eczematous dermatitis of eyelid (373.31), contact and allergic dermatitis of eyelid (373.32), xeroderma of eyelid (373.33) and discoid lupus erythematosus of eyelid (373.34).

Symptoms

- Irritation
- Itching
- Tearing.

Signs

- Chemosis (Figs 1A and B)
- Watery discharge
- Punctate keratopathy
- Lid crusting
- Lid swelling
- Scaling
- Lichenification.

Investigations

- History of exposure to potential irritants
- History of atopic disease (e.g. asthma)
- *Slit-lamp examination*: to rule out conjunctival papillary responses (atopic keratoconjunctivitis with upper tarsal conjunctival macropapillae or "cobblestones"), discharge, corneal changes or anterior-chamber reaction.
- *For atopic types*: history of food allergy or respiratory allergy; elevated immunoglobulin E (IgE) levels
- *For seborrheic dermatitis (blepharitis)*: see chapter on Blepharitis and blepharoconjunctivitis
- *Patch testing*: for allergic contact dermatitis (ACD); somewhat controversial for eyelid ACD, as patch testing by allergy specialists is usually performed on skin much thicker than the delicate skin of the eyelids.

Pearls and Considerations

- Treatment of periorbital dermatoses with steroids carries a risk for serious side effects (e.g. glaucoma, cataract) with prolonged use. Care should be taken to choose a steroid with minimal penetration.
- A recent review of agents responsible for contact dermatitis of the eyelids found common culprits to include fragrances, metals (e.g. nickel), neomycin, oleamidopropyl dimethylamine, tosylamide formaldehyde resin, cinnamic alcohol, benzalkonium chloride, other preservatives, balsam of Peru, bronopol and bacitracin.

Referral Information

If allergy or lupus is the believed culprit, consider referral to allergy and immunology specialist, or rheumatologist for further management.

Cause

- *Contact dermatitis*: results from exposure to a wide variety of environmental substances, including dyes, resins, drugs and metals; certain eye medications (neomycin, atropine, brimonidine, bacitracin) act as sensitizing agents.
- *Irritant type*: results from substances with irritant properties that cause excessive moisture; there is no allergy response in this type.
- *Seborrheic type*: considered as dermatitis of well-oiled skin; may be pruritic in its eruptive phase.
- *Allergic type*: occurs in sensitized individuals and involves T cell-mediated responses.

Epidemiology

Atopic response is most likely in younger individuals.

Immunology

- Allergic types require prior sensitization and T cell-mediated responses
- Atopic reactions have high IgE levels.

TREATMENT

Diet and Lifestyle

Avoid inciting agents, if any (see Pearls section).

Pharmacologic Treatment

- For ACD, low- to midpotency topical corticosteroids to eczematous regions
- Dermatologists occasionally administer systemic prednisone (0.5–1.0 mg/kg/d) for eruptive phase (5–7 days), then reduce the dose by 50% for resolution phase (7–10 days)
- Cromolyn drops (for atopic types)
- Antihistamines.

Nonpharmacologic Treatment

- Caution against rubbing of eyes after exposure to potentially irritating substances, such as chemicals, soaps, detergents, dyes and plants
- Apply cold compresses QID (or in severe cases, 10 minutes on, and then 10 minutes off while awake) for symptomatic relief.

Treatment Aims

To alleviate irritation and remove inciting agent

Prognosis

- Removal of the noxious stimulus and supportive care usually results in resolution. However, superinfection of irritated skin may result and should be monitored for.
- Chronic periorbital and eyelid eczema may be associated with conjunctival scarring and symblepharon, which may require surgical management.

Follow-up and Management

Avoid known allergens or irritants; topical treatments prevent scarring.

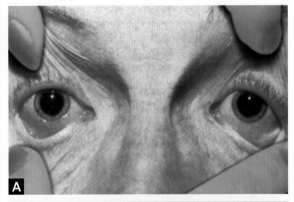

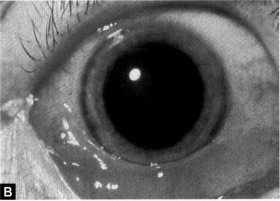

Figs 1A and B: Chemosis and mild eyelid erythema in patient with allergy to dilating drops.

GENERAL REFERENCES

Amin KA, Belsito DV. The aetiology of eyelid dermatitis: a 10-year retrospective analysis. Contact Dermatitis. 2006;55:280-5.

Beltrani VS. Eyelid dermatitis. Curr Allergy Asthma Rep. 2001;1:380-8.

Fraunfelder F, Roy F (Eds). Current Ocular Therapy. Philadelphia: Saunders; 2000.

Hornblass A. Oculoplastic, Orbital, and Reconstructive Surgery, vol. 2. Baltimore: Lippincott Williams & Wilkins; 1990.

Mughal AA, Kalavala M. Contact dermatitis to ophthalmic solutions. Clin Exp Dermatol. 2012;37:593-8.

Tan MH, Lebwohl M, Esser AC, et al. Penetration of 0.005% fluticasone propionate ointment in eyelid skin. J Am Acad Dermatol. 2001;45(3):392-6.

Foreign Body, Intraocular (871.6)

DIAGNOSIS

Definition

An object embedded within the internal space of the eye

Synonyms

None

Symptoms

- Pain
- Floaters
- Decreased vision
- Red eye
- Lid swelling.

Signs

- Entrance wound on the cornea, sclera (see Fig. 1). Sometimes wounds may be covered with blood or even appear to have self-sealed
- Subconjunctival hemorrhage
- Iris transillumination defect
- Cataract
- Peaked pupil
- Vitreous hemorrhage
- *Evidence of an intraocular foreign body*: when viewing the anterior segment or posterior segment of the eye.

Investigations

- History
- *Careful slit-lamp examination*: looking for an entrance site. Need to inspect cornea and sclera closely, in order not to miss small, self-sealing entrance sites
- *Seidel test*: to check for a wound leak
- *B-scan ultrasound*: if the view of the fundus is obscured by cataract or corneal pathology or vitreous hemorrhage
- *Computed tomography*: if metallic foreign object is suspected (see Fig. 2)
- *Magnetic resonance imaging*: if looking for glass, wood, or other vegetable matter.

Differential Diagnosis

Ruptured globe secondary to blunt trauma

Cause

Mechanisms of injury include:
- Hammering metal on metal
- Projectile weapon
- Explosion
- Auto accident with shattered glass
- Machine tool
- Gardening accident
- Tree branch
- Metal dart.

Epidemiology

- Most intraocular foreign bodies are secondary to hammering metal on metal.
- Most patients retain a final visual acuity of 20/40 or better.

Classification

Classification is based on location:
- Corneal
- Anterior chamber
- Iris
- Vitreal
- Retinal (See Fig. 3).

Diagnosis continued on p. 172

TREATMENT

Diet and Lifestyle

Safety glasses

Pharmacologic Treatment

- *Topical antibiotics*: e.g. moxifloxacin or gatifloxacin
- *Topical cycloplegics*: e.g. atropine sulfate 1%
- *Intravitreal antibiotics*: if endophthalmitis is suspected; usually amikacin and vancomycin are used; if the foreign body is vegetable matter, be concerned about fungus. *Bacillus cereus* is more common in traumatic endophthalmitis and should be treated with vancomycin.
- *Topical steroids*: to decrease inflammation
- Consider IV fluoroquinolone, cephalosporin or vancomycin.

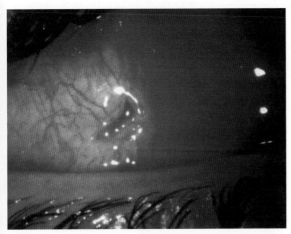

Fig. 1: Entrance wound on the sclera of a patient secondary to intraocular glass fragment from a motor vehicle accident.

Treatment Aims

To remove foreign body promptly

Prognosis

- Prognosis is good if the foreign body is removed promptly and is small. The larger the foreign body, the more potential damage to intraocular contents, which will affect final visual outcome.
- Prognosis is more guarded if secondary endophthalmitis ensues.

Follow-up and Management

Frequent follow-up visits in the postoperative period to look for signs of endophthalmitis, retinal detachment or other possible complications.

Pearls and Considerations

- Although often difficult, visual acuity should be recorded at initial presentation of ocular trauma patients. It is a valuable indicator of long-term visual prognosis.
- Patients must be thoroughly educated regarding the importance of protecting the fellow eye.

Treatment continued on p. 173

Foreign Body, Intraocular (871.6)

DIAGNOSIS—cont'd

Complications

- *Endophthalmitis*: about 10.7%.
- Cataract formation
- Retinal detachment
- Uveal prolapse
- Vitreous loss
- Choroidal rupture, hemorrhage or detachment
- Optic nerve damage
- Secondary glaucoma
- Loss of vision
- Loss of eye
- Phthisis
- *Toxic reaction to metal*: copper alloy metals at high concentration: calchosis, Kayser-Fleischer ring, sunflower cataract; copper pure: massive reaction, endophthalmitis; iron ionizes: siderosis bulbi; zinc and lead: chronic nongranulomatous reaction; gold, silver, aluminum and glass: almost inert, little or no reaction.

Referral Information

Refer for appropriate imaging and surgical intervention as each patient requires.

TREATMENT—cont'd

Nonpharmacologic Treatment

Emergency surgery: to remove foreign body from the eye; if the foreign body is metallic, a rare-earth magnet is often used at surgery to localize the foreign body and aid in its removal. General anesthesia is indicated and retrobulbar anesthesia is contraindicated due to risk of worsening the open globe by increasing the retrobulbar pressure.

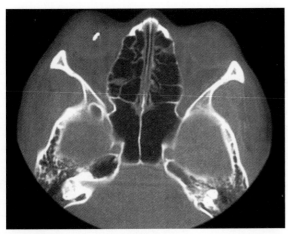

Fig. 2: Computed tomography scan of a patient with an intraocular metallic foreign body caused by an injury related to a gunshot wound.

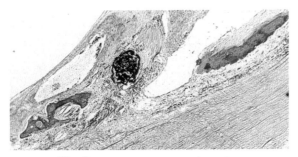

Fig. 3: Iron foreign body in the retina (hematoxylin-eosin stain).

GENERAL REFERENCES

Flynn H. Current management of endophthalmitis. Int Ophthalmol Clin. 2004;44 (4):115-37.

Hartstein ME, Fink SR. Traumatic eyelid injuries. Int Ophthalmol Clin. 2002;42(2): 123-34.

Lit ES, Young LH. Anterior and posterior segment intraocular foreign bodies. Int Ophthalmol Clin. 2002;42(3):107-20.

Rubsamen PE. Posterior segment ocular trauma. In: Yanoff M, Duker JS (Eds). Ophthalmology. St Louis: Elsevier; 2006.

Fourth-Nerve Palsy (Trochlear) (378.53)

DIAGNOSIS

Definition
Paralysis or paresis of the fourth cranial nerve (CN IV, trochlear)

Synonyms
None

Symptoms
- Vertical diplopia
- Head tilt
- Reading material held down and out
- Patient reads into the next line of print.

Signs
Hyperphoria or tropia: increases across from the higher eye or on ipsilateral head tilt.

Investigations (Figs 1A to F)
- *Measurement of the hyperphoria/hypertropia*: in cardinal positions of gaze
- *Measurement of subjective cyclotorsion*: with Maddox rods and Bagolini striated lenses
- *Assessment of objective cyclotorsion*: with ophthalmoscopy or fundus photographs
- *Old photographs*: to identify head tilt
- Neuroimaging
- Vasculopathic workup.

Differential Diagnosis
- Loss of vertical fusional reserves
- Skew deviation
- Myasthenia gravis
- Graves' orbitopathy
- Contralateral third-nerve palsy.

Cause
Adults
- Trauma
- Idiopathic
- Ischemic
- Neoplastic
- Aneurysm.

Children
- Trauma
- Congenital.

Classification
Knapp's Classification

Class I: hypertropia is greatest in the action of the overacting inferior oblique muscle.
Class II: hypertropia is greatest in the action of the paretic superior oblique muscle.
Class III: hypertropia is the same in the entire opposite field.
Class IV: hypertropia is the same in the entire opposite field and in downgaze (L-shaped pattern).
Class V: hypertropia is the same across downgaze.

Associated Features
See Table 1.

Diagnosis continued on p. 176

TREATMENT

Diet and Lifestyle

No special precautions are necessary.

Pharmacologic Treatment

No pharmacologic treatment is recommended.

Nonpharmacologic Treatment

Surgical Treatment by Knapp's Classification

Class I: inferior oblique muscle weakening.

Class II: superior oblique muscle tuck.

Class III: superior oblique tuck and inferior oblique weakening.

Class IV: superior oblique tuck, inferior oblique myectomy, and resection of ipsilateral inferior rectus muscle.

Class V: superior oblique tuck and tenectomy of contralateral superior oblique muscle.

Treatment Aims

- To restore and maintain single, simultaneous, binocular vision in primary position at distance and near
- To eliminate head tilting.

Prognosis

- Vasculopathic fourth-nerve palsies resolve in 3 months
- Traumatic fourth-nerve palsies may require 12 months
- No surgical intervention should be undertaken in a traumatic fourth-nerve palsy for 1 year unless secondary contracture is occurring.

Table 1: Anatomic localization of a "complicated" fourth-nerve palsy: the checklist examination

What to Look for	Anatomic Localization	Cause
Contralateral Horner's sign	Locus ceruleus (nuclear)	Trauma, neoplasm
Contralateral internuclear ophthalmoplegia	Medial longitudinal fasciculus (nuclear)	Infarct
Ipsilateral relative afferent pupillary defect	Brachium of superior colliculus (fascicular)	Tumor
Dorsal midbrain syndrome (vertical gaze palsy, eyelid retraction, tectal pupils, convergence-retraction nystagmus)	Anterior medullary velum (fascicular)	Trauma
Bilateral fourth-nerve palsies	Anterior medullary velum	Trauma, tumor, infarct
Truncal ataxia and ipsilateral dysmetria	Superior cerebellar peduncle	Trauma
Ipsilateral third and sixth nerves, CN VI, and oculosympathetic nerves	Cavernous sinus	Tumor

Treatment continued on p. 177

Fourth-Nerve Palsy (Trochlear) (378.53)

DIAGNOSIS—cont'd

Pearls and Considerations

- *To distinguish from ipsilateral inferior oblique fibrosis*: vertical deviation of a patient with fourth-nerve palsy will worsen in downgaze, and vertical imbalance of a patient with inferior rectus fibrosis will worsen in upgaze.
- Except in cases of trauma, trochlear nerve (CN IV) palsy is much less common than oculomotor (CN III) or abducens (CN VI) palsy.

Referral Information

Surgical referral for extraocular muscle (EOM) realignment only in select patients.

TREATMENT—cont'd

Nonsurgical Treatment

- Base-down prism before the hypertropic eye
- Eye patch.

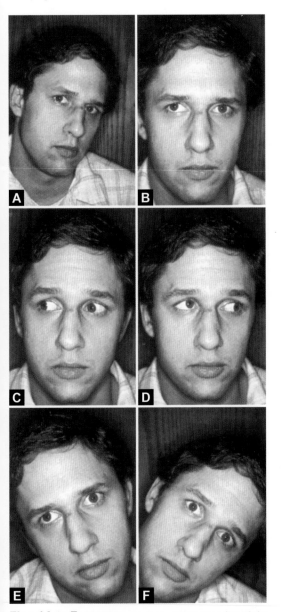

Figs 1A to F: (A) This man has a long-standing right fourth-nerve paresis with a left head tilt; (B) Head straightened; (C and D) Right hypertropia diminishes in right gaze and increases in left gaze; (E) Significant right hypertropia on right head tilt; (F) Minimal hypertropia on left head tilt.

GENERAL REFERENCES

Bielschowsky A. Etiology, prognosis, and treatment of ocular paralyses. Am J Ophthalmol. 1943;22:723-34.

Chen CH, Hwang WJ, Tsai TT, et al. Midbrain hemorrhage presenting with trochlear nerve palsy. Chung Hua Hsueh Tsa Chih/Chinese Med J. 2000;63(2): 138-43.

Glaser JS, Siatkowski RM. Infranuclear disorders of eye movement. In: Tasman W et al. (Eds). Duane's Clinical Ophthalmology (CD·ROM). Baltimore: Lippincott Williams & Wilkins; 2004.

Yanoff M, Duker J (Eds). Ophthalmology. St Louis: Elsevier; 2003.

Fuchs' Heterochromic Iridocyclitis (364.21)

DIAGNOSIS

Definition

An uncommon form of anterior uveitis. Generally, there is unilateral low-grade inflammation of the iris and ciliary body leading to iris depigmentation with fine keratic precipitates and secondary cataract.

Synonyms

Fuchs' heterochromic uveitis, Fuchs' syndrome

Symptoms

Decreased vision: most patients are asymptomatic in the early stages; cataract is typically seen in Fuchs' heterochromic iridocyclitis and will result in decreased vision; in patients with glaucoma, decreased vision may be noticed if the glaucoma is far advanced at presentation; unlike in many other forms of uveitis, hyperemia, pain and photophobia are not reported.

Heterochromia: the patient or a family member may notice the difference in iris color between the two eyes.

Age at onset: the disease is usually diagnosed in young and middle-aged adults; most cases are advanced at diagnosis, so onset must be considerably earlier; rarely diagnosed in children or adolescents.

Signs

Heterochromia: the involved iris is typically lighter (Fig. 1), although patients who already have very lightly pigmented iris may have the darker iris on the involved side.

Keratic precipitates: numerous characteristic "stellate-shaped" keratic precipitates are seen diffusely on the corneal endothelium.

Anterior-chamber flare and cells: a mild to moderate, chronic anterior-chamber reaction is seen; characteristically, this reaction is unresponsive to topical steroids; unlike in many other forms of anterior uveitis, posterior synechiae do not form.

Fine vessels in the anterior-chamber angle: fine blood vessels are seen in the angle on gonioscopy; they may bleed, producing a hyphema after intraocular surgery; rarely they may bleed spontaneously.

Investigations

Uveitis workup: the diagnosis of Fuchs' heterochromic iridocyclitis is usually obvious, and extensive laboratory and radiologic testing is not necessary.

Complications

Cataract: a cataract usually develops in the involved eye with long-standing disease; the cataract usually begins as a cortical or subcapsular opacity that generally progresses to a mature or hypermature state.

Glaucoma: common, but not an inevitable complication: 25–50% of patients with Fuchs' heterochromic iridocyclitis develop glaucoma.

Differential Diagnosis

The differential diagnosis includes other forms of uveitis that are typically unilateral, including:
- Glaucomatocyclitic crisis
- Herpes simplex
- Herpes zoster.

Other causes of heterochromia include:
- Horner's syndrome
- Iris tumors
- Hereditary heterochromia
- Trauma
- Neovascularization
- Siderosis.

Cause

- The cause is unknown. Some evidence indicates sympathetic denervation in involved eyes, suggesting an abiotrophy (late manifestation of a congenital defect).
- Possible role of herpes simplex virus (HSV) infection and ocular toxoplasmosis.

Epidemiology

- The disease is relatively rare and usually sporadic
- Most patients are diagnosed between 35 and 40 years of age.

Associated Features

Reported association with certain neural tube abnormalities (e.g. status dysraphicus, syringomyelia).

Immunology

High incidence of seropositivity for antibodies against certain corneal epithelial proteins, but the significance of this is unclear.

Pathology

Atrophy of the iris stroma with loss of melanocytes. A nongranulomatous inflammatory reaction in the trabecular meshwork, iris and ciliary body is characterized by lymphocytic and plasma cell infiltration.

TREATMENT

Diet and Lifestyle

No special precautions are necessary.

Pharmacologic Treatment

Corticosteroids

One of the characteristic features of Fuchs' heterochromic iridocyclitis is nonresponsiveness to treatment with corticosteroids. Because steroids carry a significant risk of side effects and are of no benefit, their use in patients with this disease is contraindicated.

Aqueous Suppressants and Prostaglandin Analogs

In patients with glaucoma, medical treatment is often very effective. As with most other forms of uveitis, miotics should be avoided. Aqueous suppressants should be the first line of treatment. The role of prostaglandin analogs in glaucoma associated with inflammation is unclear because of the possible increase in inflammation, which is theoretically possible with prostaglandin treatment. Until more is known, prostaglandin analogs should probably be avoided.

Nonpharmacologic Treatment

Cataract surgery: in patients with a visually significant cataract, surgery with lens implantation is indicated and usually produces good results; the risk of postoperative inflammation or increased intraocular pressure is higher than in the usual cataract patient; intraoperative or postoperative intraocular hemorrhage is a significant risk.

Laser trabeculoplasty: usually not effective in the glaucoma associated with Fuchs' heterochromic iridocyclitis and is contraindicated because of the risk of increased inflammation.

Filtering surgery: aqueous shunt devices usually have good results; because of the chronic inflammatory response, antifibrotic agents such as 5-fluorouracil or mitomycin-C should be used.

Treatment Aims

The inflammatory response in Fuchs' heterochromic iridocyclitis cannot be suppressed with currently available treatments. Thus, unlike for most other forms of uveitis, suppression of inflammation is not a treatment goal. In patients with cataract, the aim of treatment is to restore useful vision. In patients with glaucoma, preservation of vision and control of intraocular pressure are the main treatment aims.

Prognosis

The prognosis in most patients is good. Cataract surgery is usually successful, and the glaucoma can often be controlled with treatment to prevent severe vision loss.

Follow-up and Management

- Patients not showing evidence of cataract or glaucoma may be followed annually without treatment to watch for the development of complications.
- Patients with cataract or chronic glaucoma should be managed as any other patient with these conditions.

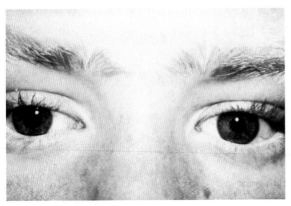

Fig. 1: Fuchs' heterochromic iridocyclitis. The lighter-colored iris indicates the involved eye.

GENERAL REFERENCES

Barequet IS, Li Q, Wang Y, et al. Herpes simplex virus DNA identification from aqueous fluid in Fuchs' heterochromic iridocyclitis. Am J Ophthalmol. 2000; 129(5):672-3.

Jones NP. Fuchs' heterochromic uveitis: an update. Surv Ophthalmol. 1993;37: 253-72.

La Hey E, de Vries J, Langerhorst CT, et al. Treatment and prognosis of secondary glaucoma in Fuchs' heterochromic iridocyclitis. Am J Ophthalmol. 1993; 116:327-40.

Glaucoma Associated with Congenital Anomalies (365.44)

DIAGNOSIS

Definition

Elevated intraocular pressure (IOP) or optic neuropathy as a symptom of an underlying congenital anomaly (systemic disease).

Synonyms

None; associated anomalies include neurofibromatosis and Sturge-Weber syndrome.

Symptoms

Glaucoma Associated with Neurofibromatosis

Children with plexiform neuromas involving the lids often present with a unilateral congenital or childhood glaucoma. Occasionally, there may be bilateral involvement. Other congenital anomalies [e.g. iris neuromas (Lisch nodules), congenital ectropion uveae, anterior-chamber anomalies] may be present.

Glaucoma Associated with Sturge-Weber Syndrome

Cosmetic blemish: the most noticeable manifestation is the large hemangioma involving the face (*see* Fig. 1).

Signs

Glaucoma Associated with Neurofibromatosis

See Symptoms.

Glaucoma Associated with Sturge-Weber Syndrome

Port-wine hemangioma of the face: typically present at birth, unilateral, and in the distribution of the trigeminal nerve.

Dilated episcleral and conjunctival veins: easily seen with the slit lamp and often visible grossly.

Choroidal hemangioma: will be visible ophthalmoscopically.

Heterochromia: involvement of the iris with the uveal hemangioma may produce darker iris on the involved side.

Congenital glaucoma: in ~50% of patients in whom the facial hemangioma involves the ophthalmic and maxillary branch of the trigeminal nerve, glaucoma will be present; typical features include corneal and ocular enlargement, elevated IOP and optic disk cupping.

Investigations

Glaucoma Associated with Neurofibromatosis

Children with neurofibromatosis should have a complete medical and neurologic evaluation. Central nervous system (CNS) tumors and a variety of other systemic anomalies may be found.

Glaucoma Associated with Sturge-Weber Syndrome

Examination under anesthesia: *see* Glaucoma, congenital.

Neurologic evaluation: vascular CNS anomalies are common; evaluation by a pediatrician or pediatric neurologist is indicated.

Differential Diagnosis

With Neurofibromatosis
• Other hamartomas with ocular involvement
• Orbital and lid tumors
• Primary congenital glaucoma.

With Sturge-Weber Syndrome
None

Cause

With Neurofibromatosis

Most cases of neurofibromatosis are inherited as autosomal dominant. The glaucoma is thought to result from incomplete development of the angle, with persistence of embryonic tissue, as well as maldevelopment of Schlemm's canal.

With Sturge-Weber Syndrome

The cause is unknown, but heredity does not seem to be a factor in most cases. The mechanism of the glaucoma is controversial. In infants, the mechanism appears to be caused by a developmental anomaly of the angle, as in congenital glaucoma. In older patients, elevated episcleral venous pressure may play a role.

Epidemiology

With Neurofibromatosis

Neurofibromatosis is estimated to occur in 1:2500–3300 births.

With Sturge-Weber Syndrome

Most cases are spontaneous without any apparent familial, racial or gender preference. The condition is uncommon but not rare.

Classification

With Neurofibromatosis

Two forms have been described:
1. Neurofibromatosis *type 1* is more common and is characterized by proliferation of neuromas and astrocytes, with mainly cutaneous and peripheral nerve involvement. The gene has been localized to chromosome 17.
2. Neurofibromatosis *type 2* is characterized by the proliferation of many cell types and involves mainly the CNS. The gene has been localized to chromosome 22.

Diagnosis continued on p. 182

TREATMENT

Diet and Lifestyle

No special precautions are necessary.

Pharmacologic Treatment

Glaucoma Associated with Neurofibromatosis

Pharmacologic treatment for any chronic glaucoma should be tried. In children with congenital glaucoma, pharmacologic treatment is often not effective.

Glaucoma Associated with Sturge-Weber Syndrome

The severity of the glaucoma in Sturge-Weber syndrome varies greatly. If ocular enlargement is not present, medical treatment may be successful in controlling IOP. Drugs that suppress aqueous production are generally most useful.

Nonpharmacologic Treatment

Glaucoma Associated with Neurofibromatosis

In patients with severe lid and ocular involvement, surgery is often unsuccessful. Filtering surgery, tube-shunt devices, or cyclodestructive procedures may be considered in severe cases, depending on the extent of lid and ocular involvement with neurofibromas.

Glaucoma Associated with Sturge-Weber Syndrome

Argon or selective laser trabeculoplasty: some success has been reported in adult patients with late onset of glaucoma; in young children, however, trabeculoplasty is usually not effective.

Trabeculotomy, goniotomy: these procedures may be tried in infants with congenital glaucoma, but success rates are lower in Sturge-Weber syndrome than in primary congenital glaucoma.

Filtering surgery: some success has been reported with trabeculectomy; in younger patients, mitomycin-C or 5-fluorouracil may be used; cyclophotocoagulation or aqueous tube-shunt devices may be tried in recalcitrant cases, but there is little reported experience with the modalities; all surgery in these cases carries a risk of choroidal hemorrhage.

Treatment Aims

With Neurofibromatosis

• To control IOP
• To preserve visual function.

In patients with plexiform neuromas, cosmesis is often a severe problem, and surgery to improve the patient's appearance may be indicated.

With Sturge-Weber Syndrome

• To control IOP
• To preserve vision.

Prognosis

With Neurofibromatosis

In patients with plexiform neuroma of the lid and glaucoma, the prognosis is quite poor, and most patients have marked loss of visual function.

With Sturge-Weber Syndrome

The prognosis depends on the age of onset and severity of the glaucoma. Generally, the later in life the glaucoma develops, the better the prognosis. Patients with extensive choroidal, iris, and angle hemangiomas tend to have a worse outcome.

Follow-up and Management

With Neurofibromatosis

Careful, lifelong follow-up as for any chronic childhood glaucoma is required.

With Sturge-Weber Syndrome

As with any juvenile glaucoma, careful and frequent follow-up throughout life is required. Patients should be carefully monitored for the development of CNS manifestations. Patients with known cerebral or spinal meningeal hemangiomas are at significant risk from general or spinal anesthesia for any surgical procedure.

Treatment continued on p. 183

Glaucoma Associated with Congenital Anomalies (365.44)

DIAGNOSIS—cont'd

Complications

Glaucoma Associated with Neurofibromatosis

Involvement of the iris, angle, limbus, or choroid may make filtering surgery difficult.

Glaucoma Associated with Sturge-Weber Syndrome

Loss of vision: a risk in any child with a congenital glaucoma; fortunately, Sturge-Weber syndrome is usually unilateral, and the contralateral eye is rarely involved.

Exudative retinal detachment: may develop over the choroidal hemangioma.

Expulsive choroidal hemorrhage: patients with large choroidal hemangiomas have a significant risk of expulsive hemorrhage after intraocular surgery.

Pearls and Considerations

Topic too broad for specific recommendations.

Referral Information

Refer to appropriate subspecialist based on etiology and underlying systemic disease.

TREATMENT—cont'd

Other Treatments

Glaucoma Associated with Sturge-Weber Syndrome

A variety of laser treatments for the skin are available to improve the patient's appearance by blanching the port-wine hemangioma on the face.

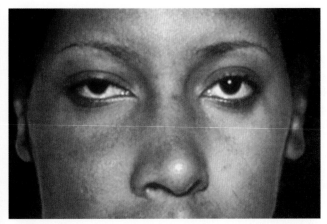

Fig. 1: Sturge-Weber syndrome showing facial hemangioma.

GENERAL REFERENCES

Iwach AG, Hoskins HD, Hetherington J, et al. Analysis of surgical and medical management of glaucoma in Sturge-Weber syndrome. Ophthalmology. 1990; 97:904-9.

Weiss JS, Ritch R. Glaucoma in the phakomatoses. In: Ritch R, Shields MB, Krupin T (Eds). The Glaucomas, 2nd edition. St Louis: Mosby; 1996. pp. 899-907.

Glaucoma Suspect: Open Angle with Borderline Findings, High Risk (365.05) and Low Risk (365.01)

DIAGNOSIS

Definition

A person who has one or more risk factors that may lead to the development of glaucoma.

Synonym

Preglaucoma

Symptoms

Patients will present with some feature that places them at greater risk for the development of glaucoma, but most are asymptomatic.

Signs

Glaucoma-like disks: patients have some features that suggest early glaucomatous change in the optic disks (e.g. asymmetry, early cup enlargement) but also have normal intraocular pressure (IOP) and visual fields.

Investigations

Complete eye examination with gonioscopy: to rule out the presence of any other form of glaucoma or another cause for the optic disk changes.

Intraocular pressure: should be measured on several occasions and at different times of the day to rule out the presence of early open-angle glaucoma.

Pachymetry: should be performed to determine central corneal thickness (CCT). Thinner corneas underestimate IOP, and thicker corneas overestimate IOP.

Perimetry: should be performed initially and at regular intervals to detect the development of an early visual field defect, indicating the development of definitive glaucomatous damage.

Optic disk and red-free photography of the retinal nerve fiber layer: should be performed to better detect any changes that may occur in the future; alternatively, computerized image analysis of the optic disk and nerve fiber layer may be performed.

Pearls and Considerations

Risk factors for glaucoma include age, race, family history, systemic health, elevated IOP, and enlarged or asymmetric cup-to-disk (C/D) ratio.

Referral Information

None; monitor these patients regularly for signs of progression to glaucoma.

Differential Diagnosis

- Primary open-angle glaucoma (in which visual field defects and elevated IOP have not been detected)
- Early chronic angle-closure glaucoma
- Other causes of optic neuropathy and congenital optic disk anomalies should be ruled out.

Classification

- The reason for the glaucoma suspicion should be documented
- *Glaucoma suspect with glaucoma-like disks*: implies normal IOP and visual fields
- *Glaucoma suspect with ocular hypertension*: implies normal visual field and optic disks
- Glaucoma suspect with historical risk factors (e.g. family history, black, high myopia).

TREATMENT

Diet and Lifestyle

No special precautions are necessary.

Pharmacologic Treatment

No pharmacologic treatment is recommended. Glaucoma suspects without definitive evidence of optic disk damage do not require treatment.

Nonpharmacologic Treatment

No nonpharmacologic treatment is recommended.

Treatment Aims

To monitor for progression to glaucoma and begin appropriate treatment when indicated.

Prognosis

The prognosis is good. Most patients with glaucoma-like disks do not develop glaucoma, although their risk is somewhat higher than in the general population.

Follow-up and Management

After obtaining visual fields and baseline photographs of the optic disk and nerve fiber layer, these patients should be followed annually.

GENERAL REFERENCES

Airaksinen PJ, Tuulonen A, Werner EB. Clinical evaluation of the optic disk and retinal nerve fiber layer. In: Ritch R, Shields MB, Krupin T (Eds). The glaucomas, 2nd edition. St Louis: Mosby; 1996. pp. 617-57.

Miglior M, Bozzini S, Ratiglia R. Glaucomatous and glaucoma-like optic neuropathy. Metab Pediatr Syst Ophthalmol. 1990;13:119-28.

Peigne G, Schwartz B, Takamoto T. Differences of retinal nerve fiber layer thickness between normal and glaucoma-like (physiologic cups) matched by optic disc area. Acta Ophthalmol Scand. 1993;71:451-7.

Schwartz B, Tomita G, Takamoto T. Glaucoma-like discs with subsequent increased ocular pressures. Ophthalmology. 1991;98:41-9.

Glaucoma Associated with Anterior-Chamber Anomalies (365.41)

DIAGNOSIS

Definition

Glaucoma resulting from congenital malformations within the anterior chamber

Synonyms

None; often associated with Axenfeld's and Rieger's anomalies.

Symptoms

- As in most chronic glaucomas, patients are usually asymptomatic
- *Decreased vision*: depending on the age of onset and severity of the glaucoma, some patients will note decreased vision
- *Ocular and skeletal deformities*: some patients or parents of patients may note the ocular or skeletal deformities in severe cases.

Signs

- *Cornea*: prominent and anteriorly displaced Schwalbe's line (posterior embryotoxon)
- *Anterior-chamber angle*: prominent, large iridocorneal adhesions attached to Schwalbe's line; between these adhesions, the angle appears to be open
- *Iris*: may appear normal in Axenfeld's anomaly (743.44); in Rieger's anomaly (743.44), there may be areas of stromal thinning and atrophy, hole formation (polycoria), or distortion and displacement of the pupil (corectopia) (Fig. 1)
- *Glaucoma*: Fifty to sixty percent of patients with Axenfeld's or Rieger's anomaly will develop glaucoma with elevation of intraocular pressure and typical optic disk cupping and visual field loss; age of onset varies from infancy to adulthood, with most cases developing during childhood or adolescence.

Investigations

- *Complete eye examination including gonioscopy*: patients with glaucoma who are old enough should have perimetry and optic disk imaging
- *Pediatric evaluation*: children should be examined by a pediatrician to rule out any systemic anomalies.

Associated Features

Some patients with Rieger's anomaly will have dental abnormalities or hypoplasia of the facial bones; this is called *Rieger's syndrome.* Other systemic anomalies involving the pituitary, central nervous system, heart, ears, umbilicus, and genitourinary system have been reported.

Pearls and Considerations

- Other anterior-chamber anomalies that may result in glaucoma include aniridia and Peters' anomaly
- Often, Axenfeld's and Rieger's anomalies are grouped together under the term *Axenfeld-Rieger syndrome*
- When Axenfeld's anomaly is associated with glaucoma, it is called *Axenfeld's syndrome.*

Referral Information

- Refer to pediatrician to rule out further systemic anomalies
- Refer for glaucoma surgery as appropriate.

Differential Diagnosis

- Iridocorneal epithelial syndrome
- Posterior polymorphous corneal dystrophy
- Peters' anomaly
- Aniridia, congenital iris hypoplasia, oculodentodigital dysplasia, ectopia lentis et pupillae, congenital ectropion uvea and previous uveitis with peripheral anterior synechiae.

Cause

It is thought that there is a developmental arrest of structures in the anterior segment derived from neural crest cells. As a result, there is retention of the primordial endothelium and the basement membrane, which leads to iris and angle changes and obstructs the outflow of aqueous. Many pedigrees demonstrate an autosomal dominant mode of inheritance. Spontaneous cases are often associated with chromosomal anomalies.

Pathology

Schwalbe's line is unusually prominent. Peripheral iris strands are adherent to the corneoscleral junction. A cellular layer with a basement membrane is seen over the iris. The iris stroma is hypoplastic in some areas. Trabecular meshwork is attenuated and hypocellular. Schlemm's canal is not developed completely.

TREATMENT

Diet and Lifestyle

No precautions are necessary.

Pharmacologic Treatment

- Any of the medications available for treating chronic glaucoma may be used
- As in many childhood glaucomas, medical treatment is often ineffective.

Nonpharmacologic Treatment

Filtering Surgery

Many patients with severe glaucoma require filtering surgery. Because such surgery often fails in children or young adults, 5-fluorouracil or mitomycin-C is often used. If filtration surgery fails, an aqueous tube-shunt device may be tried. In severe, recalcitrant cases, cyclodestruction may become necessary. Laser trabeculoplasty is ineffective in these cases.

Treatment Aims

- To control the intraocular pressure
- To preserve visual function.

Prognosis

Depends on the severity of the glaucoma. In the absence of glaucoma or severe congenital anomalies, the Axenfeld-Rieger anomaly causes only cosmetic problems. If the glaucoma can be controlled, the prognosis is quite good. In severe cases, treatment is often not effective, and severe loss of visual function ensues.

Follow-up and Management

Patients are managed as any chronic glaucoma patient, with regular optic disk evaluations and perimetry.

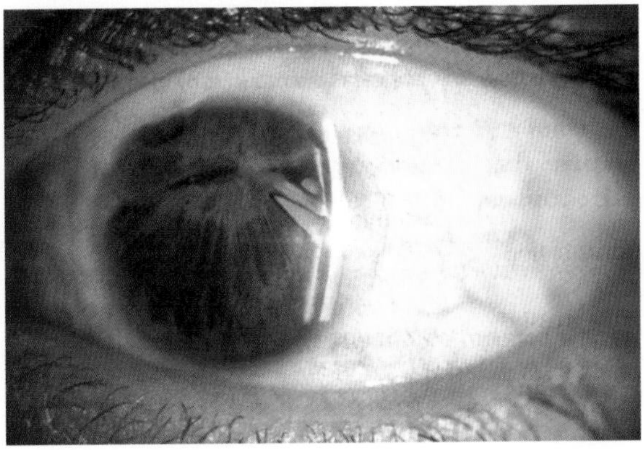

Fig. 1: Rieger's anomaly.

GENERAL REFERENCES

Beck AD, Lynch MG. Pediatric glaucoma. Focal points clinical modules for ophthalmologists. San Francisco: American Academy of Ophthalmology; 1997.

Shields MB, Buckley E, Klintworth GK, et al. Axenfeld-Rieger syndrome: a spectrum of developmental disorders. Surv Ophthalmol. 1985;29:387-409.

Waring GO III, Rodrigues MM, Laibson PR. Anterior chamber cleavage syndrome: a stepladder classification. Surv Ophthalmol. 1975;20:3-27.

Glaucoma Associated with Elevated Episcleral Venous Pressure (365.82)

DIAGNOSIS

Definition

Elevated intraocular pressure (IOP) and optic neuropathy caused by increased pressure in the episcleral veins, inhibiting uveoscleral aqueous outflow.

Synonyms

None

Symptoms

In milder cases with slow onset, the patient may be asymptomatic.

Pain: depending on the cause of the elevated episcleral venous pressure and the rapidity of onset, patient may have pain that varies from mild to severe.

Decreased vision: in acute conditions (e.g. carotid-cavernous fistulae), significant loss of vision may occur at the onset of the episcleral venous pressure elevation; in chronic conditions, the glaucomatous damage to the optic nerve may progress to symptomatic visual loss.

Tinnitus: with arteriovenous (AV) shunting, the patient may be aware of a pulsatile tinnitus corresponding to the heartbeat.

Signs

Hyperemia: elevated episcleral venous pressure, whether from venous obstruction or AV shunting, is associated with dilation of the episcleral venous plexus.

Elevated IOP

Blood in Schlemm's canal: the increased venous pressure results in increased blood in Schlemm's canal visible by gonioscopy.

Optic disk cupping and visual field loss: may be seen in the presence of chronic elevations of IOP.

Proptosis, limitations of eye movements: some causes of episcleral venous pressure elevation are associated with orbital neoplastic, inflammatory or vascular diseases that may produce proptosis or extraocular muscle restriction.

Audible bruit: some AV shunts may be associated with an audible vascular bruit over the orbit or temple.

Investigations

Measurement of episcleral venous pressure: several devices are available for measurement of episcleral venous pressure on the surface of the eye; this may be useful for diagnosis in doubtful cases.

Orbital imaging: radiography, computed tomography scan, magnetic resonance imaging and ultrasound are often useful in diagnosing orbital processes associated with elevated episcleral venous pressure.

Arteriography: carotid and cerebral angiography may also be useful for diagnosing carotid-cavernous fistulae and other conditions.

Differential Diagnosis

Conditions associated with ocular hyperemia and glaucoma (e.g. uveitis, keratitis, scleritis).

Cause

Aqueous leaves the eye through the aqueous collector channels that drain aqueous from Schlemm's canal to the episcleral venous plexus on the surface of the eye. In order for aqueous to flow from the anterior chamber into the venous system, IOP must be greater than episcleral venous pressure. The relationship between IOP and episcleral venous pressure is expressed by Goldmann's equation, $P_i = F/C + P_{ev}$ (where P_i is intraocular pressure, F is aqueous flow rate, C is the facility of outflow, and P_{ev} is the episcleral venous pressure). This equation shows that elevation of episcleral venous pressure will elevate the IOP independently of aqueous production or outflow, and that IOP cannot fall below episcleral venous pressure in the intact eye.

Associated Features

The associated features will depend on the underlying cause.

Diagnosis continued on p. 190

TREATMENT

Pharmacologic Treatment

Because the effects of episcleral venous pressure are largely independent of aqueous dynamics, medical treatment is often unsuccessful. In milder, more chronic cases, aqueous suppressants have shown some success.

Nonpharmacologic Treatment

Treatment of the underlying disease: as noted in the Classification section, many cases of episcleral venous pressure elevation are secondary to another disease process; in many patients, the glaucoma will resolve after treatment of the underlying disease.

Treatment Aims

- To treat the underlying disease (e.g. carotid-cavernous fistulae; orbital, neck or thoracic tumors): a priority
- To control IOP and preserve visual function.

Prognosis

- The prognosis depends on the nature of the underlying cause, the severity and time course of the onset, and the duration of the glaucoma. Patients with a chronic elevation of episcleral venous pressure that cannot be relieved generally have a poor long-term prognosis.
- Relatively abrupt onset of elevated episcleral venous pressure (as in carotid-cavernous fistula or thyroid ophthalmopathy) may produce acute irreversible injury to the optic nerve.

Follow-up and Management

Patients with a chronic glaucoma should be followed with frequent and regular optic disk and visual field evaluation.

Treatment continued on p. 191

Glaucoma Associated with Elevated Episcleral Venous Pressure (365.82)

DIAGNOSIS—cont'd

Complications

Optic neuropathy: elevated episcleral venous pressure may damage the optic nerve by two mechanisms: (1) in the presence of elevated IOP, cupping may develop as in any glaucoma; and (2) many conditions are associated with compressive effects in the orbit that may produce a picture resembling ischemic or compressive optic neuropathy.

Classification

Causes of Episcleral Venous Pressure Elevation

- Venous obstruction
- Orbital tumors
- Thyroid ophthalmopathy
- Superior vena cava syndrome
- Congestive heart failure
- Cavernous sinus or orbital vein thrombosis
- Episcleral or orbital vein vasculitis
- Jugular vein obstruction
- Arteriovenous shunts
- Carotid-cavernous fistula (traumatic, aneurysmal)
- Orbital varix
- Sturge-Weber syndrome
- Orbital meningeal shunt (*see* Fig. 1)
- Carotid-jugular shunt
- Intraocular vascular shunts
- Idiopathic
- Sporadic
- Familial (usually transmitted as autosomal dominant).

Pearls and Considerations

Topic is too broad for specific recommendations; each underlying cause is unique.

Referral Information

Refer for imaging and laboratory tests to determine underlying cause, and then refer to appropriate subspecialist for treatment as appropriate.

TREATMENT—cont'd

Filtering surgery: often necessary to relieve elevated IOP; there is a substantial risk of expulsive suprachoroidal hemorrhage after filtering surgery in eyes with elevated episcleral venous pressure.

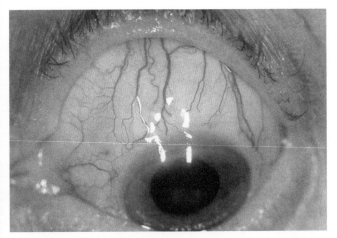

Fig. 1: Elevated episcleral venous pressure caused by orbital meningeal shunt. Note marked dilation of episcleral veins.

GENERAL REFERENCES

Fiore PM, Latina MA, Shingleton BJ, et al. The dural shunt syndrome. I. Management of the glaucoma. Ophthalmology. 1990; 97:56-62.

Grumann AJ, Boivin-Faure OL, Chapot R, et al. Ophthalmologic outcomes of direct and indirect carotid cavernous fistulas. Int Ophthalmol 2012 April; 32(2):153-9.

Moses RA, Grodzki WJ. Mechanism of glaucoma secondary to increased episcleral venous pressure. Arch Ophthalmol. 1985;103:1701-03.

Nassr MA, Morris CL, Netland PA, et al. Intraocular pressure change in orbital disease. Survey of Ophthalmology. 2009; 54(5):519-44.

Rhee DJ, Gupta M, Moncovage ML, et al. Idiopathic elevated episcleral venous pressure and open-angle glaucoma. Br J Ophthalmol 2009;93(2):231-4.

Weinreb RN, Karwatowski WSS. Glaucoma associated with elevated episcleral venous pressure. In: Ritch R, Shields MB, Krupin T (Eds). The glaucomas, 2nd edition. St Louis: Mosby; 1996. pp. 1143-55.

Glaucoma Associated with Ocular Inflammation (365.62)

DIAGNOSIS

Definition

Elevated intraocular pressure (IOP) and optic neuropathy secondary to uveitis

Synonym

Uveitic glaucoma

Symptoms

All symptoms are highly variable depending on the acuteness of the process, the severity of the inflammation, and the level and duration of IOP elevations.

Pain: most inflammatory diseases of the eye are accompanied by some degree of discomfort.

Photophobia: variable symptom that is often present in acute inflammations, but may be absent in many cases of chronic uveitis.

Loss of vision: may be profound; in some cases, loss of vision may be minimal, and patients may not complain.

Redness: most ocular inflammatory diseases are accompanied by some degree of hyperemia.

Signs

Elevated IOP: glaucomas secondary to uveitis are characterized by moderate to marked elevations of IOP.

Decreased vision and visual field loss: many patients will have decreased visual acuity; uveitis may produce loss of vision by several mechanisms; corneal, lenticular or vitreous opacities may occur; if IOP is acutely elevated, corneal edema may result; involvement of the retina or choroid may also affect vision; in patients with chronic elevations of IOP, cupping of the optic nerve with associated visual field loss will be found.

Corneal changes: corneal edema may be present; in some cases (e.g. caused by herpes simplex or zoster), epithelial or stromal keratitis may be present; keratic precipitates are often seen in cases of anterior uveitis; chronic uveitis is often associated with a band keratopathy.

Anterior-chamber flare and cells: some degree of anterior-chamber flare and cells is seen in most cases of uveitis associated with glaucoma (*see* Fig. 1).

Iris changes: posterior synechiae may be present; areas of iris atrophy, sometimes resulting in heterochromia, may be seen.

Anterior-chamber angle: the angle may be either open or closed; in some patients, the angle may appear normal; in others, inflammatory debris or excessive pigment may be seen in the angle; the angle may be partially or completely closed with peripheral anterior synechiae; in cases of iris bombé caused by extensive posterior synechiae, the angle may be closed by a secondary pupillary-block mechanism.

Differential Diagnosis

Other acute inflammatory glaucomas (e.g. acute angle-closure glaucoma, neovascular glaucoma, phacolytic and phacomorphic glaucoma)

Cause

"Uveitis" is a nonspecific term used for any inflammation involving the choroid, ciliary body or iris. In some cases, the cause of a uveitis is known (e.g. infection of herpes simplex virus). In other cases, there is an associated underlying disease (e.g. ankylosing spondylitis, Crohn disease). Uveitis can produce glaucoma by several mechanisms. Open-angle glaucoma may be caused by inflammation, edema, and dysfunction of the trabecular meshwork or by clogging of the meshwork with protein, cells or other inflammatory material. Nonpupillary-block angle closure may be seen in the presence of extensive peripheral anterior synechiae. Pupillary-block glaucoma may be seen in the iris bombé syndrome, with extensive posterior synechiae completely obstructing the flow of aqueous from the posterior chamber through the pupil into the anterior chamber.

Classification

Idiopathic Uveitis

Acute hypertensive iritis, chronic iridocyclitis.

Ocular Conditions

Fuchs' heterochromic iridocyclitis, Posner-Schlossman syndrome (glaucomatocyclitic crisis), intermediate uveitis (pars planitis), sympathetic ophthalmia, traumatic iritis.

Systemic Disease Associated with Uveitis

Rheumatologic disease (ankylosing spondylitis, Reiter syndrome, juvenile rheumatoid arthritis), sarcoidosis, Vogt-Koyanagi-Harada syndrome, Behçet disease, Crohn disease.

Infectious Diseases

- Viral [herpes simplex, herpes zoster, rubella, mumps, influenza, AIDS (HIV)]
- Bacterial (syphilis, Lyme disease, leprosy, tuberculosis)
- Protozoal and parasitic [toxoplasmosis, onchocerciasis (river blindness)].

Immunology

Most uveitis is thought to represent an autoimmune antigen-antibody response to uveal tissue.

Diagnosis continued on p. 194

TREATMENT

Diet and Lifestyle

No special precautions are necessary.

Pharmacologic Treatment

For Glaucoma

Miotics should be avoided in inflammatory glaucomas because they tend to increase vascular permeability, synechiae formation and discomfort.

Some object to the use of prostaglandin analogs in theory because prostaglandins are an important mediator of inflammation and may aggravate an existing uveitis. There are few studies, however, on the use of prostaglandin analogs in uveitis glaucoma.

Aqueous suppressants (e.g. β-blockers, α-agonists, carbonic anhydrase inhibitors) are the mainstay of glaucoma treatment in uveitis. Hyperosmotics may be useful in acute situations.

For Uveitis

Treatment of the underlying uveitis is extremely important. If a specific cause can be identified, specific treatment may be indicated. For example, herpes simplex may be treated with antivirals. Nonspecific anti-inflammatory treatment is usually required. Topical and systemic steroids, nonsteroidal anti-inflammatory agents, and immunosuppressives are the principal agents used.

Pupillary dilation with the use of cycloplegics and sympathomimetics is beneficial. Pupillary dilation aids in the prevention and breakup of posterior synechiae and possible pupillary block.

Treatment Aims

- To suppress the inflammatory response
- To control IOP
- To preserve visual function.

Prognosis

The prognosis varies depending on the nature, severity, and duration of the uveitis and the glaucoma. In some conditions (e.g. Posner-Schlossman syndrome), the prognosis for long-term retention of vision is quite good. In other conditions (e.g. juvenile rheumatoid arthritis), the prognosis is quite poor.

Follow-up and Management

As with any chronic or recurrent disease, patients with uveitic glaucoma require careful, lifelong follow-up.

Treatment continued on p. 195

Glaucoma Associated with Ocular Inflammation (365.62)

DIAGNOSIS—cont'd

Investigations

Systemic evaluation: in some patients, the cause of the uveitis may be obvious on ocular examination; other patients may not have an apparent cause for their uveitis; if the uveitis is severe, recurrent, or chronic, the patient should have a systemic evaluation to detect any underlying infectious, autoimmune, or inflammatory disease that might be associated with a uveitis.

Complications

Cataracts: many cases of uveitis are associated with the development of lenticular opacities; the chronic use of steroids may also be responsible for cataracts in some patients.

Retinal changes: chronic uveitis is often associated with cystoid macular edema.

Pathology

Uveitis may be either granulomatous or nongranulomatous. Any type of inflammatory cell infiltrate may be seen, depending on the type and duration of the uveitis.

Pearls and Considerations

- When treating the underlying inflammation, patients must be carefully monitored for additional steroid-response elevation in IOP
- Glaucoma will occur in up to 25% of patients with chronic ocular inflammation
- Glaucoma associated with uveitis may be either open angle or angle closure, with open angle the more common finding.

Referral Information

Uveitis specialist, rheumatologist, glaucoma specialist; or refer to primary care physician to rule out underlying systemic causes and infectious diseases.

TREATMENT—cont'd

Nonpharmacologic Treatment

Laser iridectomy: treatment of choice for pupillary block in the iris bombé syndrome; iridectomy may be technically difficult to perform in some of these eyes; the iridectomy may become occluded from synechiae formation on the edge of the iridectomy to the lens if the inflammation is not adequately suppressed.

Argon or selective laser trabeculoplasty: trabeculoplasty is generally ineffective in uveitic glaucoma and is contraindicated because of its tendency to increase inflammation.

Filtering surgery: has a high rate of failure in uveitic glaucomas; antifibrotics such as mitomycin-C or 5-fluorouracil are generally indicated; in severe, recalcitrant cases, aqueous tube-shunt implantation or cyclophotocoagulation may be useful.

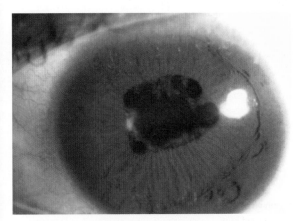

Fig. 1: Uveitic glaucoma with extensive posterior synechiae, which may lead to iris bombé.

GENERAL REFERENCES

Dunn JP. Uveitis in children. Focal Points: Clinical Modules for Ophthalmologists. San Francisco: American Academy of Ophthalmology; 1995.

Goldstein DA, Tessler HH. Complications of uveitis and their management. In: Tasman W et al (Eds). Duane's Clinical Ophthalmology (CD-ROM). Baltimore: Lippincott Williams & Wilkins; 2004.

Herndon L. Glaucoma, uveitic, 2006. [Online]. Available from www.emedicine. com.

Kass MA, Wilensky JT, Ruderman JM. Chronic uveitis and glaucoma. J Glaucoma. 1994;3:84-91.

Moorthy RS, Mermoud A, Baerveldt G, et al. Glaucoma associated with uveitis. Surv Ophthalmol. 1997;41:361-94.

Nussenblatt RB, Whitcup SM, Palestine AG. Uveitis fundamentals and clinical practice, 2nd edition. St Louis: Mosby; 1996.

Samples JR. Management of glaucoma secondary to uveitis. Focal Points: Clinical Modules for Ophthalmologists. San Francisco: American Academy of Ophthalmology; 1995.

Shields MB. Glaucoma associated with ocular inflammation. Textbook of Glaucoma, 4th edition. Baltimore: Lippincott Williams & Wilkins; 1998. pp. 308-22.

Weinreb RN. Management of uveitis and glaucoma. J Glaucoma. 1994;3: 174-6.

Glaucoma Associated with Ocular Trauma (365.65)

DIAGNOSIS

Definition

Ocular trauma is a broad topic. Trauma to the eye may be caused by contusion (blunt), penetrating or chemical injury. During the acute phase of any injury, intraocular pressure (IOP) may be elevated. Severely injured eyes may also develop chronic elevation of IOP. The management of elevated IOP in these situations is only one aspect of the overall management of the severely traumatized eye.

For the purposes of this book, the following discussion is limited to the *late-onset glaucoma* that follows a contusion injury and is associated with anterior-chamber angle recession.

Synonyms

None

Symptoms

Glaucoma associated with the late effects of a contusion injury presents as a chronic open-angle glaucoma, and patients are often asymptomatic (*see* Glaucoma, primary open-angle and normal-tension).

History of trauma: patients will usually recall an episode of blunt trauma to the eye; the trauma may have occurred many years before the detection of the glaucoma; in these cases, or when the trauma occurred in childhood, the patient may not remember.

Loss of vision: in severe cases or in cases diagnosed late in the course of the disease, the patient may become aware of a loss of visual field or central vision in the involved eye.

Signs

Elevated IOP: Intraocular pressure is typically moderately elevated, but very high pressures may also be found; most blunt injuries are unilateral, so the late glaucoma typically involves one eye; in some patients (e.g. boxers, abused spouses), bilateral trauma is more common; the IOP elevation may occur any time after the trauma, even more than 20 years later.

Asymmetry of anterior-chamber depth: the anterior chamber on the involved side may appear appreciably deeper than that of the uninvolved eye.

Optic disk cupping and visual field loss: as with any chronic glaucoma, cupping and visual field loss are found; because the disease is usually unilateral and asymptomatic, glaucomatous damage is often far advanced at diagnosis.

Gonioscopic findings: the gonioscopic appearance of the angle recession is characteristic; the ciliary body band is abnormally wide and is irregular in width (*see* Fig. 1); the iris root appears displaced posteriorly; there are often fine, gray or white linear scars in the trabecular meshwork and face of the ciliary body; there is often heavy pigment.

Differential Diagnosis

The differential diagnosis includes other forms of chronic glaucoma without signs of active inflammation:
- Primary open-angle glaucoma
- Pigmentary glaucoma
- Pseudoexfoliative glaucoma
- Chronic angle-closure glaucoma should also be considered.

Cause

When the eye is struck, aqueous is forcefully displaced toward the peripheral portion of the anterior chamber. If the force is sufficient, the trabecular meshwork and face of the ciliary body may be torn. Degenerative changes occur that eventually interfere with aqueous outflow.

Epidemiology

Ocular trauma is primarily a disease of young men; most cases of angle-recession glaucoma therefore occur in men. Populations at high risk include athletes in contact and racquet sports, abused spouses, and people living in areas where crime and violence are common. Not all cases of angle recession associated with contusion injury result in glaucoma. It is estimated that delayed-onset glaucoma occurs in only 5–20% of cases. Some evidence indicates that the fellow, uninjured eye is at greater risk for the development of primary open-angle glaucoma, suggesting that the eyes that develop angle-recession glaucoma are prone to IOP elevation.

Classification

Glaucoma associated with ocular trauma is classified by the nature of the trauma: contusion injuries, penetrating trauma, chemical injury, radiant energy.

Diagnosis continued on p. 198

TREATMENT

Diet and Lifestyle

High-risk populations should take steps to prevent ocular trauma. Athletes, particularly children and amateurs, should wear proper eye protection. Industrial workers, construction workers, and "do-it-yourselfers" who use power tools should also wear eye protection.

Pharmacologic Treatment

- Angle-recession glaucoma is treated pharmacologically similar to primary open-angle glaucoma (*see* Glaucoma, primary open-angle and normal-tension).
- In angle-recession glaucoma, outflow through the trabecular meshwork is limited. This uveal-scleral outflow plays a larger role in IOP control. Miotics decrease uveal-scleral outflow and thus are less useful.

Treatment Aims
To control IOP and preserve visual function.

Prognosis
In cases detected early or in cases with incomplete angle recessions, control of the glaucoma is often possible with treatment. In more advanced cases or in cases with 360° of angle recession, the prognosis for preservation of vision is often poor.

Follow-up and Management
Patients should be followed with regular, frequent optic disk and visual field evaluations as in any chronic glaucoma.

Treatment continued on p. 199

Glaucoma Associated with Ocular Trauma (365.65)

DIAGNOSIS—cont'd

Associated Features

Hyphema is often seen during the acute phase after blunt injury. Almost all patients with traumatic hyphema will have a detectable angle recession, but most of these do not develop glaucoma. Other signs of blunt trauma may be seen, including cataract, subluxed lens, iris sphincter tears, iridodialysis, cyclodialysis, and retinal tears or detachment. Blunt trauma resulting in orbital fractures is often associated with ocular trauma.

Pathology

The inner part of the pars plicata and the iris root are displaced posteriorly. Scar tissue is seen in the trabecular meshwork and on the anterior face of the ciliary body. There may be endothelial proliferation of the angle with production of abnormal Descemet's membrane.

Pearls and Considerations

- May occur early (acute glaucoma) or late (chronic glaucoma)
- Acute glaucoma may occur with or without a hyphema present
- Chronic glaucoma may result from a variety of processes, including angle recession, peripheral anterior synechiae (PAS), and posterior synechiae.

Referral Information

- Refer to glaucoma specialist for surgery as appropriate
- Refer to appropriate subspecialist for any other associated trauma.

TREATMENT—cont'd

Nonpharmacologic Treatment

Laser trabeculoplasty: the results are poor for angle-recession glaucoma, so it is not recommended. There have been reports of postprocedural IOP spikes.

Filtering surgery: many patients with severe disease and extensive angle recession are unresponsive to medical or laser treatment, making filtering surgery necessary.

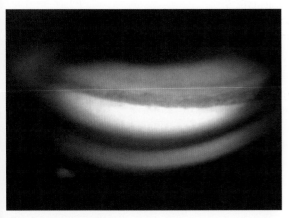

Fig. 1: Gonioscopic photograph of traumatic angle recession showing abnormally and irregularly widened ciliary body.

GENERAL REFERENCES

Berke SJ. Post-traumatic glaucoma. In: Yanoff M, Duker JS (Eds). Ophthalmology. St Louis: Elsevier; 2006.

Goldberg I. Argon laser trabeculoplasty and the open-angle glaucomas. Aust N Z J Ophthalmol. 1985;13(3):243-8.

Herschler J. Trabecular damage due to blunt anterior segment injury and its relationship to traumatic glaucoma. Ophthalmology. 1977;83:239-48.

Kaufman JH, Tolpin DW. Glaucoma after traumatic angle recession: a ten-year prospective study. Am J Ophthalmol. 1974; 78:648-54.

Mermoud A, Heuer DK. Glaucoma associated with trauma. In: Ritch R, Shields MB, Krupin T (Eds). The Glaucomas, 2nd edition. St Louis: Mosby; 1996. pp. 1259-75.

Robin AL, Pollack IP. Argon laser trabeculoplasty in secondary forms of open-angle glaucoma. Arch Ophthalmol. 1983; 101(3):382-4.

Salmon JF, Mermoud A, Levy A, et al. The detection of post-traumatic angle recession by gonioscopy in a population-based glaucoma survey. Ophthalmology. 1994;101:1844-50.

Tesluk GC, Spaeth GL. The occurrence of primary open-angle glaucoma in the fellow eye of patients with unilateral angle-cleavage glaucoma. Ophthalmology. 1985; 92:904-11.

Glaucoma Associated with Other Anterior-Segment Anomalies (365.43)

DIAGNOSIS

Definition

Elevated intraocular pressure (IOP) and optic neuropathy secondary to deformation of the anterior segment.

Synonyms

None

Symptoms

Loss of vision: patients present in infancy with congenital corneal opacity and usually cataract; loss of vision is usually profound; patients with congenital glaucoma may have epiphora, photophobia and blepharospasm.

Signs

Central corneal opacity: patients are born with a dense central corneal opacity in both eyes associated with stromal thinning and absence of Descemet's membrane and corneal endothelium centrally *(Peters anomaly)*.

Congenital cataract: the lens is often opacified, but may be clear in mild cases.

Glaucoma: in severe cases, glaucoma is often present at birth with associated buphthalmos; in milder cases, glaucoma may not develop until later in childhood (*see* Fig. 1).

Investigations

Examination under anesthesia: as in congenital glaucoma, examination under anesthesia is usually necessary.

B-scan ultrasonography: because the fundus usually cannot be seen, B-scan ultrasonography is required to evaluate the posterior segment of the eye.

Electroretinography: may be indicated if there are concerns about the function of the retina.

Pearls and Considerations

- Other anterior-chamber anomalies that may result in glaucoma include aniridia and Peters anomaly
- Often, Axenfeld and Rieger anomalies are grouped together under the term *Axenfeld-Rieger syndrome*
- When Axenfeld anomaly is associated with glaucoma, it is called *Axenfeld syndrome.*

Referral Information

- Refer to pediatrician to rule out further systemic anomalies
- Refer for glaucoma surgery as appropriate.

Differential Diagnosis

- Congenital glaucoma
- Birth trauma
- Mucopolysaccharidoses
- Congenital hereditary corneal dystrophy
- Posterior keratoconus
- Intrauterine infections
- Congenital corneal leukoma.

Cause

The cause is unknown. Most cases are spontaneous, although some familial cases with either autosomal recessive or autosomal dominant patterns of inheritance have been reported.

Classification

Type I: not associated with keratolenticular contact or cataract; most often unilateral
Type II: associated with keratolenticular contact or cataract; most often bilateral.

Associated Features

Krause-Kivlin syndrome: systemic association of Peters anomaly with short stature, facial dysmorphism, developmental delay, and delayed skeletal maturation; autosomal recessive inheritance.
Peters-plus syndrome: Peters anomaly with syndactyly, genitourinary anomalies, brachycephaly, central nervous system anomalies, cardiac disease, or deafness; uncertain inheritance pattern.
Fetal alcohol syndrome: association with Peters anomaly.
PAX-6 mutations: found in some Peters anomaly patients.

Pathology

Descemet's membrane and corneal endothelium are absent centrally. The overlying stroma is thinned and opaque. There may be iris adhesions to the borders of the corneal defect. The lens epithelium and capsule are deficient at the anterior pole, and the lens may be adherent to the cornea. The lens often has a characteristic "top hat" shape.

TREATMENT

Diet and Lifestyle

No special precautions are necessary.

Pharmacologic Treatment

Most children with Peters anomaly are rather severely affected and require surgical treatment. Older children with a chronic glaucoma may be treated pharmacologically, as for any patient with chronic glaucoma.

Nonpharmacologic Treatment

Depending on the severity of the corneal opacity, lenticular involvement and glaucoma, children may require keratoplasty, cataract surgery and filtering surgery. In some children with glaucoma without keratolenticular contact, trabeculotomy may be effective. Otherwise, filtering surgery, a tube-shunt device or cyclodestructive procedures may be necessary.

Treatment Aims

- To restore vision by removing any corneal or lenticular opacities
- In treating the glaucoma, to control IOP and preserve visual function.

Prognosis

The prognosis depends on the severity of the anomaly. In mild to moderate cases, prognosis may be quite good. In more severely affected children, marked visual disability is common.

Follow-up and Management

- Children should be followed regularly, as in patients with congenital glaucoma (*see* Glaucoma, congenital).
- Special education and programs for blind children should be recommended.

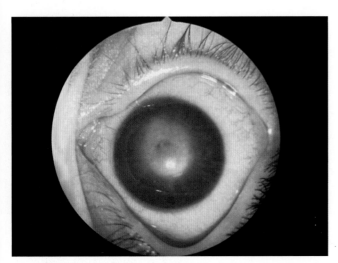

Fig. 1: Glaucoma associated with anterior-segment anomalies (Peters anomaly).

GENERAL REFERENCES

Hanson IM, Fletcher JM, Jordan T, et al. Mutations at the PAX 6 locus are found in heterogeneous anterior segment malformations including Peters' anomaly. Nat Genet. 1994;6:168-73.

Heon E, Barsoum-Homsy M, Cevrette L, et al. Peters' anomaly, the spectrum of associated ocular malformations. Ophthalmic Pediatr Genet. 1992; 13:137-43.

Mayer UM. Peters' anomaly and combination with other malformations. Ophthalmic Pediatr Genet. 1992; 13:131-5.

Miller MT, Epstein RJ, Sugar J, et al. Anterior segment anomalies associated with the fetal alcohol syndrome. J Pediatr Ophthalmol Strabismus. 1984;21:8-18.

Mirzayans F, Pearce WG, MacDonald IM, et al. Mutation of the PAX 6 gene in patients with autosomal dominant keratitis. Am J Hum Genet. 1995;57: 539-48.

Traboulsi EL, Maumenee IH. Peters' anomaly and associated congenital malformations. Arch Ophthalmol. 1992; 110: 1739-42.

Waring GO, Rodrigues MM, Laibson PR. Anterior chamber cleavage syndrome: a stepladder classification. Surv Ophthalmol. 1975;20:3-27.

Glaucoma Associated with Scleritis (365.62) and Episcleritis (379.0)

DIAGNOSIS

Definition

Elevated intraocular pressure (IOP) and optic neuropathy secondary to inflammation of the sclera or episclera

Synonyms

None

Symptoms

Pain: prominent symptom of scleral and episcleral inflammations; may vary from mild to moderate discomfort in episcleritis to severe in scleritis; the pain associated with scleritis is among the most severe of all ocular conditions.

Loss of vision: unusual in episcleritis; scleritis, particularly the necrotizing and posterior varieties, may be associated with profound vision loss; in patients who develop a secondary glaucoma, cupping and visual field loss may also produce loss of vision.

Signs

Hyperemia: marked dilation of the episcleral and conjunctival vessels is a prominent feature; episcleritis is characterized by a localized patch of hyperemia either nasally or temporally; scleritis is characterized by a diffuse, generalized hyperemia.

Tenderness: marked tenderness of the globe on palpation is a common sign.

Scleromalacia: recurrent or long-standing scleritis may produce thinning and atrophy of the sclera, allowing the underlying uvea to become visible as blue or slate-gray patches on the surface of the eye.

Elevated IOP: most patients with scleritis do not develop glaucoma; those who do, however, often have marked elevation of IOP.

Investigations

Rheumatologic evaluation: patients with scleritis often have an underlying connective tissue or autoimmune disease; a complete medical and rheumatologic evaluation is indicated.

Complications

- *Uveitis*: most patients with scleritis do not have clinical evidence of an anterior-chamber reaction; in some patients, an iridocyclitis may develop.
- *Keratitis*: stromal or sclerosis keratitis has been reported; in some cases, corneal vascularization may develop.
- Cataract.

Classification

Episcleritis: simple (379.01), nodular (379.02).

Scleritis: anterior diffuse (379.03), anterior nodular (379.03), anterior necrotizing with inflammation (379.03), anterior necrotizing without inflammation (scleromalacia perforans, 379.04), posterior (379.07).

Differential Diagnosis

Other glaucomas associated with inflammation and hyperemia (e.g. uveitic glaucoma, elevated episcleral venous pressure)

Cause

Episcleral and scleral inflammation may produce glaucoma by several different mechanisms.

Open-angle Glaucoma

- Associated with inflammation (limbal scleritis with possible involvement of trabecular meshwork, Schlemm's canal, or aqueous collector channels; uveitis, glaucoma associated with episclera vessel vasculitis)
- Elevated episcleral venous pressure
- Steroid-induced glaucoma
- Pre-existing open-angle glaucoma.

Angle-closure Glaucoma

- Acute pupillary block may occur in susceptible eyes because of pain.
- Nonpupillary block caused by edema and forward rotation of the ciliary body (sometimes with choroidal effusion).

Immunology

Scleritis is thought to represent an autoimmune reaction in which antibodies to other antigens (e.g. viruses, endogenous connective tissue) cross-react with scleral antigens. Many patients will have serum antibodies (e.g. rheumatoid factor, antinuclear antibody) that suggest immunologic abnormalities.

Pathology

Marked scleral edema and inflammation are present. The inflammation may be either granulomatous or nongranulomatous, depending on the underlying cause. In granulomatous types, marked areas of scleral thickening may develop. In other types, the sclera may become quite thin. In severe cases or in the necrotizing variety, areas of scleral necrosis may be seen.

Diagnosis continued on p. 204

TREATMENT

Diet and Lifestyle

No special precautions are necessary.

Pharmacologic Treatment

Anti-inflammatory Drugs

Episcleritis usually responds to topical steroids. Scleritis is often treated with systemic nonsteroidal anti-inflammatory drugs (e.g. indomethacin, ibuprofen). In some cases, systemic steroids may be necessary. Topical steroids may be useful, but there is a risk of scleral melting and perforation.

Immunosuppressives

In severe cases of scleritis, immunosuppressive agents (e.g. methotrexate, cyclosporine) may be necessary to suppress the inflammatory response.

For the Underlying Systemic Disease

If an underlying systemic disease can be identified, appropriate treatment may be very beneficial in resolving the scleral inflammation.

For Glaucoma

Aqueous suppressants are the drugs of choice. As in any inflammatory glaucoma, miotics and prostaglandin analogs should be avoided.

Treatment Aims

To suppress the inflammatory response, which often resolves the glaucoma.

Other Treatments

Ciliary body ablation: in severe, recalcitrant cases, laser cyclophotocoagulation may prove useful in lowering IOP.

Prognosis

The prognosis depends on the ease with which the inflammation can be controlled; if the scleritis can be adequately treated, the glaucoma can usually be well-managed.

Follow-up and Management

Patients who develop a chronic glaucoma should be followed with regular optic disk and visual field evaluations. Patients who have an underlying systemic disease or who require systemic treatment with anti-inflammatories or immunosuppressives should be followed in conjunction with a primary care physician.

Treatment continued on p. 205

Glaucoma Associated with Scleritis (365.62) and Episcleritis (379.0)

DIAGNOSIS—cont'd

Associated Features

Underlying or systemic diseases associated with scleritis include rheumatoid arthritis, relapsing polychondritis, systemic lupus erythematosus, polyarteritis nodosa, polymyalgia rheumatica, giant cell arteritis, ankylosing spondylitis, Wegener's granulomatosis, ulcerative colitis, Crohn disease, Behçet disease, herpes zoster, herpes simplex, tuberculosis, syphilis, Raynaud disease, gout, sarcoidosis, acne rosacea and psoriasis.

Pearls and Considerations

Patients treated with topical or systemic steroids must be monitored for further elevation in IOP as a side effect of this therapy.

Referral Information

- Refer to rheumatologist in all cases of scleritis to determine underlying systemic cause
- Refer to glaucoma specialist for ongoing management of IOP (surgical or pharmacologic as deemed appropriate).

TREATMENT—cont'd

Nonpharmacologic Treatment

Laser iridectomy: in the occasional patient who develops pupillary-block glaucoma in association with scleritis or episcleritis, laser iridectomy should be performed.

Filtering surgery: because of the scleral inflammation, trabeculectomy often fails. The use of mitomycin may be associated with additional scleral thinning and necrosis. In patients with scleritis-associated glaucoma who require filtration, the use of an aqueous tube-shunt device may be the safest option.

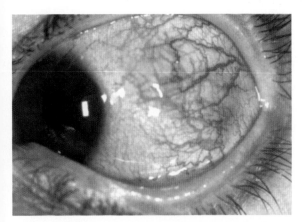

Fig. 1: Scleritis with secondary glaucomas showing marked deep and superficial hyperemia.

GENERAL REFERENCES

De la Maza MS, Foster CS, Jabbur NS. Scleritis associated with rheumatoid arthritis and with other systemic immune-mediated diseases. Ophthalmology. 1994; 101:1281-8.

De la Maza MS, Jabbur NS, Foster CS. An analysis of therapeutic decision for scleritis. Ophthalmology. 1993;100:1372-76.

De la Maza MS, Jabbur NS, Foster CS. Severity of scleritis and episcleritis, Ophthalmology. 1994;101:389-96.

Dubord PJ, Chalmers A. Scleritis and episcleritis: diagnosis and management. Focal Points: Clinical Modules for Ophthalmologists. San Francisco: American Academy of Ophthalmology; 1995.

Legmann A, Foster CS. Noninfectious necrotizing scleritis. Int Ophthalmol Clin. 1996;36:73-80.

Wilhelmus KR, Grierson I, Watson PG. Histopathologic and clinical associations of scleritis and glaucoma. Am J Ophthalmol. 1981;91:697-705.

Glaucoma, Congenital (365.14)

DIAGNOSIS

Definition

Elevated intraocular pressure (IOP) and optic neuropathy present from birth secondary to improper development of the aqueous outflow system.

Synonyms

None

Symptoms

Epiphora, blepharospasm, photophobia: infants with congenital glaucoma behave as if their eyes are painful and irritated; tearing is a frequent early symptom; blepharospasm, especially in brightly lit environments, is also common.

Enlargement of the eye: parents may observe that one or both of their infant's eyes are unusually large and prominent or that the cornea is not clear (*see* Fig. 1).

Decreased vision: infants and children may behave as if they cannot see.

Signs

Enlargement of the cornea: characteristic of congenital glaucoma; the normal newborn cornea should be less than 10.5 mm in diameter and less than 12 mm at 1 year; any corneal diameter larger than this is abnormal and may indicate glaucoma.

Enlargement of the globe: in addition to the cornea, an infant's entire eye enlarges in response to elevated IOP; in neglected or unresponsive cases, the eye may become grossly enlarged (a condition called *buphthalmos*); the abnormal enlargement of the eye is also often associated with high degrees of myopia.

Elevated intraocular pressure: intraocular pressure measurement in an infant or young child usually requires sedation or anesthesia but will normally be found to be less than 24 mm Hg; pressures greater than 24 mm Hg are unusual in normal infants and children.

Corneal edema: clouding of the cornea from stromal and epithelial edema is common in congenital glaucoma; slit-lamp examination may reveal characteristic vertical or concentric breaks in Descemet's membrane called *Haab's striae*.

Abnormal iris insertion: on gonioscopy, the iris may appear to be inserted high on the trabecular meshwork; the iris insertion may have a scalloped appearance; the trabecular meshwork appears unusually thick and seems to be covered by a membrane; in many cases of congenital glaucoma, however, the appearance of the angle cannot be distinguished from that of a normal newborn.

Cupping of the optic disk: prominent feature of all glaucomas; in congenital glaucoma, the cupping is usually concentric and often reversible if IOP is promptly brought under control.

Differential Diagnosis

- Congenital and acquired abnormalities associated with infantile glaucoma (*see* Classification section)
- Other causes of corneal clouding or enlargement (e.g. megalocornea, polysaccharidoses, neonatal infections, hereditary endothelial dystrophy, obstetric trauma)
- Other causes of epiphora or photophobia (e.g. nasolacrimal obstruction, conjunctivitis, trauma)
- Congenital optic nerve anomalies.

Cause

The disease is believed to have a genetic basis. Although most cases are sporadic, familial cases are common, usually showing an autosomal recessive inheritance pattern.

Epidemiology

Congenital glaucoma is uncommon, estimated to occur in about 1:10,000 live births. It is a significant cause of blindness in children, estimated to account for ~10% of patients in institutions for the blind. Approximately two thirds of affected patients are male.

Classification

- Isolated congenital glaucoma
- *Glaucomas associated with other congenital abnormalities*: Aniridia, Sturge-Weber syndrome, neurofibromatosis, Marfan syndrome, Pierre Robin syndrome, homocystinuria, goniodysgenesis, Lowe syndrome, microcornea, microspherophakia, rubella, chromosomal abnormalities (including trisomy 21), broad thumb syndrome, persistent hypoplastic vitreous.
- *Acquired glaucoma in infants*: Retinopathy of prematurity, tumors (retinoblastoma, juvenile xanthogranuloma), intrauterine and neonatal infections and inflammations (especially rubella), trauma.

Pathology

The iris, ciliary body and anterior-chamber angle have the appearance of arrested development, resembling that of a fetus of 6–8 months of gestation rather than that of a normal newborn. The iris and ciliary body are anteriorly placed and overlap the posterior portion of the trabecular meshwork.

Most cases of primary congenital glaucoma occur sporadically. Most inherited cases show a recessive pattern. Two major loci of recessively inherited primary congenital glaucoma (GLC-3A and GLC-3B) have been identified.

Diagnosis continued on p. 208

TREATMENT

Diet and Lifestyle

No special precautions are necessary.

Pharmacologic Treatment

Medical treatment is generally ineffective, and surgery is the primary treatment of choice.

Nonpharmacologic Treatment

Goniotomy: performed by passing a knife through clear cornea, across the anterior chamber, and into the angle; this is done with a gonioscope lens.

Treatment Aims

To preserve vision and control IOP

Other Treatments

In severe cases diagnosed later in childhood or in patients in whom goniotomy or trabeculotomy has failed, filtering surgery may be attempted using (1) antifibrotics such as 5-fluorouracil or mitomycin-C; (2) aqueous shunt devices or; (3) ciliodestructive procedures. Treatment for amblyopia is extremely important in preserving vision after definitive surgery has been performed.

Prognosis

The prognosis is generally good in patients in whom the diagnosis has been prompt and goniotomy or trabeculotomy has achieved good results. In cases diagnosed late or in patients resistant to initial treatment, prognosis is poor, and severe vision loss often results.

Follow-up and Management

Patients must be carefully followed at regular intervals for life because corneal decompensation, cataract, and elevated IOP may occur in later years.

Treatment continued on p. 209

Glaucoma, Congenital (365.14)

DIAGNOSIS—cont'd

Investigations

Complete pediatric evaluation: primary congenital glaucoma is an isolated finding in an otherwise-healthy child and is not usually associated with other anomalies; however, many congenital anomalies and syndromes are associated with a congenital glaucoma; therefore, patients should arrange a thorough physical examination by a pediatrician experienced in the evaluation of children with congenital or hereditary abnormalities.

Examination under anesthesia: for infants suspected of having congenital glaucoma: IOP measurement before deep anesthesia, corneal diameter measurement, gonioscopy, axial length measurement, retinoscopy and fundus examination.

Complications

Corneal opacification: in severe or neglected cases, chronic corneal edema may develop with vascularization and permanent opacification of the cornea.

Buphthalmos: gross enlargement of the eye may result; thinning of the sclera may result in anterior staphyloma formation.

Amblyopia: because the disease is often asymmetric, significant anisometropia with amblyopia may result.

Pearls and Considerations

- The disease is bilateral in approximately three fourths of cases
- The classic triad of symptoms in infants with congenital glaucoma is *blepharospasm, photophobia* and *epiphora.*

Referral Information

Refer to pediatric glaucoma specialist immediately for the earliest possible intervention.

TREATMENT—cont'd

Trabeculotomy: performed by making an external incision at the limbus and identifying Schlemm's canal; a small probe is placed into the lumen of Schlemm's canal and rotated into the anterior chamber, thus rupturing the overlying trabecular meshwork; done when no clear view exists through the cornea.

Either surgical procedure may be used to cut through the abnormal trabecular meshwork and allow aqueous access to Schlemm's canal. Both procedures have high success rates, and excellent results are obtained when diagnosis and treatment are not unduly delayed.

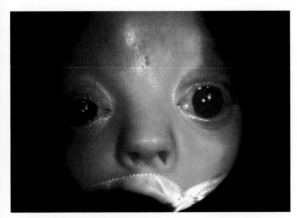

Fig. 1: Congenital glaucoma showing marked ocular enlargement, especially of the left eye.

GENERAL REFERENCES

Anderson DR. Trabeculotomy compared to goniotomy for glaucoma in children. Ophthalmology. 1983;90: 805-6.

Barsoum-Homsy M, Chevrette L. Incidence and prognosis of childhood glaucoma. Ophthalmology. 1986;93: 1323-7.

Beck AD, Lynch MG. Pediatric glaucoma. Focal Points: Clinical Modules for Ophthalmologists. San Francisco: American Academy of Ophthalmology; 1997.

Cibis GW, Urban RC, Dahl AA. (2006). Glaucoma, primary congenital. [Online]. Available from www.emedicine.com.

Glaucoma, Phacolytic (365.51)

DIAGNOSIS

Definition

Elevated intraocular pressure (IOP) resulting from ocular inflammation caused by a hypermature cataract.

Synonyms

None

Symptoms

Pain, hyperemia, loss of vision: phacolytic glaucoma typically presents as an acute inflammatory glaucoma with severe pain, redness and marked loss of vision; the patient usually has a history of a longer, gradual loss of vision for several months or years preceding the acute episode.

Signs

- Greatly elevated IOP
- *Corneal edema*: as in any acute glaucoma, corneal epithelial edema (and sometimes stromal edema) is present
- *Ocular inflammation*: there is a marked inflammatory response with conjunctival and episcleral hyperemia, a heavy anterior-chamber flare and cellular response, and a marked degree of pain and tenderness (*see* Fig. 1).
- *Loss of vision*: vision loss is usually profound, rarely better than being able to distinguish hand motions; phacolytic glaucoma is one of the few conditions in which a patient may present with no light-perception vision and yet recover vision after treatment.
- *Mature cataract*: the cataract is almost always mature or hypermature; pupil appears white; lens may appear shrunken, and there may be wrinkles in the anterior lens capsule; chunklike pieces of white material may appear on the lens capsule or in the aqueous.
- *Deep anterior chamber and open angle*: on gonioscopy, characteristic of phacolytic glaucoma.

Investigations

B-scan ultrasonography: because the fundus cannot be seen through the opaque lens, B-scan ultrasonography is indicated to rule out gross abnormalities of the vitreous or retina (e.g. retinal detachment, malignant melanoma).

Pearls and Considerations

The lens capsule may be ruptured or just abnormally leaky.

Referral Information

Refer for cataract extraction.

Differential Diagnosis

- Other acute lens-induced glaucomas (e.g. phacomorphic or subluxed lens, acute angle-closure glaucoma)
- Other acute inflammatory glaucomas (e.g. uveitis, iris bombé, neovascular glaucoma).

Cause

As the lens proteins degenerate in a maturing cataract, they become soluble and leak into the aqueous through the intact lens capsule. In the aqueous, these proteins provoke an inflammatory response characterized by macrophages that phagocytize the lens proteins and collect in the trabecular meshwork. The macrophages laden with lens protein obstruct the outflow of aqueous.

An alternative theory is that the soluble high-molecular-weight lens protein itself can obstruct the meshwork without being phagocytized by macrophages. The theory is that there is an acute phase with only leakage of proteins and then a more chronic phase with macrophages.

Epidemiology

The condition is the result of neglected cataracts. Two or three decades ago, phacolytic glaucoma was much more common, and it is still seen frequently in medically underserved parts of the world. In modern North America, where cataracts are rarely allowed to develop beyond the early stage without surgery, phacolytic glaucoma has become quite unusual.

Immunology

The lens is an immunologically privileged site. The lens proteins are isolated by the lens capsule and are not recognized by the body's immune system. When lens proteins are released into the ocular fluids, they generally provoke an immunologic response that leads to inflammation. After cataract surgery, in which lens material is not completely removed from the eye, a condition similar to phacolytic glaucoma called *lens-particle glaucoma* may be seen. *Phacoanaphylaxis*—a severe, granulomatous, foreign body-type inflammatory reaction—may occur after trauma to the lens.

Pathology

Fragmentation and globule formation are seen in the lens cortex, consistent with a mature cataract. Macrophages filled with eosinophilic lens material are seen in the aqueous and trabecular meshwork.

TREATMENT

Diet and Lifestyle

No special precautions are necessary.

Pharmacologic Treatment

- Oral or intravenous hyperosmotics should be given to lower IOP acutely before surgery
- Treatment with agents that suppress aqueous formation are also useful acutely to lower IOP
- Topical steroids and atropine should be given to suppress the inflammatory response
- Because phacolytic glaucoma is often an extremely painful condition, analgesics (including narcotics, if necessary) are indicated for relief of pain.

Nonpharmacologic Treatment

Cataract extraction: immediate removal of the lens on an emergency basis is usually the definitive treatment; if the condition has not been neglected for a long time, the resolution of the pain, inflammation, and elevated IOP is usually dramatic.

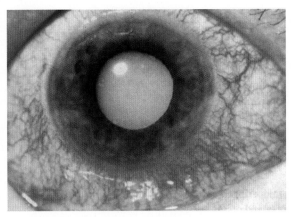

Fig. 1: Phacolytic glaucoma caused by a completely mature cataract with lens material in anterior chamber.

Treatment Aims

To eliminate the lens, which is the source of the protein provoking the inflammatory response.

Prognosis

The prognosis depends on the duration of the disease. In patients treated within 24 hours, the prognosis for resolution of inflammation and restoration of vision is good. With longer duration, the risk of permanent damage to the trabecular meshwork or optic nerve increases.

Follow-up and Management

Once the lens has been removed, the major problem is visual rehabilitation. If an intraocular lens was implanted at the original surgery, visual rehabilitation is usually accomplished with a simple refraction. If not, aphakic correction with spectacles or a contact lens may be required. Secondary lens implantation is also an option. If the IOP is controlled after lens extraction, subsequent problems with glaucoma are unusual.

GENERAL REFERENCES

Lane SS, Kopietz LA, Lindquist TD, et al. Treatment of phacolytic glaucoma with extracapsular cataract extraction. Ophthalmology. 1988;95:749-53.

Layden WE. Cataract and glaucoma. In: Tasman W et al (Eds). Duane's Clinical Ophthalmology (CD-ROM). Baltimore: Lippincott Williams & Wilkins; 2004.

Mavrakanas N, Axmann S, Issum CV, et al. Phacolytic glaucoma: are there 2 forms? J Glaucoma. 2012;21(4):248-9.

Richter CU. Lens-induced open-angle glaucoma. In: Ritch R, Shields MB, Krupin T (Eds). The Glaucomas, 2nd edition. St Louis: Mosby; 1996. pp. 1023-31.

Glaucoma, Pigmentary (365.13)

DIAGNOSIS

Definition

Elevated intraocular pressure (IOP) secondary to accumulation of pigment granules on the inner surface of the anterior chamber.

Synonyms

None

Symptoms

Most patients are asymptomatic and unaware of any ocular problem.

Decreased vision: if the disease is far advanced at diagnosis, the patients may be aware of the loss of vision.

Blurred vision with exercise: some patients will complain of blurred vision after vigorous exercise because of pigment shedding in the anterior chamber.

Signs

Elevated intraocular pressure: usually significantly elevated and often extremely asymmetric.

Optic disk cupping: indistinguishable from other forms of open-angle glaucoma.

Visual field loss: resulting from defects in the nerve fiber bundle, as in other forms of open-angle glaucoma.

Excessive pigment dispersion in the anterior segment: pigment on the endothelial surface of the cornea assumes a triangular or spindle shape (Krukenberg's spindle); pigment dotting on the anterior surface of the iris is seen; gonioscopy shows heavy pigment on the trabecular meshwork as well as pigment on Schwalbe's line and the endothelial surface of the peripheral cornea; the uniform, homogeneous trabecular pigment helps differentiate pigment dispersion from pseudoexfoliation, which has patchy trabecular pigment; pharmacologic dilation of the pupil often produces shedding of a large amount of pigment into the aqueous; pigment may also be seen on the lens zonules and on the equator of the lens (Scheie's line) by performing gonioscopy with a widely dilated pupil.

Iris transillumination and backward bowing: slitlike defects occurring in the midperiphery of the iris pigment epithelium can be seen to transilluminate the anterior chamber and often appear unusually deep; the peripheral iris appears bowed posteriorly.

Myopia: most patients have moderate to high degrees of myopia.

Investigations

B-scan ultrasound biomicroscopy: may reveal areas of iris-zonular or iris-ciliary process contact.

Complications

See Glaucoma, primary open-angle and normal-tension.

Differential Diagnosis

Other conditions in which loss of iris pigment, heavy pigmentation of the trabecular meshwork, and glaucoma may be seen:
- Uveitis
- Exfoliative glaucoma
- Post-traumatic glaucoma
- Ocular melanosis
- Postsurgical glaucomas
- Iris or ciliary body cysts and melanomas.

Cause

The disease is thought to result from abnormal posterior displacement of the peripheral iris. The iris rubs on the lens zonules or ciliary processes. The pigment in the iris pigment epithelium is released into the anterior segment. The trabecular meshwork is phagocytized by the trabecular endothelial cells. The pigment-laden endothelial cells do not function normally, and the IOP becomes elevated.

Epidemiology

- Pigmentary glaucoma is thought to represent 1–2% of all glaucomas in Europe and North America. The disease is most often diagnosed in young adults. Important risk factors include myopia and male gender. White patients are also at risk, and the disease is uncommon in nonwhite populations.
- Twenty five to fifty percent of patients with pigment dispersion syndrome develop pigmentary glaucoma.
- Autosomal dominant inheritance.

Pathology

- Reverse pupillary block mechanism
- Iris pigment epithelial cells and pigment are absent in areas corresponding to the transillumination defects. Trabecular meshwork endothelial cells are heavily laden with phagocytized pigment and show signs of degeneration and disintegration. There is collapse of the trabecular beams, loss of intertrabecular spaces, and collection of cellular debris in the outflow pathway.

Diagnosis continued on p. 214

TREATMENT

Diet and Lifestyle

No special precautions are necessary.

Pharmacologic Treatment

Treatment is similar to that for open-angle glaucoma (*see* Glaucoma, primary open-angle and normal-tension). Because these patients are younger than most glaucoma patients, miotics may produce more side effects of brow ache, ciliary spasm and blurred vision. Use of pilocarpine gel or Ocuserts (Alza Pharmaceuticals, Palo Alto, Calif) is often helpful.

Treatment Aims

To control IOP and prevent loss of visual function

Prognosis

Prognosis with adequate treatment is usually good. Pigment dispersion tends to decrease with age; thus, the need for treatment may diminish as the patient grows older.

Follow-up and Management

Patients should be followed at regular intervals with optic disk evaluation and perimetry as for open-angle glaucoma (*see* Glaucoma, primary open-angle and normal-tension). The frequency of the follow-up will depend on the severity of the disease.

Treatment continued on p. 215

Glaucoma, Pigmentary (365.13)

DIAGNOSIS—cont'd

Classification

Pigment Dispersion Syndrome

Characterized by signs of pigment dispersion without elevated IOP evidence of optic nerve damage.

Active phase: evidence of active pigment shedding, or increasing iris transillumination over time.

Inactive phase: no evidence of active pigment shedding, or decreasing iris transillumination over time.

Pigmentary Glaucoma

Pigmentary glaucoma is characterized by signs of pigment dispersion syndrome with evidence of elevated IOP and signs or risk of optic nerve damage.

Pearls and Considerations

- Pigmentary glaucoma is thought to be an autosomal dominant inherited condition
- Active pigment dispersion usually ceases in these patients at 45–50 years of age
- Pigmentary glaucoma is considered to be an "ocular-only" disease, meaning that it has no associated underlying systemic conditions.

Referral Information

Refer for glaucoma surgery as appropriate.

TREATMENT—cont'd

Nonpharmacologic Treatment

Argon laser trabeculoplasty: often successful in pigmentary glaucoma; these patients are exceptions to the general rule that laser trabeculoplasty is less effective in younger patients.

Selective laser trabeculoplasty: repeatable alternative to argon laser trabeculoplasty.

Laser iridectomy/iridotomy: has been proposed to eliminate the backward bowing of the iris and consequent rubbing of the pigment epithelium on the lens zonules by eliminating the reverse pupillary block and equalizing the pressure in the anterior and posterior chambers; there are no long-term, large studies showing the benefit of this treatment, so it remains experimental at present.

Filtering surgery: indications are the same as for open-angle glaucoma (*see* Glaucoma, primary open-angle and normal-tension).

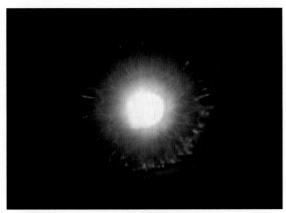

Fig. 1: Pigmentary glaucoma showing typical iris transillumination pattern.

GENERAL REFERENCES

Ball SF. Pigmentary glaucoma. In: Yanoff M, Duker JS (Eds). Ophthalmology. St Louis: Elsevier; 2006.

Campbell DG. Pigmentary glaucoma: mechanism and role for laser iridotomy. J Glaucoma. 1994;3:173-4.

Farrar SM, Shields MB. Current concepts in pigmentary glaucoma. Surv Ophthalmol. 1993;37:233-52.

Sawada A, Yamada H, Yamamoto T. Two Japanese cases of pigmentary glaucoma followed for 15 and 16 years following laser peripheral iridotomy. Jpn J Ophthalmol. 2012;56(2):134-7. Epub 2012 Jan 17.

Wilensky JT. Diagnosis and treatment of pigmentary glaucoma. Focal Points: Clinical Modules for Ophthalmologists. San Francisco: American Academy of Ophthalmology; 1987.

Glaucoma, Primary Open-Angle (365.11) and Normal-Tension (365.12)

DIAGNOSIS

Definition

A chronic and progressive form of optic neuropathy with a characteristic acquired loss of optic nerve fibers.

Synonyms

Common abbreviations include POAG (primary open-angle glaucoma) and NTG (normal-tension glaucoma).

Symptoms

Most patients are asymptomatic and unaware of any vision problem.

Decreased vision: patients with far-advanced disease at diagnosis may complain of decreased vision; some may be aware of defects in their field of vision earlier in the course of the disease; many who do not volunteer symptoms note a variety of visual problems, such as with night driving, fluctuating vision, with reading or close work, and going from brightly lit to dim environments.

Side effects of treatment: a variety of complaints are related to effects of treatment.

Signs

Optic Disk Cupping and Loss of Retinal Nerve Fiber Layer

Glaucoma produces a characteristic optic neuropathy in which there is loss of the neuroretinal rim of the optic disk with associated enlargement of the optic cup, an increase in the area of pallor of the disk, excavation of the neuroretinal rim, and exposure and backward bowing of the lamina cribrosa. This is accompanied by loss of the retinal nerve fiber layer (NFL) (*See* Fig. 1).

Two patterns of damage to the optic nerve and NFL are recognized: *diffuse* (concentric loss of neuroretinal rim, cup enlargement, thinning of retinal NFL) and *focal* (preferential loss of neuroretinal rim and cup enlargement in one area, marked defect in one area of NFL).

Visual Field Loss

The most common form of visual field loss is the *nerve fiber bundle defect*. In its early stages, the defect is characterized by the tendency to respect the horizontal midline, especially in the nasal portion of the visual field. Defects are generally located in the Bjerrum or arcuate area, which extends from 1° or 2° from fixation to 20° from fixation. Defects also tend to have an arcuate shape, being wider circumferentially than radially. The nerve fiber bundle defect is not specific for glaucoma and may be seen in many other optic nerve diseases.

Afferent Pupil Defect

In any glaucoma with asymmetric damage to the optic nerve, an afferent pupil defect may be seen in the eye with the greater degree of cupping.

Elevated Intraocular Pressure

Most patients with open-angle glaucoma have an intraocular pressure (IOP) greater than 21 mm Hg at least some of the time. Different studies have shown that 10–40% of patients with open-angle glaucoma do not have an elevated IOP; such patients are said to have *normal-tension glaucoma*. IOP in many glaucoma patients is highly variable and may show considerable diurnal fluctuation.

Differential Diagnosis

Other Forms of Glaucoma
- Chronic angle-closure glaucoma
- Chronic secondary open-angle glaucomas (e.g. pigmentary, exfoliative, post-traumatic).

Nonglaucomatous Optic Neuropathies
- Compressive lesions of the optic nerve and chiasm
- Arteritic and nonarteritic forms of ischemic optic neuropathy
- Congenital anomalies of the optic nerve
- Degenerative optic neuropathies (e.g. optic disk drusen).

Cause

Unknown, but may be genetic, resulting from degenerative changes in the extracellular matrix of the trabecular meshwork, or from poor circulation that can produce chronic ischemia.

Epidemiology

The prevalence of open-angle glaucoma varies with the population being studied. The Baltimore Eye Survey found a prevalence of ~1.0% in the adult white population and ~4.2% in the adult black population. The prevalence increases greatly with age. Significant risk factors for the presence of open-angle glaucoma include IOP, race, age, family history, optic nerve cupping and central corneal thickness.

Classification

It is thought that open-angle glaucoma represents a final common pathway of several causative factors. Classifications have been proposed on the basis of the presence or absence of these factors, including normal-tension and high-tension glaucoma, vasospastic or nonvasospastic glaucoma, and focal ischemic or senile sclerotic glaucoma.

New additional coding classification based on severity of disease:

365.70 – Glaucoma stage, unspecified
365.71 – Mild stage glaucoma
365.72 – Moderate stage glaucoma
365.73 – Severe stage glaucoma
365.74 – Intermediate stage glaucoma

Diagnosis continued on p. 218

TREATMENT

Diet and Lifestyle

- Recent studies have shown that regular aerobic exercise is associated with a long-term reduction in IOP. Patients in the appropriate physical condition should be encouraged to exercise
- Some evidence indicates that smoking is associated with glaucomatous damage, and patients who smoke should be encouraged to quit.

General Treatment

Target Pressure

Before beginning treatment, the clinician should establish a *target pressure,* a theoretical pressure level at which progression of the glaucomatous damage will no longer occur. There is no way to determine this precisely for each patient, but most clinicians establish an initial target pressure of 30–50% below the pretreatment pressure level. Patients with more advanced disease or who appear to be progressing more rapidly require a lower target pressure. If the target pressure is not achieved with the initial therapy, additional therapeutic modalities are indicated.

Pharmacologic Treatment

Treatment is usually initiated with medication. Some drugs lower IOP by enhancing the outflow of aqueous. Other drugs act by reducing the production of aqueous by the ciliary body. Most clinicians would try two medications, one from each group. If the combination of two drugs does not achieve the target pressure, or the clinician may add a third drug or recommend a laser or surgical procedure. The miotics and prostaglandin analogs enhance aqueous outflow. Epinephrine and dipivefrin appear to have dual action on both outflow and production. The other agents inhibit the formation of aqueous.

Nonpharmacologic Treatment

Argon Laser Trabeculoplasty

Using an argon laser, small-diameter laser burns are placed on the trabecular meshwork. This lowers the IOP in ~70–80% of the patients treated. The mechanism by which laser trabeculoplasty lowers IOP is unknown. Laser trabeculoplasty is indicated when the target pressure cannot be achieved with medication. Although laser trabeculoplasty produces good initial results in most open-angle glaucoma patients, the effect seems to diminish with time; after 5 years, less than half of all patients continue to show good IOP control.

Selective Laser Trabeculoplasty

Similar to argon laser trabeculoplasty (ALT) but is repeatable and results in less damage to the trabecular meshwork compared with ALT.

Treatment Aims

To preserve vision by lowering IOP below the target pressure.

Prognosis

Without treatment, open-angle glaucoma is a progressive disease and will produce some degree of visual disability in most patients. With proper treatment, it is estimated that less than 5% of open-angle glaucoma patients will become blind as a result of their disease.

Follow-up and Management

Open-angle glaucoma is a chronic, progressive, lifelong illness. Regular follow-up with optic-disk evaluation and visual field testing is required. The treatments for glaucoma have a high failure rate over time and often produce adverse effects. Once the target pressure has been achieved and the disease appears stabilized, patients should be seen every 3–6 months, with detailed optic disk evaluation and perimetry every 6–12 months. Patients with more advanced disease will require more frequent follow-up.

Treatment continued on p. 219

DIAGNOSIS—cont'd

Investigations

Imaging of the optic disk and NFL: stereophotography of the optic disk and red-free photography of the NFL should be performed to aid in the detection of glaucomatous damage and to provide a baseline record of the appearance of the optic disk at diagnosis. In some settings, computerized image analysis may be available.

Automated static perimetry: to detect and monitor visual field defects.

Serial tonometry: in some patients, especially those with lower IOP levels, serial tonometry or diurnal tension curves may be useful in defining the role of IOP and the effect of treatment.

Pachymetry: the Ocular Hypertensive Treatment Study showed that central corneal thickness (CCT) is a factor in the progression to primary open-angle glaucoma. Thinner CCT is a significant risk factor for progression. Goldmann's applanation tonometry assumes a CCT of 500 μm. The IOP is underestimated in thin corneas and overestimated in thick corneas.

Neuroimaging; carotid flow studies; systemic, vascular and neurologic evaluation: these types of studies may be indicated in some patients with atypical features (e.g. low IOP levels); younger patients; and patients with rapidly progressive visual loss, greatly asymmetric disease, atypical patterns of visual field loss, or changes in the optic disk.

Pearls and Considerations

- Glaucoma is a leading cause of irreversible blindness, second only to macular degeneration
- The Ocular Hypertension Treatment Study has demonstrated a reduced risk of glaucoma development in ocular hypertension patients who are started on pre-emptive IOP-lowering therapy.

Referral Information

Refer for glaucoma surgery as appropriate.

Pathology

There is degeneration of the collagen of the trabecular beams, degeneration and loss of trabecular endothelial cells, and collapse of the intertrabecular spaces. There is a reduction in the pore density and number of giant vacuoles in the endothelium of Schlemm's canal. The optic nerve shows loss of nerve fibers, capillaries and glial cells. There is thinning and backward bowing of the lamina cribrosa and undermining of the disk margin, producing the characteristic "bean pot" appearance.

TREATMENT—cont'd

Filtering Surgery

Glaucoma filtering surgery creates a fistula from the anterior chamber to the subconjunctival space. This allows aqueous to flow out of the eye, lowering the IOP. Filtering surgery is indicated in patients whose glaucoma is progressive and in those who are at high risk for progression despite the use of medical and laser treatments. In most glaucoma patients who have not had prior surgery, glaucoma filtering surgery has a success rate of ~75–90%. Risk factors for failure of filtering surgery include younger age, black African ancestry, previous ocular surgery, long-term use of glaucoma medications, and intraocular inflammation, membrane growth, or neovascularization. In these patients, filtering surgery may be modified by the use of antifibrotic agents (e.g. 5-fluorouracil, mitomycin-C) or an aqueous tube-shunt device (e.g. Molteno tube).

Complications

Blindness: the major complication of neglected open-angle glaucoma.

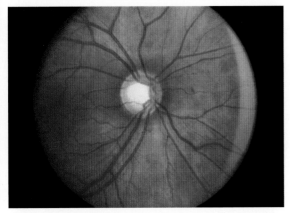

Fig. 1: Primary open-angle glaucoma showing typical glaucomatous cupping of the optic nerve.

GENERAL REFERENCES

Bell JA, Noecker RJ. (2006). Primary open angle glaucoma. [Online]. Available from www.emedicine.com.

Shields MB. Open-angle glaucomas. Textbook of Glaucoma, 4th edition. Baltimore: Lippincott Williams & Wilkins; 1998. pp. 153-76.

Thomas JV, Belcher CD, Simmons RJ. Glaucoma Surgery. St Louis: Mosby; 1992.

Werner EB. Normal-tension glaucoma. In: Ritch R, Shields MB, Krupin T (Eds). The Glaucomas, 2nd edition. St Louis: Mosby; 1996. pp. 769-97.

Wilson MR, Martone JF. Epidemiology of chronic open-angle glaucoma. In: Ritch R, Shields MB, Krupin T (Eds). The Glaucomas, 2nd edition. St Louis: Mosby; 1996. pp. 753-68.

Glaucoma, Pseudoexfoliative (365.52)

DIAGNOSIS

Definition

Elevated intraocular pressure (IOP) and optic neuropathy secondary to flakes of granular material on the inner surface of the anterior chamber

Synonyms

Pseudoexfoliation glaucoma, pseudoexfoliation syndrome

Symptoms

Most patients are asymptomatic and unaware of any problem with their vision.

Loss of vision: if the disease is far advanced when diagnosed, the patient may be aware of the loss of vision; many patients with pseudoexfoliation syndrome also develop cataracts and may present with loss of vision on that basis. *See also* Pseudoexfoliation of the lens (366.11).

Signs

Elevated intraocular pressure: usually significantly elevated and often extremely asymmetric; often very labile in pseudoexfoliative glaucoma.

Optic disk cupping: indistinguishable from other forms of open-angle glaucoma.

Visual field loss: visual field defects of the nerve fiber bundle are seen as in other forms of open-angle glaucoma (*see* Glaucoma, primary open-angle and normal-tension).

Deposit of whitish fibrillar material (Fig. 1): deposition of a flaky, white material on the anterior lens capsule looks as though it is arising from the surface of the lens; typically there is a disk-shaped deposit centrally, a mid-peripheral clear zone, and additional material deposited on the peripheral portion of the lens; the clear zone corresponds to the area of the lens in contact with the pupillary margin of the iris; additional deposits of this whitish material may be seen on the pupillary margin, anterior iris stroma, corneal endothelium and trabecular meshwork.

Pigment dispersion: some degree of pigment dispersion in the anterior segment is usually seen, with corneal endothelial pigment, pigment dotting of the anterior iris stroma, and heavy pigment in the trabecular meshwork (quite common); a pigment line is often seen anterior to Schwalbe's line on gonioscopy (Sampaolesi's line).

Iris transillumination: atrophy and transillumination defects of the peripupillary iris are often seen.

Shallow anterior chamber: the anterior chamber is shallower and the angle is narrower than average in many patients with pseudoexfoliation.

Differential Diagnosis

True capsular delamination: usually the result of trauma, exposure to infrared radiation, uveitis, pigmentary glaucoma or primary amyloidosis.

Cause

The cause of pseudoexfoliation syndrome is unknown. The glaucoma is thought to result from obstruction of aqueous outflow by collection of the exfoliation material in the trabecular meshwork and by the effects of the excess pigment on the trabecular endothelial cells.

Epidemiology

Pseudoexfoliation is common in certain ethnic groups and uncommon in others. The highest prevalences are reported in individuals of Scandinavian ancestry, particularly in Finland and Iceland. Pseudoexfoliation syndrome is often seen as an incidental finding in the absence of glaucoma. The frequency of the disease increases with age and is rare in younger individuals.

About 10% of patients with pseudoexfoliation syndrome develop glaucoma.

Associated Features

Cataract is more common in patients with pseudoexfoliation syndrome than in the general population. Although shallow anterior chambers and narrow angles are more common in pseudoexfoliation syndrome, angle-closure glaucoma is unusual. Iris rigidity and ischemia are common findings and result in poor pupil dilation.

Pathology

There is extensive atrophy and depigmentation of iris pigment epithelial cells. The pseudoexfoliation material is fibrillar and appears to be derived from basement membrane. In addition to being found on the anterior lens capsule, the material is widely deposited on all the structures of the anterior segment. It is also found in association with blood vessels in the iris, ciliary body and conjunctiva. The material has been reported in the skin and even in the liver.

Diagnosis continued on p. 222

TREATMENT

Diet and Lifestyle

No special precautions are necessary.

Pharmacologic Treatment

Pharmacologic treatment is similar to that for open-angle glaucoma (*see* Glaucoma, primary open-angle and normal-tension). Although it is often less effective and labile, poorly controlled IOP often persists.

Treatment Aims

To control IOP and preserve visual function

Prognosis

The prognosis is somewhat worse than with open-angle glaucoma because of the increased difficulty in controlling IOP. The high prevalence of cataract and the increased risk of complications after cataract surgery also contribute to a poorer visual prognosis.

Follow-up and Management

Patients should be followed with optic disk evaluation and perimetry at regular intervals, as in open-angle glaucoma. The frequency of follow-up will depend on the severity of the disease.

Treatment continued on p. 223

Glaucoma, Pseudoexfoliative (365.52)

DIAGNOSIS—cont'd

Investigations

Special investigations other than those for open-angle glaucoma are not required (*see* Glaucoma, primary open-angle and normal-tension).

Complications

Subluxation of the lens: one of the characteristic changes in pseudoexfoliation syndrome is laxity and degeneration of the lens zonules; as a result, dehiscence of the zonules and spontaneous subluxation of the lens may occur.

Difficulties with cataract surgery: the weakness of the zonules increases the risk of capsule rupture and vitreous loss during cataract surgery; the pupil of patients with pseudoexfoliation often dilates poorly, making cataract surgery more difficult.

Pearls and Considerations

- Pseudoexfoliation is rarely seen in patients under 50 years of age
- Often presents unilaterally, but will eventually involve the fellow eye in up to 40% of cases
- May be associated with abdominal aneurysm in 10% of cases.

Referral Information

Refer for glaucoma surgery as appropriate.

TREATMENT—cont'd

Nonpharmacologic Treatment

Argon laser trabeculoplasty: produces results similar to or better than those seen in open-angle glaucoma.

Selective laser trabeculoplasty: indications similar to those for open-angle glaucoma.

Filtering surgery: indications similar to those for open-angle glaucoma.

See Glaucoma, primary open-angle and normal-tension.

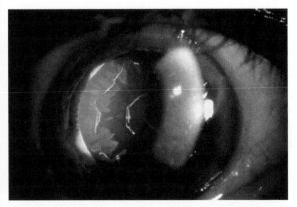

Fig. 1: Pseudoexfoliative glaucoma showing deposition of white material on the anterior lens surface.

GENERAL REFERENCES

Konstas AG, Jay JL, Marshall GE, et al. Prevalence, diagnostic features and response to trabeculectomy in exfoliation glaucoma. Ophthalmology. 1993;100: 619-27.

Lumme P, Laatikainen L. Exfoliation syndrome and cataract extraction. Am J Ophthalmol. 1993;116:51-5.

Pons ME, Eliassi-Rad B. (2006). Glaucoma, pseudoexfoliation. [online]. Available from www.emedicine.com.

Prince AM, Streeten BW, Ritch R, et al. Preclinical diagnosis of pseudoexfoliation syndrome. Arch Ophthalmol. 1987; 105:1076-82.

Ritch R. Exfoliation syndrome: the most common identifiable cause of open-angle glaucoma. J Glaucoma. 1994;3:176-8.

Threlkeld AB, Hertzmark E, Strum RT, et al. Comparative study of the efficacy of argon laser trabeculoplasty for exfoliation and primary open-angle glaucoma. J Glaucoma. 1996;5:311-6.

Glaucoma, Pupillary Block Angle-Closure (365.2)

DIAGNOSIS

Definition

An acute elevation in intraocular pressure (IOP) resulting from the iris pushing forward and decreasing or halting aqueous outflow.

Synonyms

None

Symptoms

Blurred vision: acute (365.22) and *intermittent* (365.21) forms are characterized by rapid onset of blurred vision; *chronic* angle-closure glaucoma (365.23) is usually asymptomatic unless far advanced with severe visual field loss.

Colored haloes: occasionally, a patient may note colored haloes around lights caused by the diffraction effect of the corneal edema.

Pain: *acute* angle-closure glaucoma is a very painful condition; the rapid increase in IOP is accompanied by significant inflammation and ischemia, both of which will produce pain; the pain may be so severe that it completely disables the patient and produces vomiting; *intermittent* angle-closure glaucoma is characterized by episodes of mild to moderate pain that the patient may describe as a "headache" and may not localize to the eye; *chronic* angle-closure glaucoma is typically painless.

Signs

Elevated intraocular pressure: marked elevation of IOP is typically seen in all forms of angle-closure glaucoma; because the disease often presents in only one eye, the pressure in the fellow eye may be normal.

Closed angle: on gonioscopy, the angle will be closed, usually in all quadrants.

Dynamic indentation gonioscopy: should be performed to determine if appositional versus synechial closure; indentation gonioscopy may help break the attack.

Hyperopia: most eyes with angle-closure glaucoma are hyperopic.

Differential Diagnosis

Includes other forms of angle closure not thought to result from primary pupillary block:

- Plateau iris syndrome, ciliary block (malignant) glaucoma
- Angle closure in association with retinopathy of prematurity
- Phacomorphic glaucoma
- Nanophthalmos.

Also includes other forms of acute glaucoma that may or may not be caused by angle closure:

- Neovascular glaucoma
- Uveitis
- Posner-Schlossman syndrome
- Phacolytic glaucoma
- Schwartz-Matsuo syndrome.

Cause

Eyes at risk for developing pupillary-block angle-closure glaucoma are smaller than normal. The area of contact between the pupillary margin and the anterior surface of the lens is greater than normal. This increases the resistance to aqueous flow from the posterior to the anterior chamber at the pupil. If this pupillary block is great enough, the aqueous pressure in the posterior chamber may exceed that in the anterior chamber enough to cause the peripheral iris to bow forward until it comes into contact with the trabecular meshwork, thereby obstructing the outflow of aqueous.

Epidemiology

Most studies of Western populations have shown a prevalence of critically narrow angles of 0.5–1.0%. The prevalence of angle-closure glaucoma is 0.1–0.2%. The majority of patients with angle-closure glaucoma have the chronic forms. The acute form is somewhat less common.

Classification

- Acute angle-closure glaucoma (365.22)
- Intermittent (subacute) angle-closure glaucoma (365.21)
- Primary angle closure without glaucoma damage (365.06)
- Chronic angle-closure glaucoma (365.23).

Diagnosis continued on p. 226

TREATMENT

Diet and Lifestyle

No special precautions are necessary.

Pharmacologic Treatment

Acute Angle-Closure Glaucoma

The first line of treatment is hyperosmotics. If the patient's general health will permit intravenous mannitol or oral isosorbide, either should be given to lower IOP as soon as possible. Aqueous suppressants (e.g. β-adrenergic blockers, α-adrenergic agonists, or carbonic anhydrase inhibitors) are also useful as initial treatment. If the patient is having severe pain, analgesics (including narcotics, if necessary) should be given. Once the IOP begins to decrease, a weak miotic (e.g. 1% or 2% pilocarpine) should be given to constrict the pupil and open the angle, which facilitates laser iridectomy. Pilocarpine should also be placed in the fellow eye at the time of diagnosis to prevent angle closure and to facilitate a prophylactic iridectomy.

Long-Term Treatment (All Forms)

Many patients with angle-closure glaucoma will fail to achieve complete IOP control after laser iridectomy and may require long-term medical treatment. The agents and indications are similar to those for open-angle glaucoma (see Glaucoma, primary open-angle and normal-tension).

Investigations

Gonioscopy of the fellow eye: the fellow eye of a patient with pupillary-block angle-closure glaucoma will almost always have an anatomically narrow angle (see Anatomically narrow angle).

Complications

Permanent corneal edema: severe cases may damage the corneal endothelium, resulting in permanent corneal edema.

Iris atrophy: permanent dilation of the pupil may result in troublesome glare and blurred vision.

Cataract: cataract formation is more common following an episode of acute angle-closure glaucoma.

Optic nerve damage: ischemic optic neuropathy or glaucomatous cupping may result in permanent loss of visual function.

Pearls and Considerations

Angle-closure glaucoma can result in bilateral blindness within 2–3 days of onset.

Referral Information

Refer immediately for peripheral iridotomy.

Treatment Aims

To control IOP and preserve visual function

Other Treatments

Dynamic indentation gonioscopy may occasionally open a closed angle and break an attack quickly. Chamber-deepening procedures, which involve hyperinflating the anterior chamber, may open an angle closed with synechiae and avoid the need for filtering surgery. Rarely, a laser iridectomy cannot be performed, and surgical iridectomy may be necessary.

Prognosis

The prognosis depends on the duration of angle closure. In patients with acute attacks who are treated promptly, the angle usually can be opened, and long-term pharmacologic treatment is not required. In neglected acute attacks or advanced cases of chronic angle-closure glaucoma, long-term pharmacologic treatment or filtering surgery will usually be needed.

Follow-up and Management

Once the iridectomy has been completed and the IOP brought under control, the patient should be followed as any other chronic glaucoma patient, with regular optic disk evaluation and perimetry at intervals determined by the severity of the disease.

Treatment continued on p. 227

Glaucoma, Pupillary Block Angle-Closure (365.2)

DIAGNOSIS—cont'd

Corneal edema: in acute angle-closure glaucoma, the cornea is usually edematous because of the rapid increase in IOP; the appearance of the cornea has been described as "steamy", resembling a bathroom mirror after a hot shower.

Dilated pupil: the pupil in acute angle closure is usually fixed in the mid-dilated position and typically appears vertically oval; the pupil may remain permanently dilated, and areas of iris stromal atrophy may develop; the pupil is usually normal in the intermittent and chronic forms.

Ocular inflammation: a marked degree of inflammation with hyperemia and anterior-chamber flare and cells typically is seen in *acute* angle-closure glaucoma; in *intermittent* angle-closure glaucoma, milder degrees of inflammation may be present; inflammation is not present in *chronic* angle-closure glaucoma.

Glaukomflecken: in severe cases of acute angle-closure glaucoma, small, white, comma-shaped opacities may be seen in the anterior subcapsular region of the lens (*see* Fig. 1).

Optic disk changes: in acute angle-closure glaucoma, the sudden increase in IOP may cause an ischemic optic neuropathy with disk edema and permanent loss of a portion of the visual field; after the acute phase, a flat optic atrophy may be seen; recurrent attacks of intermittent angle-closure and chronic angle-closure glaucoma are generally associated with more typical glaucomatous cupping of the optic disk.

TREATMENT—cont'd

Nonpharmacologic Treatment

Laser iridectomy: the definitive treatment for pupillary block; should be performed as soon as the cornea is clear enough and as the patient's condition permits; there is no need to wait for the IOP to become normal before performing iridectomy; the fellow eye should be treated at the same sitting to prevent angle closure; by placing a hole in the iris, aqueous is allowed to flow freely from the posterior to the anterior chamber, thus eliminating pupillary block.

Filtering surgery: in many cases, iridectomy alone followed by pharmacologic treatment will not control IOP; the trabecular meshwork may be damaged, or the angle may be permanently closed with peripheral anterior synechiae; filtering surgery may then be necessary; the indications are much the same as for open-angle glaucoma (*see* Glaucoma, primary open-angle and normal-tension).

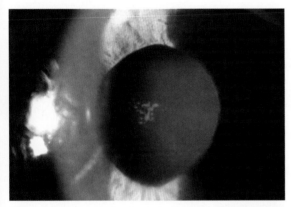

Fig. 1: Acute angle-closure glaucoma showing the partially dilated pupil and white anterior lens opacities known as glaukomflecken.

GENERAL REFERENCES

American Academy of Ophthalmology, Preferred Practice Pattern Committee. Primary angle-closure glaucoma. San Francisco: The Academy; 1996.

Erie JC, Hodge DO, Gray DT. The incidence of primary angle-closure glaucoma in Olmstead County, Minnesota. Arch Ophthalmol. 1997;115:177-81.

Kim YY, Jung HR. Clarifying the nomenclature for primary angle closure glaucoma. Surv Ophthalmol. 1997;42:125-36.

Lowe RF. A history of primary angle closure glaucoma. Surv Ophthalmol. 1995;40:163-70.

Simmons RB, Montenegro MH, Simmons RJ. Primary angle closure glaucoma. In: Tasman W et al. (Eds). Duane's Clinical Ophthalmology (CD-ROM), Baltimore: Lippincott Williams & Wilkins; 2004.

Glaucomatocyclytic Crisis (Posner-Schlossman Syndrome) (364.22)

DIAGNOSIS

Definition

An acute unilateral elevation in intraocular pressure (IOP) of uncertain pathogenesis

Synonym

Posner-Schlossman syndrome

Symptoms

Pain: glaucomatocyclitic crisis is a syndrome characterized by unilateral attacks of marked elevation of IOP and minimal to mild signs of an anterior uveitis; patients usually complain of a mild degree of ocular discomfort and photophobia.

Blurred vision, haloes: patients usually complain of some blurred vision and may describe colored haloes around lights.

Signs

Elevated intraocular pressure: during attacks, IOP typically is greatly elevated; pressures greater than 40 mm Hg and even greater than 60 mm Hg are not unusual.

Hyperemia: typically the eye is white during an attack, but a mild ciliary flush may be seen.

Corneal edema: corneal epithelial bedewing may be present.

Anterior-chamber reaction: flare and cells are characteristically absent during an attack; a rare cell may be seen; keratic precipitates are either absent or few in number, but very fine keratic precipitates may be seen, especially in the peripheral cornea and angle.

Heterochromia: iris stromal atrophy with hypochromia may be seen after recurrent attacks.

Gonioscopic findings: the angle is generally widely open; keratic precipitates may be visible gonioscopically in patients even though none are seen with the slit lamp.

Investigations

Optic disk imaging: the appearance of the optic disk should be well-documented with photography or other imaging techniques to monitor the development of cupping.

Perimetry: as with any glaucoma, perimetry should be carried out at regular intervals to detect the development of visual field loss.

Complications

Persistent elevation of intraocular pressure: recurrent attacks may lead to persistent elevation of IOP and development of open-angle glaucoma.

Optic disk cupping and visual field loss: caused by recurrent attacks or persistent elevation of IOP.

Pearls and Considerations

Recurrences and elevated IOP are common.

Referral Information

Refer unresponsive patients for glaucoma surgery.

Differential Diagnosis

Any anterior uveitis associated with an elevated IOP may resemble glaucomatocyclitic crisis. Inflammatory signs in glaucomatocyclitic crisis are minimal or absent altogether. Typically, the hyperemia and anterior-chamber reaction increase after treatment for the elevated IOP. Most other types of uveitis will have more prominent signs of inflammation. Because of its unilateral nature and heterochromia, glaucomatocyclitic crisis may resemble Fuchs' heterochromic iridocyclitis; however, Fuchs' is characterized by constant signs of anterior-chamber reaction.

Cause

The cause is unknown. The mechanism of the marked elevation in IOP is thought to be either an inflammatory response localized to the trabecular meshwork (trabeculitis) or the result of the release of chemical mediators (e.g. prostaglandins, cytokines) into the aqueous.

Epidemiology

Most cases are spontaneous and occur in young adults 20–50 years of age. A few familial cases have been described.

Pathology

There are no reports of the histopathology of glaucomatocyclitic crisis.

TREATMENT

Diet and Lifestyle

No special precautions are necessary.

Pharmacologic Treatment

Anti-inflammatory Drugs

Moderate doses of topical corticosteroids are usually very effective in controlling the inflammation and shortening the attack. In patients at risk for complications of topical steroids, systemic nonsteroidal anti-inflammatory agents (e.g. indomethacin) have been effective.

Aqueous Suppressants

α-Adrenergic agonists (e.g. apraclonidine, brimonidine) seem to be particularly effective, but β-blockers or carbonic anhydrase inhibitors may also be used. As with any inflammatory glaucoma, miotics and prostaglandin analogs should be avoided.

Nonpharmacologic Treatment

Filtering surgery may be indicated in severe or recalcitrant cases, but this is rare. Laser trabeculoplasty is ineffective.

Treatment Aims

- To control inflammation and IOP to shorten the attack
- There is no known treatment that will prevent attacks.

Prognosis

Glaucomatocyclitic crisis is usually a self-limited disease. Attacks tend to diminish and disappear after age 50 years.

Follow-up and Management

Patients should be advised to seek medical attention at the onset of an attack. Cooperative patients who understand their condition may be given medication to use at the onset of an attack if it is not possible to see a physician promptly. As with any glaucoma, regular follow-up and evaluation of the optic disk and visual field are essential.

GENERAL REFERENCES

Krupin T, Feitl ME, Karalekas D. Glaucoma associated with uveitis. In: Ritch R, Shields MB, Krupin T (Eds). The glaucomas, 2nd edition. St Louis: Mosby; 1996. pp. 1235-7.

Posner A, Schlossman A. Syndrome of unilateral recurrent attacks of glaucoma with cyclitic symptoms. Arch Ophthalmol. 1948;39:517-28.

Shazly TA, Aljajeh M, Latina MA. Posner-Schlossman glaucomatocyclitic crisis. Semin Ophthalmol. 2011;26(4-5):282-4.

Wang RC, Rao NA. Idiopathic and other anterior uveitis syndromes. In: Yanoff M, Duker JS (Eds). Ophthalmology. St Louis: Elsevier; 2006.

Graves Disease (Thyroid Eye Disease, Graves Ophthalmopathy) (242.0)

DIAGNOSIS

Definition

Orbital inflammation or increase in volume of the orbital tissue associated with thyroid disease that may lead to decreased ocular mobility, exposure keratitis, optic neuropathy and exophthalmos.

Synonyms

Thyroid eye disease, Graves ophthalmopathy.

Symptoms

- Exophthalmos
- Diplopia
- Tearing and lacrimation
- Conjunctival hyperemia
- Eyelid retraction
- Spontaneous subluxation of globe.

Signs

- *Upper eyelid retraction*: most reliable sign
- *Eyelid lag*: unreliable sign
- *Swollen eyelids*: finger-like or jelly roll-like edema; diurnal improvement
- Lagophthalmos
- Decreased blinking (or increased if irritated)
- *Exophthalmos*: eye is displaced in the direction of the tethered muscle
- Resistance of the globe to retrodisplacement
- *Restricted motility*: noncomitant strabismus that can be diurnally variable (*see* Fig.1)
- *Head-moving strategy*: makes patients appear to have a visual field defect
- *Inferior rectus muscle infiltration*: develops 60–70% of the time, creating (1) an elevation deficit that simulates a superior rectus muscle paresis; (2) the absence of a Bell's phenomenon, promoting greater corneal exposure; (3) elevated intraocular pressure (IOP) in attempted upgaze because of the inferior tethering of the globe; and (4) an inferiorly displaced globe because of an infiltrated inferior rectus muscle that restrains the globe.
- *Medial rectus muscle infiltration*: occurs 25% of the time and creates an abduction deficit (pseudo-sixth-nerve palsy)
- *Superior rectus muscle infiltration*: occurs in 10% of Graves disease patients and creates a depression deficit simulating inferior rectus palsy
- *Dysthyroid optic neuropathy*: occurs as the result of severe crowding of the orbital apex in 2–5% of patients with Graves' ophthalmopathy; dysthyroid optic neuropathy has an insidious and acute onset; older diabetic men seem to be at greatest risk; there is greater risk in later-onset ophthalmopathy and with a globe that decompresses posteriorly with limitation of motility
- *Red eye*: occurs because of injection over the recti muscles, exposure from exophthalmos, and infrequent blinking; can lead to keratitis, ulcer, and corneal melt
- *Frequency of rectus muscle involvement*: inferior > medial > superior > lateral.

Differential Diagnosis

Idiopathic orbital pseudotumor, lymphoid tumor, sarcoid, amyloidosis, Wegener's syndrome, optic nerve sheath and sphenoid wing meningiomas, carotid-cavernous fistula, orbital cellulitis, orbital cysts, neoplasms, vascular anomalies, eye prominence.

Cause

- Graves ophthalmopathy occurs within 18 months of the onset of hyperthyroidism
- Graves disease is a multisystem disorder of unknown cause characterized by hyperthyroidism, infiltrative ophthalmopathy and infiltrative dermopathy
- Graves disease can occur in isolation without the hyperthyroidism.

Epidemiology

- Genetically preselected population with immunogenetic predisposition; HLA-DR3 and HLA-D8 have been identified as genetic markers
- Ratio of female to male is 3.2:1.0. The mean age of onset for men and women is ~44 years.

Immunology

- T lymphocytes fail to prevent proliferation of randomly mutating B lymphocytes. The B lymphocytes spawn autoantibodies that attack EOM fibers and connective tissue
- Poorly functioning or absent T-suppressor lymphocytes allow influx of cytotoxic T lymphocytes, contributing to further destruction.

Pathology

- The EOMs are infiltrated by lymphocytes, plasma cells and mast cells. Hydrophilic mucopolysaccharides and collagen formation create degenerative changes in the EOMs. Fibroblasts produce hydrophilic glycosaminoglycans that accumulate in the retro-ocular tissues. This contributes to the edema of the orbital connective tissue and EOMs.
- Late findings: fibrosis and fatty infiltration.

230

Diagnosis continued on p. 232

TREATMENT

Diet and Lifestyle

Patients should stop smoking, sleep with head elevated, and apply cold compresses to relieve eyelid edema.

Pharmacologic Treatment

Treatment of the underlying thyroid gland dysfunction will improve symptoms. The development, improvement or worsening of Graves disease is unrelated to the mode of therapy.

- Artificial tear substitutes and ointments
- Steroids: prednisone, 30–120 mg
- Immunosuppressives: cyclosporine.

Treatment Aims

- To protect the cornea
- To monitor and prevent dysthyroid optic neuropathy
- To lessen or eliminate diplopia.

Prognosis

- Remission of the signs of Graves ophthalmopathy is unpredictable
- In Graves disease, eyelid retraction may spontaneously remit in ~50% of patients
- Exophthalmos tends to remain unchanged.
- There is a high incidence of spontaneous remission of diplopia
- Dysthyroid optic neuropathy is unpredictable.

Follow-up and Management

- Monitor for dysthyroid optic neuropathy.
- Routinely observe optic nerve function with the following:
  - Snellen acuity test
  - Threshold visual field test
  - Relative afferent pupillary test
  - Contrast sensitivity test
  - Ophthalmoscopy and fundus photos
  - Motility measurements.

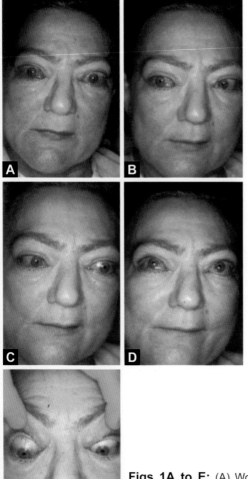

Figs 1A to E: (A) Woman with severe Graves disease and almost complete limitation of bilateral eye movement; (B and C) Restricted right and left gaze; (D and E) Limited upgaze and downgaze. Note the typical injection over the medial and lateral rectus muscles, particularly visible in the right eye.

231

Treatment continued on p. 233

Graves Disease (Thyroid Eye Disease, Graves Ophthalmopathy) (242.0)

DIAGNOSIS—cont'd

Investigations

- Palpebral fissure measurement, corneal evaluation, quantitation of motility and exophthalmos, retrodisplacement, optic nerve function
- *Orbital magnetic resonance imaging (MRI) or computed tomography (CT)*: not every patient with Graves disease requires orbital imaging
- *Extraocular muscles (EOMs)*: EOM enlargement with sparing of tendons (*see* Fig. 2)
- Serum thyroid-stimulating hormone (TSH), calculated free thyronine (T_4) index, thyroid-stimulating immunoglobulins, antithyroid antibodies, serum triiodothyronine (T_3), acetylcholine receptor antibody
- A small percentage of patients fail to demonstrate any laboratory thyroid abnormality
- Ten percent of patients with Graves disease have hypothyroidism or autoimmune thyroiditis
- Associated with myasthenia gravis.

Complications

- Dysthyroid optic neuropathy
- Subluxation of globe.

Pearls and Considerations

Computed tomography scanning is more useful than MRI for viewing the bony landmarks when evaluating Graves disease.

Referral Information

- Refer to endocrinologist for treatment of the underlying disease
- Refer for surgical evaluation if orbital decompression is indicated.

TREATMENT—cont'd

Nonpharmacologic Treatment

Prism, patches, tape, eye exercises

Sequence of Surgical Interventions

- Orbital decompression
- Ocular muscle surgery
- Adjustment of eyelid margin
- Blepharoplasty
- Retrobulbar radiation therapy (up to 2000 cGy).

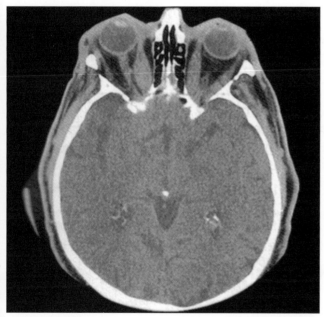

Fig. 2: Magnetic resonance image of orbits in Graves disease demonstrating enlargement of extraocular muscles with sparing of muscle tendons.

GENERAL REFERENCES

Bartalena L, Marcocci C, Pinchera A. Orbital radiotherapy for Graves ophthalmopathy. J Clin Endocrinol Metab. 2004; 89(1):13-4.

Kusuhara T, Nakajima M, Imamura A. Ocular myasthenia gravis associated with euthyroid ophthalmology. Muscle Nerve. 2003;28(6):764-6.

Terris DJ, Levin P. (2003). Orbital decompression for Graves' disease. [Online] Available from www.emedicine.com.

Wiersinga WM, Prummel MF. An evidence-based approach to the treatment of Graves' ophthalmopathy. Endocrinol Metab Clin North Am. 2000;29(2):297-319, vi-vii.

Yeh S, Foroozan R. Orbital apex syndrome. Curr Opin Ophthalmol. 2004;15(6):490-8.

Hypertension, Ocular (365.04)

DIAGNOSIS

Definition

Increased intraocular pressure (IOP) in the absence of any clinical evidence of nerve fiber layer (NFL) damage.

Synonyms

None; typically abbreviated OHT (ocular hypertension)

Symptoms

Ocular hypertension is a condition in which IOP is repeatedly greater than 21 mm Hg, the anterior-chamber angle is open, and the optic disk, retinal NFL, and visual field are normal. Patients are asymptomatic.

Signs

Elevated intraocular pressure: IOP is greater than 21 mm Hg on more than one measurement made at different times.

Investigations

Optic disk and NFL photography or imaging: elevated IOP is often associated with evidence of glaucomatous damage to the optic nerve and NFL. A normal optic disk must be documented to support the diagnosis of OHT.

Perimetry: the visual field must be shown to be normal.

Pachymetry: Goldmann's applanation tonometer was calibrated based on a central corneal thickness (CCT) of 500 μm. The IOP may be underestimated with thinner corneas and overestimated with thicker corneas. The Ocular Hypertension Treatment Study (OHTS), a multicenter clinical trial, showed that OHT patients have thicker-than-average CCT.

Complications

Glaucomatous damage to the optic nerve: elevated IOP is the principal risk factor for the development of glaucoma; patients with OHT have approximately a tenfold greater risk of developing glaucoma than the normal population.

Differential Diagnosis

The differential diagnosis includes other conditions in which elevated IOP may be seen without producing symptoms, including:

- Open-angle glaucoma
- Chronic angle-closure glaucoma
- Certain secondary glaucomas (e.g. pigmentary glaucoma, pseudoexfoliative glaucoma, post-traumatic glaucoma).

Cause

The cause is unknown, but the IOP is believed to be genetically controlled. Because IOP tends to increase with age in most populations, age-related changes in the trabecular meshwork may play a role.

Epidemiology

- Five to ten percent of the adult population have OHT, with the percentage increasing with age. An estimated 1% of these patients per year develop evidence of glaucomatous damage to the optic nerve.
- Significant risk factors for the progression to glaucoma found in the OHTS were CCT, age, pattern standard deviation, cup-to-disk ratio and IOP.
- Race and family history are other well-described risk factors.

234

TREATMENT

Diet and Lifestyle

No special precautions are necessary.

Pharmacologic Treatment

For Lowering Intraocular Pressure (see Glaucoma, Primary Open-Angle and Normal-Tension)

The 5-year OHTS results have cleared some of the controversy concerning treatment of OHT. The study reported a reduction in progression of glaucoma in the treated group. The progression rate in the treated OHT patients was 4.4% versus 9.5% in the untreated group. Of note is the significance of CCT on risk of glaucoma progression. The risk of progression increases to 36% for untreated OHT with CCT less than 555 µm and IOP greater than 25.75.

Nonpharmacologic Treatment

Laser and surgical treatment is generally not indicated in OHT.

Treatment Aims

To reduce or eliminate the risk of developing glaucomatous damage; at present, the best way to achieve this goal is not known.

Prognosis

Approximately 10% of asymptomatic patients with open angles and elevated IOP show evidence of glaucomatous damage to the optic nerve; the others have OHT. Of these, long-term longitudinal studies show a good prognosis, with only 10–20% of OHT patients developing glaucomatous damage over a 10-year period.

Follow-up and Management

Because OHT patients are at risk for glaucoma and because it is impossible to predict which patients will develop damage, all OHT patients should be followed at regular intervals with careful optic disk evaluation and perimetry. Examination once or twice per year is probably adequate, with optic disk imaging and perimetry every 12–18 months.

GENERAL REFERENCES

American Academy of Ophthalmology Glaucoma Panel: Preferred Practice Pattern Guidelines. Primary Open-Angle Glaucoma Suspect. San Francisco, CA: American Academy of Ophthalmology, 2010.

Gordon MO, Beiser JA, Brandt JD, et al. The Ocular Hypertension Treatment Study: baseline factors that predict the onset of primary open-angle glaucoma. Arch Ophthalmol. 2002; 120(6):714-20, 829-30 (discussion).

Kass MA, Heuer DK, Higgenbotham EJ, et al. The Ocular Hypertension Treatment Study: a randomized trial determines that topical ocular hypotensive medication delays or prevents the onset of primary open-angle glaucoma. Arch Ophthalmol. 2002;120(6):701-13, 829-30 (discussion).

Kass MA. The Ocular Hypertension Treatment Study. J Glaucoma. 1994;3: 97-100.

Shields MB. Glaucoma screening. Textbook of Glaucoma, 4th edition. Baltimore: Lippincott Williams & Wilkins; 1998. pp. 137-41.

Shields MB. Intraocular pressure and tonometry. Textbook of Glaucoma, 4th edition. Baltimore: Lippincott Williams & Wilkins; 1998. pp. 46-51.

Hypertensive Retinopathy (362.11)

DIAGNOSIS

Definition

Retinal complications of elevated systemic blood pressure.

Synonyms

None

Symptoms

- Patients are asymptomatic in early stages
- Later stages can have blurry, distorted vision or even significant loss of visual acuity.

Signs

- Focal narrowing and straightening of retinal arterioles (*see* Fig. 1)
- "Nicking of the retinal veins": arteriovenous crossing changes
- Increased light reflex and loss of transparency of blood column
- Arteriolar and venous tortuosity
- Cotton-wool spots
- Dot and blot hemorrhages
- Retinal edema
- Optic nerve edema
- Venous-venous collaterals.

Investigations

- Blood pressure measurement
- Visual acuity testing
- Slit-lamp and dilated fundus examinations
- *Fluorescein angiography*: to look for evidence of impedance to blood flow, local areas of nonperfusion, and leakage from dilated capillaries.

Complications

- Vascular occlusive disease (venous and/or arteriolar)
- Macroaneurysm formation
- Optic neuropathy
- Optic nerve edema
- Blindness.

Pearls and Considerations

The Scheie classification system identifies the following stages of hypertensive retinopathy:

- *Stage 0:* normal
- *Stage 1:* broadening of the light reflex from the arteriole, with minimal or no arteriovenous compression
- *Stage 2:* light reflex changes and crossing changes are more prominent
- *Stage 3:* arterioles have a "copper wire" appearance, with more arteriovenous compression
- *Stage 4:* arterioles have a "silver wire" appearance, and arteriovenous crossing changes are most severe.

Referral Information

Refer to internist for evaluation, management and control of hypertension.

Differential Diagnosis

- Congenital venous tortuosity
- Involutional sclerosis (atherosclerosis associated with aging).

Cause

Acute and/or chronic systemic hypertension.

Epidemiology

Ten to fifteen percent of the adult population have hypertensive retinal changes.

Classification

- Essential hypertensive retinal changes as described in Signs section
- Malignant hypertension (which includes the findings of essential hypertension plus exudative retinal detachment and optic nerve edema).

Associated Features

- Heart failure
- Renal failure
- Stroke
- Peripheral vascular disease.

Pathology

Retinal arterioles develop thickening of their walls as a result of intimal hyalinization, medial hypertrophy and endothelial hypertrophy.

TREATMENT

Diet and Lifestyle

- Lose weight and exercise
- Monitor sodium intake.

Pharmacologic Treatment

Control blood pressure with medication supervised by the patient's primary care physician.

Nonpharmacologic Treatment

No nonpharmacologic treatment is recommended.

Treatment Aims

To normalize systemic blood pressure.

Prognosis

Good

Follow-up and Management

Yearly dilated eye examinations to monitor blood vessel changes.

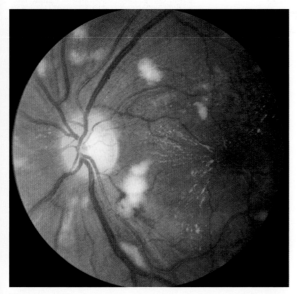

Fig. 1: Left eye from patient with marked hypertension and Grade III hypertensive retinopathy. Note cotton-wool spots (areas of axoplasmic flow backup) and macular star (exudates in Henle's outer plexiform layer of neural retina).

GENERAL REFERENCES

Hayreh SS, Servais GE, Virdi PS, et al. Fundus lesions in malignant hypertension. III. Arterial blood pressure, biochemical, and fundus changes. Ophthalmology. 1986;93:45-59.

Leishman R. The eye in general vascular disease: hypertension and arteriosclerosis. Br J Ophthalmol. 1957;41:641-701.

Murphy RP, Larn LA, Chew EY. Hypertension. Retina, 4th edition. St Louis: Elsevier; 2006.

Hyphema (361.41)

DIAGNOSIS

Definition

Bleeding into the anterior chamber.

Synonyms

None

Symptoms

Most patients present with pain, and children may be somnolent.

Signs

Tearing, photophobia, squinting

Investigations

- Careful history eliciting mechanism of injury
- Visual acuity
- Intraocular pressure with minimal globe manipulation
- Measurement of clot and grading of hyphema
- Funduscopic examination
- Blood studies as indicated (blood cell dyscrasias).

Complications

- *Corneal blood staining*: endothelial decompensation
- Cataract
- *Glaucoma*: from trabecular meshwork blockage
- *Central retinal artery occlusion*: from glaucoma in patient with sickle cell disease, trait, or HbSC.

Differential Diagnosis

Cause

- Most commonly as a result of trauma
- Spontaneous causes include juvenile xanthogranuloma, retinoblastoma, and herpes zoster.

Epidemiology

- Most commonly caused by blunt ocular injury
- Greatest risk for rebleeding is within 72–96 hours
- Highest rate of rebleeding in African Americans, lowest in Scandanavians
- Increased risk in children and individuals on blood thinners.

Pathology

- Shearing rupture of the ciliary muscle after a contusion
- Secondary bleeds result from fibrinolysis and clot retraction from fragile vessels.

Diagnosis continued on p. 240

TREATMENT

Diet and Lifestyle

No special precautions are suggested.

Pharmacologic Treatment

- Sedation as required
- Laxatives during period of increased rebleeding risk
- Cycloplegia (typically atropine)
- Topical steroids (prednisolone acetate 1%, every 2–6 hours)
- Antiemetic as needed
- Antiglaucoma medications (beta-blockers as first line)
- Antifibrinolytic agents.

Treatment Aims

- Resolution of hyphema
- Clearing the cornea
- Preventing glaucoma.

Prognosis

- Most small hyphemas resolve in a few days without any surgical intervention
- Varies depending on size of hyphema, intraocular pressure, and risk of rebleeding.

Follow-up and Management

- Daily evaluations until period of rebleeding has passed
- Long-term follow-up for risk of developing glaucoma secondary to angle recession.

Treatment continued on p. 241

DIAGNOSIS—cont'd

Pearls and Considerations

Hyphema can mask more severe trauma and possible globe compromise.

Commonly Associated Conditions

- Posterior globe rupture with hypotony and total hyphema
- Glaucoma and corneal blood staining
- If severe, macular injury may be associated.

Referral Information

Inpatient hospitalization is required in many cases.

TREATMENT—cont'd

Nonpharmacologic Treatment

- Hospitalization
- Bed rest (head of bed elevated to 30°)
- Daily examinations for first 4 days
- Eye shield
- Surgical evaluation for clot clearing.

GENERAL REFERENCES

Ashaye AO. Traumatic hyphaema: a report of 472 consecutive cases. BMC Ophthalmol. 2008;8:24.

Bagnis A, Lai S, Iester M, Bacino L, et al. Spontaneous hyphaema in a patient on warfarin treatment. Br J Clin Pharmacol. 2008;66(3):414-5. Epub 2008 Jul 15.

Cho J, Jun BK, Lee YJ, et al. Factors associated with the poor final visual outcome after traumatic hyphema. Korean J Ophthalmol. 1998;12(2):122-9.

Shepard J, Williams PB. (2005) Hyphema; [online] Available from www.emedicine.com.

Wilson FM. Traumatic hyphema: pathogenesis and management. Ophthalmology. 1980;687:910-9.

Internuclear Ophthalmoplegia (378.86)

DIAGNOSIS

Definition

A lesion of the medial longitudinal fasciculus (MLF) resulting in paresis of adduction and dissociated nystagmus.

Synonyms

None; abbreviated INO (internuclear ophthalmoplegia).

Symptoms

- Blurred vision
- Double vision (vertical and horizontal)
- Oscillopsia.

Signs

Adduction deficit that varies from the absence of adduction to a mild decrease in the velocity of adduction without any limitation in the extent of movement: a "slowness" of adduction is seen more often than abducting nystagmus of the fellow eye; internuclear ophthalmoplegia is named "right" or "left" by the adduction deficit; the lesion is located on the same side as the adduction deficit; to "flush out" the adduction deficit, the patient must make large-amplitude horizontal saccades or be tested with optokinetic tape.

Abducting nystagmus with an inward drift with an outward corrective saccade that may be hypermetric, hypometric or orthometric: the nystagmus intensity will decrease if the patient fixates with the eye with nystagmus.

Hypertropic eye: on the side of the adduction deficit, representing ocular skew torsion

Convergence failure: suggests that the lesion involves the MLF in the midbrain; this is labeled an "anterior" INO

Intact convergence: implies that the lesion has involved the MLF more caudally in the pons, sparing the medial rectus subnucleus; this is termed a "posterior" INO.

Investigations

- Magnetic resonance imaging (MRI): T2-weighted images, with attention to the brainstem
- Anti-Ach Ab; Tensilon (edrophonium) test: to rule out myasthenia gravis.

Differential Diagnosis

- Inferior-division third-nerve palsy
- Orbital disease
- End-position nystagmus
- Myasthenia gravis, Guillian-Barré syndrome (pseudo-INO)
- Miller-Fisher syndrome (involves oculomotor dysfunction, potentially with INO, ataxia, and diminished or absent reflexes).

Cause

- Unilateral disease (INO) is caused more often by brainstem infarction and observed more frequently in older males. The onset is apoplectic and associated with an ocular skew torsion sign in approximately 50% of cases.
- Bilateral disease (BINO) is likely caused by demyelinating disease, is more common in younger patients, and has an equal gender incidence. It has a more progressive onset.
- Convergence is present in 80% of both INO and BINO patients
- Less common causes include:
  - Arnold-Chiari malformation with associated hydrocephalus and syringobulbia
  - Meningoencephalitis
  - Tuberculous meningitis
  - Paraneoplastic encephalomyelitis
  - Human immunodeficiency virus (HIV)-related cytomegalovirus (CMV) encephalitis
  - Head trauma
  - Drug intoxications
  - Systemic lupus erythematosis
  - Migraine
  - Syphilis
  - Supratentorial arteriovenous malformation
  - Intracranial tumors
  - Nutritional (e.g. Wernicke's encephalopathy, pernicious anemia), degenerative and metabolic disorders.

Pathology

- Damage to MLF
- Explanations for the abducting nystagmus include:
  - Increased convergence tone
  - Disinhibition of the medial rectus muscle on the opposite side of the lesion
  - Interruption of descending internuclear fibers that project to the fourth-nerve nucleus
  - Gaze-evoked nystagmus
  - Adaptation to the contralateral medial rectus muscle weakness.

Diagnosis continued on p. 244

TREATMENT

Diet and Lifestyle

No special precautions are necessary.

Pharmacologic Treatment

- Treatment of multiple sclerosis, if applicable
- Botulinum toxin A injection (botox) into one or more extraocular muscles has shown promise in treatment of diplopia, appearance, and head posture.

Nonpharmacologic Treatment

- Prisms and patches are sometimes helpful
- Strabismus surgery can be considered for symptomatic patients. Recession-resection procedures have been used for this purpose, though a variation of the Jensen transposition procedure combined with ipsilateral lateral rectus recession for surgical correction of INO in patients with large angle exotropia and adduction weakness has recently shown promise for maintaining long-term balance.

Treatment Aims

To diagnose the underlying disease, and to alleviate diplopia and appearance.

Treatment continued on p. 245

Internuclear Ophthalmoplegia (378.86)

DIAGNOSIS—cont'd

Classification

- Variations of INO include binocular internuclear ophthalmoplegia (BINO, *see* Figs 1A to E), "wall-eye" BINO (WEBINO), and the "one-and-a-half" syndrome (1 & 1/2)
- Binocular internuclear ophthalmoplegia is an INO in each eye, i.e. bilateral adduction deficits with bilateral abducting nystagmus (*see* Figs 1A to E)
- "Wall-eye" BINO is a BINO with a manifest exotropia in primary position; the eye opposite the side of the lesion is deviated outward
- One-and-a-half is gaze palsy in one direction and INO in the opposite direction; paramedian pontine reticular formation (PPRF) or cranial nerve (CN) VI nucleus and ipsilateral MLF lesions
- Midbrain lesion (more rostral disease): Cogan's anterior INO convergence is affected because of CN III nuclei involvement.

Pearls and Considerations

- Internuclear ophthalmoplegia can be unilateral or bilateral
- The most common cause of INO (especially bilateral) in young adults is multiple sclerosis, whereas the most common cause of INO in an older patient (and the most common cause overall) is ischemic infarction.

Referral Information

Refer for extensive systemic workup to rule out brain tumors, demyelinating disease, and other systemic etiologies.

TREATMENT—cont'd

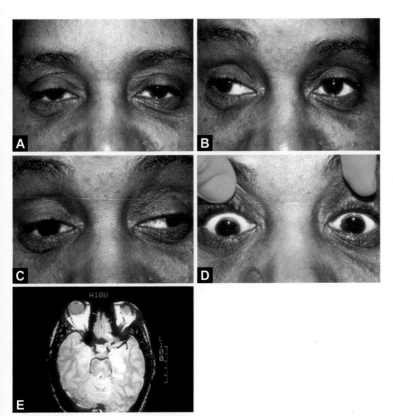

Figs 1A to E: (A) Woman with multiple sclerosis who has binocular internuclear ophthalmoplegia in primary position; (B) In right gaze, she has a left adduction deficit; (C) In left gaze, she has a right adduction deficit. She has both right-eye and left-eye abducting nystagmus; (D) Convergence is defective, suggesting that the lesion is anterior or in the midbrain; (E) Corresponding T2-weighted axial MRI scan through the midbrain with high signal in the medial longitudinal fasciculus.

GENERAL REFERENCES

Frohman S, Galetta R, Fox R. Pearls & oysters: the medial longitudinal fasciculus in ocular motor physiology. Neurology. 2008;70:e57.

Gray M, Forbes RB, Morrow JI. Primary isolated brainstem injury producing internuclear ophthalmoplegia. Br J Neurosurg. 2001;15(5):432-4.

Keane JR. Internuclear ophthalmoplegia: unusual causes in 114 of 410 patients. Arch Neurol. 2005;62(5):714-7.

Leigh RJ, Daroff RB, Troost BT. Supranuclear disorders of eye movements. In: Tasman W et al (Eds). Duane's Clinical Ophthalmology (CD-ROM). Philadelphia: Lippincott Williams & Wilkins; 2004.

Levin A, Arnold A. Neuro-ophthalmology. New York: Thieme Medical Publishers; 2005.

Murthy R, Dawson E, Khan S, et al. Botulinum toxin in the management of internuclear ophthalmoplegia. J Am Assoc Pediatr Ophthalmol Strabismus. 2007;11(5):456-9.

Nathan NR, Donahue SP. Transposition surgery for internuclear ophthalmoplegia. J Am Assoc Pediatr Ophthalmol Strabismus. 2012;16(1):e24.

Iridocyclitis, Acute and Subacute (364.0)

DIAGNOSIS

Definition

Inflammation of the uveal tract.

Synonyms

Iritis, uveitis, pars planitis.

Symptoms

- Pain
- Redness (Fig. 1)
- Photophobia
- Increased lacrimation
- Blurry vision
- Pain, decreased vision, and redness may be minimal in subacute cases.

Signs

Acute

- Ciliary injection of the conjunctiva (hyperemia around the limbus)
- Fine to large keratic precipitates (granulomatous) and fibrin dusting of the corneal endothelium
- Anterior chamber shows many cells, variable flare, and in rare cases, a hypopyon
- Dilated iris vessels and, rarely, a hyphema
- Posterior synechiae (adhesion of the pupillary iris to the lens)
- Iris nodules
- Anterior vitreous cells
- Cystoid macular edema and, rarely, a disk edema
- *Low intraocular pressure*: usually, but may be elevated.

Chronic

Variable conjunctival redness as well as anterior-chamber reaction

Investigations

- *Histories*: onset and duration of symptoms, systems review (especially of arthritic, gastrointestinal, and genitourinary disorders), insect bite, rash, sexual, drug, family back disorders (e.g. ankylosing spondylitis).
- Visual acuity testing
- Slit-lamp examination
- Intraocular pressure
- Dilated fundus examination
- *If uveitis is bilateral, granulomatous or recurrent, then consider workup*: complete blood count, erythrocyte sedimentation rate, antinuclear antibody, rapid plasma reagin, fluorescent treponemal antibody absorption, purified protein derivative (tuberculin) with anergy panel. Obtain a chest radiograph and consider HLA-B27.

Differential Diagnosis

- Rhegmatogenous retinal detachment (pigment cells in the anterior chamber)
- Leukemia
- *Retinoblastoma*: in children
- Intraocular foreign body
- Malignant melanoma
- Juvenile xanthogranuloma.

Cause

- *Idiopathic*: most common
- HLA-B27-positive iridocyclitis
- Juvenile rheumatoid arthritis
- Fuchs' heterochromic iridocyclitis
- Herpes simplex keratouveitis
- Syphilis
- Traumatic, sarcoid, and tuberculosis iridocyclitis.

Classification

- *Acute*: signs and symptoms appear suddenly and last for up to 6 weeks.
- *Chronic*: onset is gradual and inflammation lasts longer than 6 weeks.
- *Granulomatous*: insidious onset; chronic course; eye nearly white; iris nodules and large keratic precipitates (mutton fat) present; posterior segment is commonly involved.
- *Nongranulomatous*: acute onset; shorter course; red eye and intense flare present; no iris nodules
- *Infectious*: viruses, bacteria, rickettsiae, fungi, protozoa, parasites
- *Noninfectious*: exogenous (trauma, chemical injury), endogenous (immunologic types 1–4 hypersensitivities).

Associated Features

Iris heterochromia, corneal band keratopathy

Immunology

Mostly Type III hypersensitivity reaction but also Type II.

Pathology

Neutrophils, eosinophils and lymphocytes in the anterior chamber and on the corneal endothelial and iris surfaces: large keratic precipitates and iris nodules are granulomas.

Diagnosis continued on p. 248

TREATMENT

Diet and Lifestyle

No special precautions are necessary.

Pharmacologic Treatment

Cycloplegia

Standard dosage: Cyclopentolate 1–2%, three times daily for mild to moderate inflammation;
Atropine 1%, two to three times daily for moderate to severe inflammation.
Prednisolone acetate 1%, every 1–6 hours.

Special points: Consider subtenons injection of steroid or systemic steroid, if patient unresponsive to topical therapy.
Treat secondary glaucoma with topical antiglaucoma medication.
If an infectious cause is determined, then the specific management should be added to the above regimen.
Consider a rheumatology consult.

Treatment Aims
To lessen or obviate inflammatory response in the anterior chamber and anterior vitreous.

Other Treatments
Other immunosuppressive therapy may be necessary to control inflammation.

Prognosis
- Prognosis is usually good with therapy
- Patients with juvenile rheumatoid arthritis and Fuchs' heterochromic iridocyclitis have a high complication rate with cataract surgery.
- Patients with sarcoid, tuberculosis and syphilis do well with appropriate therapy.

Follow-up and Management
- Patients should be followed every 1–7 days in the acute phase and every 1–6 months when stable. Complete ocular examination should be performed at each visit.
- If the anterior-chamber reaction is improving, then the steroid should be tapered slowly for a 3-week period. In some cases, chronic low-dose steroids may be needed to prevent recurrence.

Treatment continued on p. 249

Iridocyclitis, Acute and Subacute (364.0)

DIAGNOSIS—cont'd

Complications

- Cataract
- Glaucoma
- Corneal edema
- Cystoid macular edema.

Pearls and Considerations

- Upon second presentation of idiopathic iridocyclitis, patients should be referred for full systemic workup
- Anterior chamber cells and flare are best observed at the slit lamp with a bright conic section and room lights very dim.

TREATMENT—cont'd

Nonpharmacologic Treatment

- Glaucoma surgery (e.g. tube-shunt devices): to control intraocular pressure
- *Cataract surgery*: usually not undertaken until the eye rests for at least 6 months.

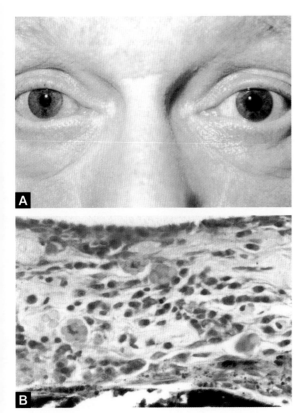

Figs 1A and B: (A) Ciliary injection and constricted right pupil caused by chronic endogenous uveitis ("acute" iritis); (B) Iris shows chronic nongranulomatous inflammation with lymphocytes, plasma cells, and Russell bodies (large, pink, globular structures).

GENERAL REFERENCES

Albert DM, Jakobiec FA (Eds). Principles and practice of ophthalmology. Philadelphia: Saunders; 1994.

American Academy of Ophthalmology. Basic and Clinical Science. San Francisco: American Academy of Ophthalmology; 2006-2007.

Kotaniemi K, Savolainen A, Karma A, et al. Recent advances in uveitis of juvenile idiopathic arthritis. Surv Ophthalmol. 2003;48:489. (major review).

Teyssot N, Cassoux N, Lehoang P, et al. Fuchs heterochromic cyclitis and ocular toxocariasis. Am J Ophthalmol. 2005;139:915.

Wright K. Textbook of ophthalmology. Baltimore: Williams & Wilkins; 1997.

Iris Atrophy, Essential or Progressive (Iridocorneal-Endothelial Syndrome) (364.51)

DIAGNOSIS

Definition

Decompensation or breakdown of the iris tissue.

Synonyms

None; abbreviated iridocorneal-endothelial (ICE) syndrome.

Symptoms

Distortion of the pupil: Patients are usually asymptomatic, but the patient or a family member may notice the distortion of the pupil (Fig. 1).

Decreased vision: If there is associated corneal edema or if the glaucoma is far advanced, the patient may complain of decreased vision in the involved eye.

Pain: Rare, but may occur in cases of severe corneal decompensation with bullous keratopathy; may be caused by angle closure.

Age at onset: Usually in young or middle-aged adults (20–50 years).

Signs

Corneal changes: The corneal endothelium assumes a characteristic "beaten metal" appearance that can be seen with the slit lamp; corneal edema may be present.

Iris atrophy and nodules: Iris changes may be atrophic or nodular; in the atrophic form, displacement of the pupil (corectopia) and atrophic defects in the iris stroma and pigment epithelium (polycoria) may be seen; in the nodular type, pigmented, pedunculated nodules are seen on the iris surface; the disease is usually unilateral.

Elevated intraocular pressure (IOP): Approximately half of patients with (ICE syndrome develop glaucoma; IOP is usually extremely elevated; significant optic nerve cupping and visual field loss are seen, depending on the duration of the elevated IOP; the glaucoma is more severe in the iris atrophy and iris nevus syndrome variations.

Anterior-chamber-angle closure: Gonioscopy may reveal angle closure by peripheral anterior synechiae (PAS) without pupillary block; the PAS extend beyond Schwalbe's line. In earlier cases, all or some of the angle may be open.

Investigations

Complete eye examination: Including gonioscopy.

Photography: Photographic documentation of the anterior segment as well as the optic nerve is useful to monitor the progression of the disease.

Perimetry: Should be performed at regular intervals.

Complications

Glaucoma and corneal edema: The glaucoma may be very difficult to control, resulting in permanent vision loss in the affected eye; persistent corneal edema may require corneal transplantation.

Referral Information

Refer for glaucoma surgery and penetrating keratoplasty as appropriate.

Differential Diagnosis

- Corneal endothelial disorders (e.g. posterior polymorphous corneal dystrophy, Fuchs' endothelial dystrophy).
- Acquired iris abnormalities (e.g. herpes virus infections, iritis, previous episodes of acute glaucoma and iris melanoma).
- Hereditary iris conditions (e.g. Axenfeld-Rieger syndrome).

Cause

The cause is unknown. The lack of family history, adult onset, and unilaterality of most cases would suggest an acquired cause. Some speculate that the cause is infectious, possibly herpes simplex virus or Epstein-Barr virus.

Epidemiology

- Iridocorneal-endothelial syndrome is rare, and most cases are sporadic
- The disease is more often seen in women.

Classification

- Essential iris atrophy is used for cases in which the iris atrophy predominates
- Chandler's syndrome is used for cases in which corneal changes predominate and iris atrophy is minimal.
- Cogan-Reese syndrome, also called the iris nevus syndrome, is used to describe cases in which iris nodules are the predominant feature.

Pathology

- Corneal changes are characterized by an abnormal endothelial cell membrane that proliferates onto the iris surface and over the anterior-chamber angle. The membrane interferes with the function of the trabecular meshwork, resulting in glaucoma. As the membrane contracts, it pulls the peripheral iris into the angle, forming PAS.
- Atrophic changes are seen in the iris with loss of both stroma and pigment endothelium, resulting in distortion, displacement of the pupil, and full-thickness holes in the iris. In the nodular type, pigmented lesions resembling nevi are seen over the anterior surface of the iris.

TREATMENT

Diet and Lifestyle

No precautions are necessary.

Pharmacologic Treatment

- Miotics are generally ineffective in treating the glaucoma associated with ICE syndrome. Aqueous suppressants and prostaglandin analogs are often successful in the early stages of the disease; as the disease progresses, however, medical treatment is less likely to achieve control of IOP.
- Hypertonic saline solutions can aid in the control of the corneal edema.

Nonpharmacologic Treatment

Laser: Laser trabeculoplasty is of no benefit in the glaucoma associated with ICE syndrome; because the angle closure is not caused by pupillary block, laser iridectomy is likewise of no benefit.

Filtering surgery: Filtering surgery or the use of aqueous shunt devices is often successful, but late failures are common because of endothelialization of the fistula. Yttrium-aluminum-garnet (YAG) laser can be used to cut the endothelial cell membrane and reopen the fistula.

Cyclodestructive procedures: When IOP cannot be controlled with medical or surgical treatment, a cyclodestructive procedure may be used.

Corneal transplantation: In patients with corneal edema that causes reduced vision, corneal transplantation may help to restore vision, although success rates are lower in ICE syndrome than in other causes of corneal edema.

Treatment Aims

To preserve vision by controlling IOP.

Prognosis

- The prognosis is poor.
- Iridocorneal-endothelial syndrome is the result of a proliferation of an abnormal cellular membrane inside the anterior chamber; there is no treatment that halts this process. As the proliferation continues, the glaucoma becomes more severe and resistant to standard treatments. Severe and permanent loss of vision in the affected eye is a common outcome.

Follow-up and Management

- Patients should be followed at regular intervals to monitor the progression of the disease; IOP and the appearance of the cornea and optic disk should be recorded at each visit.
- Visual fields should be tested frequently, depending on the severity of the glaucoma.
- Although there is no cure and the ultimate prognosis is poor, useful vision may often be preserved for a long time with careful follow-up and treatment.

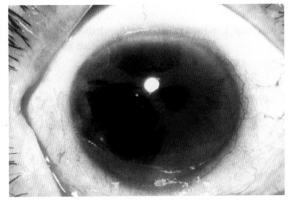

Fig. 1: Iridocorneal-endothelial (ICE) syndrome showing distortion and displacement of the pupil as well as large areas of iris atrophy.

GENERAL REFERENCES

Eagle RC, Font RL, Yanoff M, et al. Proliferative endotheliopathy with iris abnormalities in the iridocorneal endothelial syndrome. Arch Ophthalmol. 1979;97:2104-11.

Laganowski HC, Kerr Muir MG, Hitchings RA. Glaucoma and the iridocorneal endothelial syndrome. Arch Ophthalmol. 1992;110:346-50.

Ritch R, Wilson MR, Samples J. Management of iridocorneal endothelial syndrome. J Glaucoma. 1994;3:154-9.

Shields MB. Progressive iris atrophy, Chandler's syndrome, and the iris nevus (Cogan-Reese) syndrome: a spectrum of disease. Surv Ophthalmol. 1979;24:3-20.

Keratitis (370.9)

DIAGNOSIS

Definition

Inflammation of the cornea

Synonyms

Keratoconjunctivitis, keratopathy

Symptoms

- Redness
- Ocular pain
- Decreased vision
- Photophobia
- Discharge.

Signs

- *Corneal infiltrate/ulcer*: If infectious keratitis
- *Ring infiltrate*: Seen in acanthamebiasis, topical anesthetic abuse
- *Hypopyon*: More common in infectious keratitis
- Corneal edema
- *Dendrites, pseudodendrites*: If epithelial involvement in herpes simplex virus (HSV) or herpes zoster virus (HZV); may be early sign of *Acanthamoeba* infection (Fig. 1).
- *Periorbital rash*: Seen with HZV keratitis; occasionally seen with HSV keratitis
- Epithelial defect.

Investigations

- *Corneal cultures*: Bacterial and fungal cultures on all patients, consider additional cultures (Löwenstein-Jensen, nonnutrient agar with *Escherichia coli* overlay) if atypical organism suspected or history of laser-assisted in situ keratomileusis (LASIK).
- Consider cultures of contact lenses or contact lens case
- *Viral cultures*: May be performed to support diagnosis of HSV, but this is typically a clinical diagnosis
- *Corneal biopsy*: Consider if keratitis continues to progress, highly suspect infectious organisms, but routine cultures negative.

Differential Diagnosis

- Bacterial keratitis
- Fungal keratitis
- Herpes simplex keratitis
- Herpes zoster keratitis
- *Acanthamoeba*
- Sterile corneal infiltrate
- Topical anesthetic abuse
- Atypical mycobacteria.

Cause

- *Pseudomonas* most common cause of bacterial keratitis in contact lens wearers; main risk factor is sleeping with contact lenses.
- Fungal keratitis seen after outdoor or dirty ocular trauma or in patients with chronic ocular surface disease.
- *Acanthamoeba* most often seen in contact lens wearers with homemade or tap water cleaning solutions or those wearing contact lenses while swimming, fishing, or using hot tub.
- Atypical mycobacteria recognized etiology of infectious keratitis following LASIK.

Diagnosis continued on p. 254

TREATMENT

Diet and Lifestyle

- Prevent corneal ulcers by avoiding sleeping in contact lenses
- Clean contact lenses daily; use enzyme weekly
- Consider daily disposable soft contact lenses as alternative.

Pharmacologic Treatment

Infectious Keratitis

Standard dosage:

- *If bacterial keratitis*: Fortified antibiotics, broad spectrum. Typical combination includes fortified cefazolin (50 mg/mL) or fortified vancomycin (25 mg/mL) and fortified tobramycin (15 mg/mL) or fortified gentamicin (15 mg/mL). After giving a loading dose of drops every 5–15 minutes, use every 1 hour, around the clock initially. For smaller infiltrates, consider topical gatifloxacin or moxifloxacin every hour daily in place of fortified antibiotics.
- *Special points*: Fortified antibiotics need to be made by hospital or compounding pharmacy and usually have a limited shelf life of a few days to 2 weeks.
- *If fungal ulcer*: Topical natamycin 5% (especially for filamentous fungi), or amphotericin B 0.15% (especially for molds, candida) every hour; consider topical voriconazole as well.
- *If hypopyon or significant anterior-chamber reaction*: Cycloplegia. Atropine 1%, three times daily if hypopyon; scopolamine 0.25% or cyclogel 1–2%, two or three times daily for mild to moderate anterior-chamber inflammation.

Herpes Simplex Keratitis

Standard dosage:

- *For epithelial/dendritic disease*: Trifluridine every 2 hours. Can also use oral antivirals (e.g. acyclovir, 400 mg five times daily) in place of topical agents.
- *For stromal keratitis*: Topical steroids (prednisolone acetate 1%) four times daily. Need to give antiviral prophylaxis, either with trifluridine (four times daily) or oral antiviral (acyclovir, 400 mg twice daily). Also consider cycloplegia (cyclogel 1–2% or scopolamine 0.25%, two or three times daily).

Herpes Zoster Keratitis

- *Pseudodendrites or superficial punctate keratitis (SPK)*: Frequent lubrication with preservative-free artifical tears every 1–2 hours. May benefit from topical steroids as well (prednisolone acetate 1%, four times daily).
- *Stromal keratitis*: Topical steroids (prednisolone acetate 1%, initially every 2–4 hours); steroids must be tapered very slowly over months to years.

Treatment continued on p. 255

Keratitis (370.9)

DIAGNOSIS—cont'd

Complications

- Corneal scarring
- Corneal perforation
- *Elevated intraocular pressure*: Most common with HZV
- *Recurrent keratitis*: Especially with HSV.

Pearls and Considerations

Usually avoid steroids acutely, especially if fungal infection or HSV epithelial keratitis.

Referral Information

Consider referral if ulcer progresses despite treatment, or if perforation appears likely or occurs.

TREATMENT—cont'd

Nonpharmacologic Treatment

- No contact lens wear
- For herpes simplex epithelial keratitis, consider debridement of dendrites.

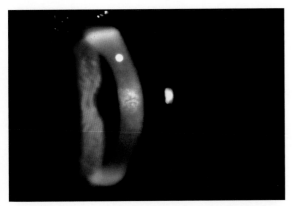

Fig. 1: Herpes simplex dendrite stained with Rose Bengal.

GENERAL REFERENCES

American Academy of Ophthalmology. Basic and Clinical Science. San Francisco: The Academy; 2006-2007.

Smolin G, Thoft RA. The Cornea: Scientific Foundation and Clinical Practice. Boston: Little, Brown. 2004.

Tasman W, Jaeger E. Duane's clinical ophthalmology, vol 4. Philadelphia: Lippincott-Raven; 2005.

Yanoff M, Fine BS. Ocular pathology: a color atlas. Philadelphia: Lippincott Williams & Wilkins; 1988.

Keratoconus (371.60)

DIAGNOSIS

Definition
Noninflammatory, usually bilateral disease of the cornea characterized by thinning of the corneal stroma and resultant protrusion of the cornea.

Synonym
Conical cornea

Symptoms
- Progressive decrease in vision
- Sudden onset of pain, redness, tearing, and blurred vision in acute hydrops.

Signs
- Central corneal ectasia with thinning (Fig. 1)
- Irregular corneal reflex on retinoscopy
- *Vogt's striae*: parallel tension lines in posterior corneal stroma
- *Fleisher ring*: iron line outlining protruding cone (Fig. 2)
- *Munson's sign*: bulging of eyelid in downward gaze
- *Hydrops*: acute break in Descemet's membrane causing significant edema and opacification of cornea. May be acutely painful.

Investigations
- Slit-lamp examination
- *Retinoscopy*: water drop or scissors reflex
- Refraction
- *Computed corneal topography*: typically shows irregular astigmatism with inferior steepening
- *Keratometry*: irregular mires and steepening.

Complications
Hydrops: see Signs.

Pearls and Considerations
Consider keratoconus in young patients who present with decreased vision and an otherwise normal examination; examine closely for signs.

Referral Information
Refer to contact lens specialist for special fitting with rigid gas-permeable contact lenses ideally with corneal topographic measurements. If there is no improvement in vision or unable to tolerate contact lenses, consider referral to a cornea subspecialist for surgical management.

Differential Diagnosis
- Pellucid marginal degeneration
- Keratoglobus.

Cause
- Unclear; traditionally thought related to chronic eye rubbing
- The most popular current hypothesis is that there is a genetic predisposition that requires a "second hit" or environmental event to elicit progressive disease in keratoconus. Eye rubbing may serve as the "second hit" in some predisposed individuals. Active research is underway to reveal possible inflammatory mediators to determine if keratoconus is truly a noninflammatory disorder.
- Associated with Down syndrome, Ehlers-Danlos syndrome, congenital rubella, atopic disease and mitral valve prolapse.

TREATMENT

Diet and Lifestyle

Patients counseled to refrain from eye rubbing.

Pharmacologic Treatment

For Acute Hydrops

Standard dosage:

- Scopolamine 0.25%, two or three times daily
- Sodium chloride 5%, drops or ointment, four times daily
- Oral analgesics as needed.

Nonpharmacologic Treatment

- Mild cases may be treated with glasses or soft contact lenses
- Moderate to advanced cases require specially-fit rigid, gas-permeable contact lenses
- Corneal transplantation, either penetrating keratoplasty or deep anterior lamellar keratoplasty (DALK), is performed when patients are intolerant of contact lenses or cannot achieve adequate vision with contact lenses.
- Keratoconus is an area of active advancements in treatment: lamellar keratoplasty has been revived with improved outcomes, and devices such as intrastromal ring segments (ICRS) with and without femtosecond laser techniques are being investigated and used to treat cases of keratoconus effectively.
- Additionally, corneal collagen cross-linking (CXL) using epithelial debridement, application of topical riboflavin drops and ultraviolet-A exposure has shown great promise in arresting the progression of corneal ectasia in primary and recurrent keratoconus. Generally, a minimum corneal thickness of 400 μm after epithelial removal is considered necessary for safe and effective CXL treatment.

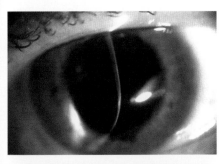

Fig. 1: Central corneal thickening and ectasia in a patient with keratoconus.

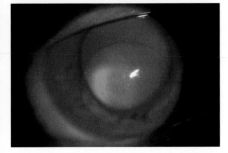

Fig. 2: Fleisher ring seen with cobalt-blue light.

Treatment Aims

To optimize visual acuity, reduce vision loss from irregular astigmatism and myopia, reduce corneal scarring, and minimize the chances of progression of corneal ectasia.

Prognosis

Prognosis for good visual acuity is excellent.

Follow-up and Management

- Every 6–12 months for patients doing well with glasses or contact lenses
- Patients with hydrops should be seen every 1–4 weeks until resolved.

GENERAL REFERENCES

Alio JL, Shah S, Barraquer C, et al. New techniques in lamellar keratoplasty. Curr Opin Ophthalmol. 2002;13:224-9.

Ashar JN, Pahuja S, Vaddavalli PK. Repeat keratoplasty for keratoconus. Ophthalmology. 2012;119(5):1088.

Basic and Clinical Science Course (BCSC): External Disease and Cornea Section 8. San Francisco: American Academy of Ophthalmology; 2006–2007.

Jhanji V, Sharma N, Vajpayee RB. Management of keratoconus: current scenario. Br J Ophthalmol. 2011;95:1044-50.

Kymionis GD, Portaliou DM, Diakonis VF, et al. Corneal collagen crosslinking with riboflavin and ultraviolet-A irradiation in patients with thin corneas. Am J Ophthalmol. 2012;153(1):24-8.

Smolin G, Thoft RA (Eds). The Cornea: Scientific Foundation and Clinical Practice. Boston: Little Brown; 2004.

Sugar J, Macsai MS. What causes keratoconus? Cornea. 2012;31:716-9.

Tasman W, Jaeger E (Eds). Duane's Clinical Ophthalmology, vol. 4. Philadelphia: Lippincott-Raven; 2005.

Uzbek AK, Müftüoğlu O. Advances in keratoconus treatment. Expert Rev Ophthalmol. 2011;6(1):95-103.

Yanoff M, Fine BS. Ocular Pathology: A Color Atlas. Philadelphia: Lippincott; 1988.

Lattice Degeneration (362.63)

DIAGNOSIS

Definition

A thinning of the peripheral retina characterized by local round, oval or linear patches of pigmented or nonpigmented thinning.

Synonym

Snail-track degeneration

Symptoms

Patients are asymptomatic.

Signs

- *Round, oval or elongated areas of retinal thinning*: with sharp borders usually located between the ora serrata and the equator; common locations are found from the 11 to 1 o' clock positions and between the 5 and 7 o' clock positions; retinal thinning found in the inferotemporal quadrant is the most common (see Fig. 1).
- Lattice often has white lines, which represent sheathed vessels. Small, round, atrophic retinal holes may be found within the lattice degeneration or adjacent to these areas.

Investigations

- Visual acuity testing
- Biomicroscopic examination
- Dilated fundus examination.

Complications

- *Retinal tears*: may occur with posterior vitreous detachments or trauma, leading to retinal detachment
- The vitreous is more firmly attached to the edges of the lattice; thus, when the vitreous separates, the retina may tear at the edge of an area of lattice.

Pearls and Considerations

Lattice degeneration must be differentiated from other forms of peripheral retinal degenerations because other forms do not predispose the patient to retinal detachment as does lattice degeneration.

Referral Information

Refer to retinal specialist if secondary detachment or tear occurs.

Differential Diagnosis
- Peripheral pigmentation
- Cystoid degeneration.

Cause
- Lattice degeneration is more common in myopic patients
- There may be an inheritance pattern of autosomal dominance.

Epidemiology
- Seven percent of the population will have lattice degeneration
- Lattice degeneration tends to be bilateral in 45% of patients
- The disease is equally distributed between the two genders
- There is no racial predilection
- In ~30% of eyes with a rhegmatogenous retinal detachment, the detachment is secondary to lattice degeneration.

Classification
Peripheral retinal degeneration.

Associated Features
May be seen in patients with pigment dispersion syndrome (who also have a tendency to be myopic).

Pathology
- There is a lack of internal limiting membrane, overlying vitreous liquefaction, vitreous condensation, and exaggerated vitreoretinal adherence at the borders of these lesions.
- There may be associated retinal pigment abnormalities (e.g. focal pigment loss, pigment migration into retina and around retinal vessels).
- Trypsin digest reveals loss of capillaries and decreased number of endothelial cells.
- There is also glial proliferation at the interface between the retina and formed vitreous.

TREATMENT

Diet and Lifestyle

- Safety glasses are recommended for sports-related activity for individuals with large patches of lattice degeneration
- In patients with a history of retinal detachment and lattice degeneration in their fellow eye, high-impact sports are not recommended.

Pharmacologic Treatment

No pharmacologic treatment is recommended.

Nonpharmacologic Treatment

- Prophylactic laser surgery or cryotherapy is indicated in patients with retinal breaks secondary to vitreoretinal traction or with a history of retinal detachment in their fellow eye. Prophylactic laser surgery is not indicated for the lattice with atrophic holes, which is asymptomatic.
- Controversy remains over whether prophylactic laser surgery should be performed in the fellow eye in patients with a history of retinal detachment; despite laser therapy, retinal tears can still develop at the edge of the laser scars.

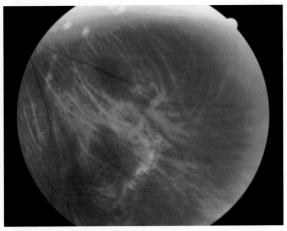

Fig. 1: Peripheral to a small nevus is an area of concentric, white lattice degeneration with small, atrophic holes. Because of its appearance, this type of lesion is termed "snail-track" lattice.

Treatment Aims

- To educate patients on signs and symptoms of retinal detachment
- Prophylactic barrier thermal laser can be done in certain patients predisposed to retinal detachment, e.g. with a retinal detachment in the fellow eye or with a strong family history of retinal detachments.

Prognosis

- Depends on degree of vitreoretinal adhesion, pigment changes, and associated round retinal holes.
- Overall, the incidence of retinal detachment is still quite low.

Follow-up and Management

- Annual dilated eye examinations
- Patients need to be educated on the signs and symptoms of a retinal detachment (flashes, floaters, peripheral shadows and loss of vision) and taught that this is an ocular emergency.
- Elongated oval area of retinal thinning, sharply outlined margins with increased pigmentation, and white, sclerosed vessels traversing the area.

GENERAL REFERENCES

Edwards AO, Robertson JE. Hereditary vitreoretinal degenerations. Retina, 4th edition. St Louis: Elsevier; 2006.

Kroll AJ, Patel SC. Retinal breaks. In: Albert DM, Jakobiec FA (Eds). Principles and Practice of Ophthalmology. Philadelphia: Saunders; 1994. pp. 1057-61.

Wesley P, Liebman J, Walsh JB, et al. Lattice degeneration of the retina and pigment dispersion syndrome. Am J Ophthalmol. 1992;114:539-43.

Leber's Hereditary Optic Neuropathy (377.39)

DIAGNOSIS

Definition

A condition found primarily in young men resulting in dyschromatopsia and bilateral reduction in visual acuity.

Synonyms

None; often abbreviated LHON (Leber's hereditary optic neuropathy).

Symptoms

- Acute, rapid, irreversible, painless central vision loss: usually in one eye, followed by second eye in days to weeks
- "Mist" or "fog" obscuring vision
- Mild dyschromatopsia
- Vision loss acute to subacute with stabilization in less than 4 months.

Signs

- *Acuity loss*: can be asymmetric; most Snellen acuities are worse than 20/200 but range from 20/20 to no light perception
- Pupillary light reflexes relatively preserved compared to the extent of visual loss
- *Color vision*: significantly affected
- *Central or cecocentral scotoma*: 25–30 degrees of absolute scotoma surrounded by a relative scotoma
- *Hyperemic nerve*: during the acute phase of visual loss; late in course of diagnosis, pale
- Dilated and tortuous vessels
- Retinal and optic disk hemorrhages
- Retinal striations
- Obscurations of the disk margin
- Circumpapillary telangiectatic microangiopathy
- Peripapillary edema of the nerve fiber layer
- Acquired cupping of the optic disk
- Arteriolar attenuation.

Differential Diagnosis

- Toxic nutritional optic neuropathy
- Optic neuritis (papillitis) and demyelinating conditions [e.g. multiple sclerosis (MS)]
- Acute disseminated encephalomyelitis
- Dominant optic atrophy (DOA)
- Normal tension glaucoma.

Cause

- Mitochondrial DNA point mutations: three DNA mutations (m.11778G>A, m.3460G>A and m.14484T>C) account for approximately 90–95% of cases of LHON.
- Thought to be due to disturbed mitochondrial function and a predominantly complex I respiratory chain defect, leading to increased susceptibility of the retinal ganglion cells (RGCs) to exogenous influences such as light exposure, smoking, and pharmacological agents with putative mitochondrial toxic effects.
- Selective loss of RGCs with the early involvement of the papillomacular bundle.

Epidemiology

- Dominance in men is 80–90%
- Occurrence rate in women at risk is 4–32%
- Onset of visual loss occurs at ages 15–35 years. However, patient age can range from 5–80 years. Over 90% of carriers who will experience visual failure do so before age 50
- Singleton cases constitute 57–90% of reported cases, but this may be due to difficulties in obtaining detailed family histories
- Minimum prevalence of LHON using Northern England data is approximately 1 in 31,000
- Up to 60% of affected individuals report other family members with a pattern of early-onset visual failure.

Diagnosis continued on p. 262

TREATMENT

Diet and Lifestyle

- Patients should avoid tobacco and excessive alcohol use
- Certain implicated medications should be avoided, if possible: chloramphenicol (rarely used), linezolid, macrolide antibiotics (e.g. erythromycin), ethambutol, certain antiretroviral agents [nucleoside analogue reverse transcriptase inhibitors (NRTIs)].

Treatment Aims

To maximize usable vision, and counsel patient regarding the unique genetic/hereditary characteristics of this condition.

Prognosis

- In most patients with LHON, the visual loss is usually permanent
- Patients less than 20 years of age have a better prognosis, with final acuities of better than 20/80
- Leber's hereditary optic neuropathy patients with the 11778 mitochondrial DNA mutation have the least chance (only 4%) of spontaneous recovery
- Leber's hereditary optic neuropathy patients with the 14484 mitochondrial DNA mutation have the greatest chance (37–65%) of spontaneous recovery
- Improvement usually occurs gradually over 6–12 months. There are reports of significant visual recovery years after onset of visual loss
- Recurrence of LHON is unlikely.

Treatment continued on p. 263

Leber's Hereditary Optic Neuropathy (377.39)

DIAGNOSIS—cont'd

Investigations

- D-15 and Farnsworth Munsell 100-hue test
- Electrocardiography
- Magnetic resonance imaging (may exhibit increased T2 signal in the optic nerves and chiasm extending to the optic tracts and lateral geniculate bodies)
- Fluorescein angiography
- Molecular genetic testing
  - Male carriers with mtDNA point mutations can be reassured that their children are not at risk of inheriting their genetic defect.
  - Female carriers will transmit the mutation to all their offsprings, but if the mutation is heteroplasmic, it is not possible to reliably predict the level of expression that will be transmitted.
- Detailed family history.

Pearls and Considerations

- Absence of dye leakage from the disk or papillary region on fluorescein angiography
- Leber's hereditary optic neuropathy is in the differential diagnosis of acute, painless loss of vision in a young patient
- If unilateral, the fellow eye is usually affected within 6–8 weeks
- In about 20% of LHON cases, the optic disk looks entirely normal
- Similar to anterior ischemic optic neuropathy (AION), a small, crowded disk may predispose carriers to higher rates of visual loss
- Exhibits incomplete penetrance and significant gender bias.

Referral Information

Genetic testing is available for relatives. Male carriers have about a 50% lifetime risk of visual failure compared with only 10% for female carriers.

Associated Features

- The 11778 mitochondrial DNA mutation has associated cardiac conduction abnormalities.
- The 3460 mitochondrial DNA mutation has the highest association with the cardiac pre-excitation syndromes (Wolff-Parkinson-White and Lown-Ganong-Levine).
- The controversial 15257 mitochondrial DNA mutation may have a maculopathy resembling Stargardt's disease.
- Leber's hereditary optic neuropathy female carriers are twice more likely to develop an MS-like demyelinating illness compared with male carriers.
- In DOA, by contrast, most affected families harbor mutations in the OPA1 gene, coding for a mitochondrial inner membrane protein.

TREATMENT—cont'd

Pharmacologic Treatment

- Treatment with the following pharmacologic agents remains controversial and/or investigational, and is likely highly influenced by favorable mutation status:
  - Coenzyme Q10
  - Succinate
  - Vitamin K_1
  - Vitamin K_3
  - Vitamin C
  - Thiamine
  - Vitamin B_2
  - Idebenone (a synthetic analog of CoQ_{10})
  - Estrogen compounds (e.g. 17b-estradiol)
  - Brimonidine
- "Mitochondrial cocktails", e.g. creatine (3g BID), CoQ10 (120 mg BID), and alpha-lipoic acid (300 mg BID)
- Gene therapy (investigational), including pronuclear transfer to prevent the transmission of mtDNA mutations in human embryos.

Note: A 2006 Cochrane review found no evidence supporting any intervention in the management of mitochondrial disease.

Nonpharmacologic Treatment

Low-vision aids

GENERAL REFERENCES

Chinnery P, Majamaa K, Turnbull D, et al. Treatment for mitochondrial disorders. Cochrane Database Syst Rev. 2006;(1): CD004426.

Koilkonda RD, Guy J. Leber's hereditary optic neuropathy-gene therapy: from benchtop to bedside. J Ophthalmol. 2011; 2011:179412.

Manastersky N, Yevseyenkov V. Technology applications in near total vision impairment associated with Leber's hereditary optic neuropathy. Optometry. 2010;81(6):277.

Man PY, Turnbull DM, Chinnery PF. Leber hereditary optic neuropathy. J Med Genet. 2002;39(3):162-9.

Mroczek-Tonska K, Kisiel B, Piechota J, et al. Leber hereditary optic neuropathy: a disease with a known molecular basis but a mysterious mechanism of pathology. J Appl Genet. 2003;44(4):529-38.

Newman NJ. Hereditary optic neuropathies. Eye. 2004;18(11):1144-60.

Newman NJ. Hereditary optic neuropathies. In: Miller NR, Newman NJ (Eds). Walsh and Hoyt's Clinical Neuro-ophthalmology. Baltimore: Williams & Wilkins; 1998.

Newman NJ. Treatment of Leber hereditary optic neuropathy. Brain. 2011;134(Pt 9):2447-50.

Sadun AA, Gurkan S. Hereditary, nutritional and toxic optic atrophies. In: Retina, 4th edition. St Louis: Elsevier; 2006.

Yu-Wai-Man P, Griffiths PG, Chinnery PF. Mitochondrial optic neuropathies–disease mechanisms and therapeutic strategies. Prog Retin Eye Res. 2011;30(2):81-114.

Leukokoria (360.44)

DIAGNOSIS

Definition

White papillary reflex.

Synonyms

"Eyeshine"

Symptoms

- Varies depending on the etiology
- Blurry vision may be reported in patients able to communicate.

Signs

White papillary reflex, often first seen in photographs or by screening pediatricians.

Investigations

- Documented eye size
- History including prematurity, trauma, or familial eye disease
- Birth history including intrauterine infections
- Complete anterior and posterior chamber evaluation, often including ultrasound.

Complications

Varies depending on etiology.

Pearls and Considerations

Most serious cause of leukokoria in children is retinoblastoma.

Cause

Varies depending on etiology.

Epidemiology

- *Retinoblastoma*: incidence is 1:20,000 live births; 94% of cases are sporadic (somatic mutations, unilateral); 6% are familial (germinal mutations, autosomal dominant inheritance, usually bilateral); no gender or race predilection; gene isolated to 13q14 locus; some patients will have 13q deletion.
- *Persistent hypertrophic primary vitreous (PHPV)*: not hereditary; no gender or race predilection.
- *Retinopathy of prematurity (ROP)*: not hereditary; no gender or race predilection.
- *Coats' disease*: not hereditary; no gender or race predilection; 90% of those affected are men.
- *Norrie disease*: X-linked recessive; gene isolated to DXS7 locus on Xp 11; no race predilection.
- *Incontinentia pigment*: X-linked dominant; lethal in males; only noted in females; no race predilection.

Pathology

Retinoblastoma: sheets of small basophilic cells, with frequent calcification in the areas removed from retinal vessels; may grow toward the vitreous, through the sclera, or both; exits the eye through the vortex veins, down the optic nerve, and from aqueous veins.
Persistent hypertrophic primary vitreous: enlarged ciliary body process invades the lens; traction bands from the lens to retina.
Retinopathy of prematurity: retinal neovascularization at junction of vascular and avascular retina attaches to lens and causes retinal detachment; engorgement and tortuosity of posterior pole retinal vessels and iris vessels.
Coats' disease: miliary aneurysms of peripheral retinal vessels; intraretinal and subretinal lipid deposition in fovea and periphery.
Norrie disease: dysplastic, detached retina with absent photoreceptors; retinal gliosis.
Incontinentia pigmenti: occlusive retinal vasculitis with detachment, optic nerve atrophy.
Toxocariasis: retinal nematode with zonular inflammatory surround of eosinophils, granulomatous cells.
Choroidal coloboma: absent retinal pigment epithelium, choriocapillaris, outer retina; inner retina is thin, acellular.

Diagnosis continued on p. 266

TREATMENT

Diet and Lifestyle

Ingestion of the ova of *Toxocara canis* or *T. catis* (usually through contact with the ova in puppy feces or fur) leads to high risk of toxocariasis in infants.

Pharmacologic Treatment

No pharmacologic treatment is recommended.

Treatment Aims

- *Retinoblastoma:* to preserve vision, life
- *Coats' disease:* to destroy abnormal retinal vessels and resolve foveal lipid
- *Toxocariasis:* to control intraocular inflammation.
- *Persistent hypertrophic primary vitreous:* to improve visual acuity; prevent phthisis.

Prognosis

- *Retinoblastoma:* approximately 70% of globes can be salvaged with some useful vision; 5% of children will die of metastatic tumor; patients with hereditary retinoblastoma (germinal mutation) have a 26% chance of dying from second cancer in 40 years.
- *Toxocariasis:* eyes require enucleation; vision compromised in most patients
- *Coats' disease:* significant recovery of visual acuity, if treated early
- *Persistent hypertrophic primary vitreous:* few eyes will develop good visual acuity even after lensectomy; some will develop glaucoma, require enucleation.
- *Norrie disease:* all children bilaterally blind
- *Incontinentia pigmenti:* varies greatly, and many children maintain useful vision; some will be bilaterally blind.

Follow-up and Management

Varies depending on cause.

Treatment continued on p. 267

Leukokoria (360.44)

DIAGNOSIS—cont'd

Differential Diagnosis/Cause

- *Premature*: retinopathy of prematurity
- *Trauma*: cataract, retinal detachment, endophthalmitis
- *Family history*: retinoblastoma, familial exudative vitreoretinopathy, incontinentia pigmenti (females only), retinal dysplasia, retinal astrocytoma
- Toxoplasma gondii, rubella virus, cytomegalovirus, herpes simplex virus (TORCHES)
- *Small eye*: persistent hyperplastic primary vitreous, retinal coloboma, retinoblastoma.

Pearls and Considerations

Leukokoria is the presenting symptom in 90% of retinoblastoma cases and is considered the classic clinical presentation for retinoblastoma.

Referral Information

Varied, dependent upon cause of the condition.

TREATMENT—cont'd

Nonpharmacologic Treatment

- *Retinoblastoma:* enucleation, external proton beam radiation, scleral plaque placement, systemic drugs as indicated in each case
- *Coats' disease:* photocoagulation of abnormal vessels
- *Toxocariasis:* topical or systemic steroids
- *Persistent hypertrophic primary vitreous:* lensectomy, removal of fibrous tissue invading lens
- *Retinopathy of prematurity:* photocoagulation or cryotherapy to avascular retina, repair of retinal detachment, management of amblyopia, strabismus, glaucoma as indicated
- *Norrie disease:* no known treatment
- *Incontinentia pigmenti:* no known treatment
- *Choroidal coloboma:* no known treatment; repair of secondary retinal detachment
- *Congenital retinal schisis:* no treatment needed, unless retinal detachment occurs.

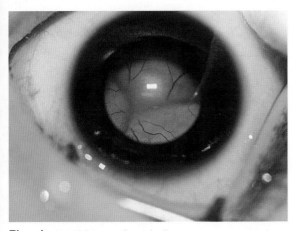

Fig. 1: In children, Coats' disease may present as leukokoria, with advanced lipid deposition and exudative retinal detachment. In this eye, the anterior chamber is shallowed slightly, and the retina is immediately behind the lens.

GENERAL REFERENCES

Balmer A, Munier F. Differential diagnosis of leukocoria and strabismus, first presenting signs of retinoblastoma. Clin Ophthalmol. 2007;1(4):431-9.

Catalano RA. Incontinentia pigmenti. Am J Ophthalmol. 1990;110:696-703.

Demirci H, Shields CL, Shields JA, et al. Leucocoria as the presenting sign of a ciliary body melanoma in a child. Br J Ophthalmol. 2001;85(1):115-6. No abstract available.

Eagle RC. Retinoblastoma and simulating lesions. In: Tasman W, et al (Eds). Duane's Clinical Ophthalmology (CD-ROM). Philadelphia: Lippincott Williams & Wilkins; 2004.

Goldberg MF, Mafee M. Computed tomography for diagnosis of persistent hyperplastic primary vitreous (PHPV). Ophthalmology. 1983;90:442-50.

Haik BK. Advanced Coats' disease. Trans Am Ophthalmol Soc. 1991;89: 371-80.

Holmes LB. Norrie's disease: an X-linked syndrome of retinal malformations, mental retardation, and deafness. N Engl J Med. 1971;284:367-74.

Jain IS, Mohan K, Jain S. Retinoblastoma: modes of presentation. J Ocul Ther Surg. 1985;4:83-7.

Patz A. Observations on the retinopathy of prematurity. Am J Ophthalmol. 1985; 100:164-72.

Sang DN, Albert DM. Retinoblastoma: clinical and histopathologic features. Hum Pathol. 1982;13:133-6.

Shields CL, Eagle RC, Shah RM, et al. Multifocal hypopigmented retinal pigment epithelial lesions in incontinentia pigmenti. Retina. 2006;26(3): 328-33.

Smirniotopoulos JG, Bargallo N, Mafee MF. Differential diagnosis of leukokoria: radiologic-pathologic correlation. Radiographics. 1994;14(5):1059-79; quiz 1081-2.

Watzke RC, Oaks JA, Folk JC. *Toxocara canis* infection of the eye: correlation of clinical observations with developing pathology in the primate model. Arch Ophthalmol. 1984;102:282-8.

Macular Degeneration, Age-Related (362.5)

DIAGNOSIS

Definition

Nonexudative form: an inherited retinal condition typified by drusen, retinal pigment epithelium (RPE) changes and visual disturbances.

Exudative form: an advanced form in which choroidal neovascular membranes develop under the RPE and leak fluid and blood, ultimately leading to a blinding, disciform scar.

Synonyms

None; typically abbreviated ARMD; nonexudative form often referred to as "dry" and exudative form as "wet".

Symptoms

- Metamorphopsia (distortion)
- Blurry vision
- Scotomas (small areas of vision missing).

Signs

- Decreased vision
- Abnormal Amsler grid
- Subretinal and intraretinal hemorrhage, fluid, and lipid exudation secondary to choroidal neovascularization (CNV): *see* Figures 1 and 2
- Pigment alteration in the macula.

Investigations

- Careful history to determine the duration of symptoms
- Visual acuity testing
- *Amsler grid testing*: look for areas of distortion, doubling of lines, and areas missing; the Amsler grid tests the central 20° of visual field
- Slit-lamp examination
- *Dilated fundus examination*: pay careful attention to the macula; best viewed with a Goldmann fundus lens

Differential Diagnosis

- Parafoveal telangiectasia
- Macroaneurysm secondary to hypertension
- Chronic central serous retinopathy
- Macular granuloma
- *Idiopathic CNV*: secondary CNV caused by ocular histoplasmosis, trauma with choroidal rupture, angioid streaks and multifocal choroiditis.

Cause

- *Dry ARMD*: Thickening of Bruch's membrane
- Drusen deposits
- Retinal pigment epithelium atrophy
- *Wet ARMD*: Growth of choroidal neovascular vessels with leakage and bleeding into neurosensory retina.

Epidemiology

- Leading cause of visual loss and blindness in people aged greater than 60 years
- More than 1.6 million Americans older than age 60 have advanced ARMD
- Age-related macular degeneration is far more prevalent among white than black people.

Classification

Dry ARMD: occurs in the majority of individuals affected by ARMD. Patients develop drusen and then pigment alteration in the macula (coalescence of drusen leads to areas of pigment atrophy). The smaller areas of atrophy coalesce with time. Patients develop gradual loss of vision with distortion and scotomas.

Wet ARMD: Ten percent of patients develop CNV characterized by serous or hemorrhagic detachment of the macula and RPE. Eventually, if untreated, subretinal fibrosis occurs leading to a disciform scar.

Pathology

Drusen: round, discrete, yellowish sub-RPE deposits of eosinophilic extracellular material (periodic acid-Schiff positive).

Basal-laminar drusen: represents focal thickening of the RPE basement membrane and the inner collagenous layer of Bruch's membrane.

Choroidal neovascular membranes: blood vessel growth from the choroid into the subretinal space with fibroblasts.

Diagnosis continued on p. 270

TREATMENT

Diet and Lifestyle

- Age-related eye disease study vitamins reduced the rate of exudative ARMD by about 25% over a 6-year period. The specific amounts of antioxidants and zinc used in the study were 500 mg vitamin C, 400 IU vitamin E, 25,000 IU vitamin A, 80 mg zinc oxide and 2 mg cupric oxide (latter added to prevent zinc-induced anemia).
- All patients with exudative disease in one eye and all patients with nonexudative ARMD should take an AREDS vitamin formula. It is not clear whether there is any benefit to the eye once exudative disease has started. Vitamins are used to prevent conversion of dry ARMD to wet ARMD.
- Patients should be counseled to stop smoking, because smoking doubles the risk of developing wet ARMD.

Pharmacologic Treatment

The treatment of choice has now become serial intravitreal injections of anti-VEGF type A medications. Currently, there is one selective VEGF-A inhibitor [pegaptanib (Macugen)] and two pan-isoform VEGF-A inhibitors [bevacizumab (Avastin) and ranibizumab (Lucentis)]. The goal of therapy is to improve, not just stabilize, vision. Ranibizumab and pegaptanib are Food and Drug Administration (FDA) approved for use in the treatment of ARMD; bevacizumab is FDA approved for colon cancer; therefore, its use in the eye is off-label. The most impressive visual results are seen with bevacizumab and ranibizumab; therefore, these two medications are now the most commonly used forms of therapy. If patients are treated soon after the onset of exudative disease, they may be able to carry on activities of daily living and lead productive lives.

Treatment Aims
To improve vision

Other Treatments
Low-vision aids

Prognosis
- Eventual decline to legal blindness is common, if not treated
- Incidence of CNV in the fellow eye is 5–14% per year.

Follow-up and Management
All patients need to be instructed to test their vision daily with an Amsler grid, looking for blurry vision or areas of distortion or missing vision. If these changes develop, patients will need to be treated as an emergency and should contact their ophthalmologist immediately.

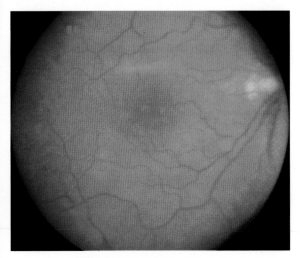

Fig. 1: Drusen in the macula.

Treatment continued on p. 271

Macular Degeneration, Age-Related (362.5)

DIAGNOSIS—cont'd

- *Fluorescein angiography (FA)*: used to determine whether there is a presence of CNV, RPE detachment or tear; if CNV is seen on FA, it is important to categorize the leakage pattern as "well defined" or "occult", as well as to define the location to determine whether the patient is eligible for extrafoveal laser treatment (Fig. 3).
- *Indocyanine angiography*: may be used as a secondary test if FA shows poorly defined leakage or if the area in question is obscured by blood
- *Optical coherence tomography (OCT)*: used to determine anatomic distortions of the retina, RPE and choriocapillaris. Best method of determining intraretinal edema, thickness and scarring. Useful in determining response to antivascular endothelial growth factor (anti-VEGF) therapy.

Complications

- Decreased vision
- *Vitreous hemorrhage*: secondary release of subretinal blood into the vitreous cavity
- *Optical coherence tomography*: used in determining retinal thickness and response to treatment. Resolution of edema is now documented better with OCT than with FA (Figs 4 and 5).

Diagnosis continued on p. 272

TREATMENT—cont'd

Nonpharmacologic Treatment

- Thermal laser is currently reserved for the small minority of patients with extrafoveal well-defined lesions (i.e. patients in whom the lesion is far enough away from the center of the macula not to induce scotomas or threaten the fovea with treatment).
- Photodynamic therapy was the mainstay of therapy for subfoveal lesions until the advent of anti-VEGF medications. Because it only results in visual improvement approximately 10% of the time, it is now used infrequently as the initial treatment of choice.

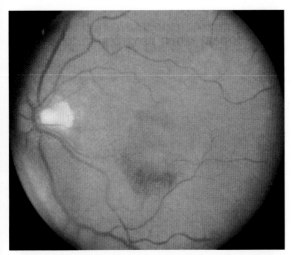

Fig. 2: Choroidal neovascularization with drusen, subretinal fluid and hemorrhage.

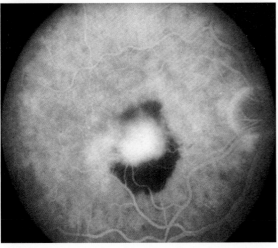

Fig. 3: Fluorescein angiogram of the same patient as in Fig. 2 showing central poorly defined leakage with a surrounding area of hypofluorescence caused by blockage from blood.

Treatment continued on p. 273

Macular Degeneration, Age-Related (362.5)

DIAGNOSIS—cont'd

Pearls and Considerations

- According to the International Classification Guidelines, ARMD cannot be diagnosed in patients less than 50 years old
- Retinal pigment epithelium atrophy that progresses to larger areas is termed geographic atrophy
- Age-related macular degeneration is the leading cause of blindness in patients greater than 50 years of age in the United States
- Although ARMD is an accepted genetic disorder, smoking has been demonstrated to double the patient's risk for the disease
- Age-related eye disease study (AREDS) formula vitamins come in both smokers' and nonsmokers' formulations. The smokers' formulations are β-carotene free.

Referral Information

Monitor dry form, and refer for immediate retinal treatment when progression to the exudative form is suspected.

TREATMENT—cont'd

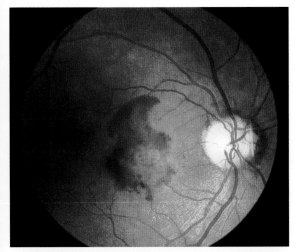

Fig. 4: Classic subfoveal choroidal neovascular membrane with surrounding intraretinal hemorrhage.

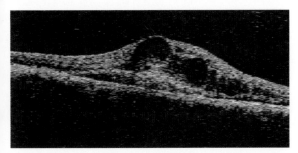

Fig. 5: Optical coherence tomography (OCT) of the same patient as in Fig. 4 demonstrating intraretinal growth of choroidal neovascular membrane with associated intraretinal cystic fluid and thickening of neurosensory retina.

GENERAL REFERENCES

Age-Related Eye Disease Study Research Group. A randomized, placebo-controlled, clinical trial of high-dose supplementation with vitamins C and E, beta carotene, and zinc for age-related macular degeneration and vision loss: AREDS report no. 8. Arch Ophthalmol. 2001;119:1417-36.

Avery RL, Pieramici OJ, Rabena MD, et al. Intravitreal bevacizumab (Avastin) for neovascular age-related macular degeneration. Ophthalmology. 2006;113:363-72.e5.

Gragoudas ES, Adamis AP, Cunningham ET, et al. VEGF Inhibition Study in Ocular Neovascularization Clinical Trial Group. Pegaptanib for neovascular age-related macular degeneration. N Engl J Med. 2004;351:2805-16.

Rosenfeld PJ, Brown OM, Heier JS, et al. Ranibizumab for neovascular age-related macular degeneration, N Engl J Med. 2006;355:1419-31.

273

Macular Edema, Cystoid (Postoperative) (362.53)

DIAGNOSIS

Definition

Fluid-filled spaces within the central macular neurosensory retina.

Synonyms

None; typically abbreviated CME.

Symptoms

* *Gradual, painless loss of central vision*: usually starting within 1 month after eye surgery
* Ocular irritability.

Signs

* May be seen after uncomplicated cataract surgery without any anterior signs
* Ruptured anterior hyaloid face
* Vitreous incarceration in the wound
* Iris incarceration in the wound
* Poor pupillary dilation
* Peaked pupil secondary to adherent vitreous
* Fovea may be normal in appearance
* Obvious intraretinal cysts are often seen clinically. In chronic cases, alteration in the pigment layer may occur.

Investigations

* *Careful slit-lamp examination*: look for evidence of vitreous in the wound or anterior chamber, and for a rent in the lens capsule
* *Close inspection of the fovea*: a contact lens may show the changes better than a handheld lens
* *Fluorescein angiography*: shows early symmetric leakage from the perifoveal capillaries; the pattern of leakage is classically "petalloid" in shape (Figs 1 and 2A & B); the degree of leakage does not necessarily correspond to the level of visual acuity; there may also be evidence of leakage without clinical evidence of edema
* *Optical coherence tomography*: shows intraretinal cystoid spaces. Neurosensory retina is thickened. There is loss of the normal foveal indentation.

Complications

Permanent visual loss: most cases, however, usually resolve spontaneously within a few weeks to months.

Pearls and Considerations

Cataract extraction is the most common cause of, although any intraocular surgery can produce, CME.

Referral Information

Optometrists comanaging postcataract patients should refer a patient immediately to the performing surgeon on suspicion of CME.

Differential Diagnosis

* Hypotony maculopathy
* Pre-existing macular degeneration
* Edema associated with other conditions, e.g. diabetes, vein occlusion, hypertension, retinal telangiectasia uveitis, macular pucker, and epinephrine use in aphakia.

Causes

* Most often occurs after uncomplicated cataract surgery
* Less common after extracapsular surgery than intracapsular surgery
* Iris-supported intraocular lenses are associated with a high incidence of CME
* More common in patients with vitreous loss or disruption of the anterior hyaloidal face.

Epidemiology

* One percent of postcataract surgery patients have clinical evidence of CME
* Ten to twenty percent of patients will have angiographic evidence of CME, but most are asymptomatic.

Associated Features

* Cystoid macular edema is more common in older patients
* If one eye develops CME, the other is thought to be at risk.

Pathology

Accumulation of watery, proteinaceous material within the inner and outer plexiform layers; the edema can greatly distort the neural elements; loss of photoreceptors occurs in chronic cases.

TREATMENT

Diet and Lifestyle

No special precautions are necessary.

Pharmacologic Treatment

- Topical nonsteroidal drops such as ketorolac tromethamine (Acular), nepafenac (Nevanac), and bromfenac (Bromday) have been shown to reduce angiographic evidence of CME and improve vision
- Continued topical prednisolone acetate 1%, 4 times daily, may decrease inflammation, which may be contributing to the edema
- Oral acetazolamide (250 mg qid) and/or posterior subtenon's injection of steroids have shown limited success
- Intravitreal injection of triamcinolone can produce a dramatic improvement in vision and reduction in fluid as measured by optical coherence tomography (OCT). This is typically done after a failed trial of topical nonsteroidal anti-inflammatory drugs (NSAIDs).

Nonpharmacologic Treatment

- Pars plana vitrectomy has occasionally been effective in patients with chronic CME with vision of 20/80 or less of at least 2–3 months' duration.
- Neodymium:yttrium-aluminum-garnet (Nd:YAG) vitreolysis of strands adherent to the cataract wound has shown a positive effect in resolving CME.

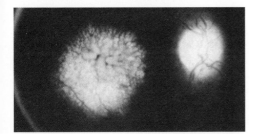

Fig. 1: Fluorescein angiogram showing petalloid leakage pattern in the macula with hyperfluorescent leakage off the optic nerve (Irvine-Gass syndrome).

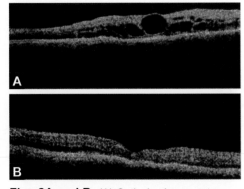

Figs 2A and B: (A) Optical coherence tomography shows cystoid macular edema pre-intraocular steroid injection; (B) Postinjection. Edema fluid resolved.

Treatment Aims

- Decrease inflammation
- Lysis of vitreous adhesions
- Restore vision.

Prognosis

Good, because most cases resolve spontaneously over weeks to months.

Follow-up and Management

Each treatment attempted should be given at least 3–4 weeks to show an effect before altering therapy.

GENERAL REFERENCES

Blair NP, Kim SH. Cystoid macular edema after ocular surgery. In: Albert DM, Jakobiec FA (Eds). Principles and Practice of Ophthalmology. Philadelphia: Saunders; 1994. pp. 898-904.

Fung WE. Vitrectomy for chronic aphakic cystoid macular edema: results of a national collaborative, prospective, randomized investigation. Ophthalmology. 1985;92:1102-11.

Tolentino Fl, Schepens CL. Edema of the posterior pole after cataract extraction: a biomicroscopic study. Arch Ophthalmol. 1965;78:781.

Wright PL, Wilkinson CP, Balyeat HD, et al. Angiographic cystoid macular edema after posterior chamber lens implantation. Arch Ophthalmol. 1988;106:740-4.

Macular Hole, Idiopathic (362.83)

DIAGNOSIS

Definition

A discontinuity in the foveal retina from the internal limiting membrane to the outer photoreceptor layer.

Synonyms

None

Symptoms

- *Decreased vision*: to the 20/200 range; patients may not appreciate the visual loss until they cover their other eye
- Visual distortion.

Signs

- *Central scotoma*: abnormal Amsler grid
- *Full-thickness hole*: in the fovea, ranging in size from 200 μm to 400 μm
- Halo of fluid: often present (Fig. 1)
- *Yellow deposits in the base of the hole*: *see* Figure 1
- Small, overlying retinal operculum
- Macular pucker.

Investigations

- *Careful history*: to determine previous trauma or eye surgery
- Visual acuity
- Amsler grid testing
- Slit-lamp examination
- Dilated fundus examination
- *Watkze-Allen test*: interruption of the vertical slit beam of light or "pinching" of the light beam implies an interruption in retinal tissue because of the hole
- *Fluorescein angiography (FA)*: will show a round, hyperfluorescent spot in the center of the fovea from secondary changes in the retinal pigment epithelium (RPE)
- *Optical coherence tomography (OCT)*: is better than FA. Will show tenting of neurosensory retina (a cyst) or a full-thickness defect in the neurosensory retina (a hole; Fig. 2).

Complications

Retinal detachment: rare

Pearls and Considerations

- Although most macular holes are idiopathic, they can also be related to trauma, laser treatment, cystoid macular edema, retinal vascular disease, retinal pucker, or hypertensive retinopathy. Patients presenting with macular hole should have these underlying conditions ruled out.
- Up to 10% of patients may develop a cyst or a hole in the fellow eye.

Referral Information

Refer to retinal specialist for surgical intervention.

Differential Diagnosis

- *Pseudohole with an associated epimacular membrane*: usually the vision is better.
- Pseudohole associated with severe macular edema.

Cause

Unknown

Epidemiology

- Occurs primarily in women in their 6th decade of life
- Bilateral in 10% of cases
- 5–15% of cases are caused by trauma.

Classification

Stage IA: yellow spot in the center of the fovea with loss of foveal depression
Stage IB: transition from stage IA to a small, yellow halo in the fovea. Cyst seen on OCT
Stage 2: full-thickness macular hole less than 200 μm in size; it may begin eccentrically. Best seen with OCT
Stage 3: full-thickness macular hole greater than 200 μm in size; usually includes a cuff of fluid, yellow deposits in the base, overlying operculum, and cystoid edema. Can be seen clinically quite readily.
Stage 4: full-thickness macular hole with posterior vitreous detachment.

Associated Features

It may be associated with vitreoretinal traction or partial separation of the posterior vitreous.

Pathology

- *Full-thickness retinal defect*: in the fovea with rounded edges; the edges may be detached from the RPE because of subretinal fluid
- *Cystoid spaces*: may be seen in the retina
- Overlying epiretinal membrane
- Variable photoreceptor atrophy
- *Yellow deposits in the hole*: represent xanthophyll-laden macrophages.

TREATMENT

Diet and Lifestyle

No precautions are necessary.

Pharmacologic Treatment

No pharmacologic treatment is recommended.

Nonpharmacologic Treatment

Pars plana vitrectomy, separation of the posterior vitreous from the surface of the retina, peeling of the internal limiting membrane, and fluid-gas exchange with face-down positioning for at least 5 days

- Surgical intervention for stage 1 macular holes was no better than natural history
- Surgical intervention for stages 2–4 macular holes resulted in significantly better vision at 6 months after surgery compared with natural history.

Treatment Aims

- To seal the macular hole
- To improve vision by at least two lines of Snellen acuity with surgery.

Prognosis

- Eighty percent of patients with stage 2 macular holes will progress to stage 3 or 4 holes within 6 months with considerable loss of vision.
- Most patients with successful closure of the macular hole with surgery will have significantly better vision at 6 months compared with natural history.
- There is a significant risk of cataract formation after vitrectomy for macular holes.

Follow-up and Management

Amsler grid testing of the fellow eye to detect early stage 1 or 2 holes.

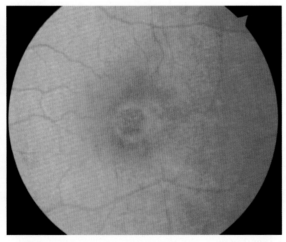

Fig. 1: Stage 3 macular hole with a rim of fluid and yellow deposits in the base of the hole.

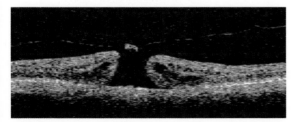

Fig. 2: Optical coherence tomography demonstrating full-thickness macular hole with operculum in overlying posterior vitreous.

GENERAL REFERENCES

de Bustros S. Vitrectomy for prevention of macular holes. Results of a randomized multicenter clinical trial. Vitrectomy for Prevention of Macular Hole Study Group. Ophthalmology. 1994;101:1055-9.

Gass JD. Idiopathic senile macular hole. Its early stages and pathogenesis. Arch Ophthalmol. 1988;106:629-39.

Hughes BM, Valero SO. (2012). Macular hole. [online] Available from http://emedicine.medscape.com/article/1224320-overview, 2006, VI/WW.emedicine.com [Accessed April, 2013].

Kim JW, Freeman WR, Azen SP, et al. Prospective randomized trial of vitrectomy or observation for stage 2 macular holes. Am J Ophthalmol. 1996;121:605-14.

Green WR. The macular hole. Histopathologic studies. Arch Ophthalmol. 2006;124:317.

Macular Pucker and Idiopathic Preretinal Macular Fibrosis (362.56)

DIAGNOSIS

Definition
Wrinkling of the retinal surface secondary to traction from an epiretinal membrane.

Synonyms
Surface-wrinkling retinopathy, cellophane retinopathy, epiretinal membrane.

Symptoms
- Blurry vision
- Distorted vision (metamorphopsia)
- Monocular diplopia
- Macropsia (larger image size) or micropsia (smaller image size).

Signs (Figs 1 and 2)
- Wrinkling of macular surface
- Fibrosis of the retina in the macula
- *Displacement of the fovea*: from tractional forces
- *Posterior vitreous detachment*: seen in 90% of cases.

Investigations
- Visual acuity
- Amsler grid testing
- *Dilated slit-lamp and fundus examinations*: a characteristic abnormal sheen to the retinal surface in the macular area suggests a membrane; sometimes obvious striae and superficial fibrosis are present; this may be more obvious with the green-filtered light on slit-lamp examination of the retina
- *Fluorescein angiography (FA)*: shows distortion of retinal vasculature caused by areas of traction from the membrane. Late phases may show cystoid macular edema (CME)
- *Optical coherence tomography (OCT)*: often shows areas of adherence of vitreoretinal interface. Sometimes, if only horizontal traction, will only show thickening of internal limiting membrane with associated intraretinal thickening and loss of foveal depression.

Complications
- Decreased vision
- Distorted vision.

Pearls and Considerations
- Macular pucker can be a complication of retinal reattachment surgery
- Amsler grid is the most useful take-home tool for patients to monitor their level of visual involvement.

Referral Information
Refer to retinal specialist for surgical peel as appropriate for symptomatic patients.

Differential Diagnosis
Macular hole

Causes
Abnormal proliferation of glial cells on the retinal surface can be seen after retinal cryotherapy, retinal laser, trauma, vitreous hemorrhage, and ocular surgery.

Epidemiology
- Disease usually occurs bilaterally
- Approximately 75% of eyes retain good vision of 20/50 or better.

Pathology
Some have suggested that migration of glial cells from the retina through the internal limiting membrane may be a natural component of aging. Most membranes are probably composed of a variety of cells capable of developing myofibroblastic properties that are responsible for contraction.

TREATMENT

Diet and Lifestyle

No precautions are necessary.

Pharmacologic Treatment

No pharmacologic treatment is recommended.

Nonpharmacologic Treatment

If the vision drops below 20/40, and the patient is bothered by decreased or distorted vision, surgical peeling of the membrane can be performed. There is a small risk of recurrence after vitrectomy. Although recovery time is quicker, long-term visual outcomes appear to be similar for 20 gauge versus 25 gauge (sutureless) surgical techniques.

Treatment Aims

- To improve vision
- To decrease distortion.

Prognosis

Good, because most cases of macular pucker do not progress, and vision remains better than 20/40.

Follow-up and Management

- Yearly dilated eye examinations
- Amsler grid testing at home by the patient to detect increasing distortion.

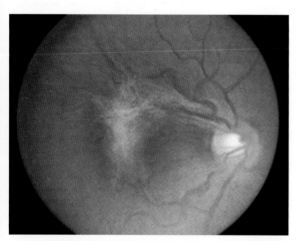

Fig. 1: Extensive preretinal fibrosis.

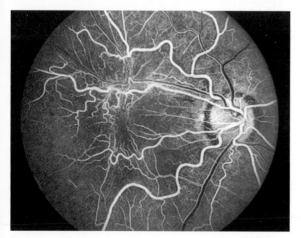

Fig. 2: Fluorescein angiogram of the patient in Figure 1, showing dislocation of the fovea superiorly and straightening of retinal vessels.

GENERAL REFERENCES

Green WR, Sebag J. Vitreoretinal interface. Retina, 4th edition. St Louis: Elsevier; 2006.

Kadonosono K, Yamakawa T, Uchio E, et al. Comparison of visual function after epiretinal membrane removal by 20-gauge and 25 gauge vitrectomy. Am J Ophthalmol. 2006;142:513-5.

Michels RG. Vitrectomy for macular pucker. Ophthalmology. 1984;91: 1384-8.

Sidd RJ, Fine SL, Owens SL, et al. Idiopathic preretinal gliosis. Am J Ophthalmol. 1982;94:44-8.

Wallow IH, Stevens TS, Greaser ML, et al. Actin filaments in contracting preretinal membranes. Arch Ophthalmol. 1984;102:1370-5.

Marcus-Gunn (Jaw-Winking) Syndrome (374.73)

DIAGNOSIS

Definition

A congenital, synkinetic ptosis involving intermittent elevation of the ptotic lid with coinciding contraction of the mastication muscles, resulting in a "winking" movement during eating or chewing (Figs 1A and B).

Synonyms

- Gunn syndrome
- Gunn phenomenon
- Marcus-Gunn phenomenon.

Symptoms

- *Ptosis*: some patients exhibit a chin-up posture to maintain binocular vision
- Aesthetic deformity in many patients.

Signs

- The severity of the ptosis and the amplitude of the wink are proportionately related. Measurable levator function is variable or decreased
- The upper eyelid crease is usually intact
- Hypotropia and other forms of strabismus may be seen in the jaw-winking syndrome
- Affected upper lid elevates when mandible is depressed or moved to opposite side (external pterygoid muscle contracts): less often, affected upper lid elevates when patient clenches teeth (internal pterygoid muscle)
- *Ptosis*: in many patients when mandible is closed (6% of patients with congenital ptosis have this syndrome)
- *Lid synkinesis*: most noticeable in infancy when patient sucking bottle, in older children when chewing food or gum
- Syndrome may be unilateral or bilateral and may be extremely asymmetric if bilateral.

Investigations

- Observing the parent provide a bottle for the child
- Observing the child chew gum or move the mandible side to side
- Documenting any chin-up posture
- Measuring eyelid response to phenylephrine
- Measuring ptosis with mandible closed as well as lid excursion with lid moving side to side.

Complications

- Amblyopia and possible anisometropia
- Neck deformity from chin-up posture
- Lagophthalmos after sling procedures.

Pearls and Considerations

- Present at birth
- The wink often becomes less noticeable with age, as patients learn to limit oral movements that stimulate the synkinesis.

Referral Information

Oculoplastics referral for ptosis surgery in severe cases.

Differential Diagnosis

- Aberrant regeneration of the third cranial nerve may lead to varying lid positions as the globe moves, but lid position is not dependent on mandible position, and patients often have strabismus and pupillary involvement.
- *Cyclic oculomotor spasm*: during spastic phase, the pupil constricts, the eye adducts, and the ptotic lid elevates; during paralytic phase, the pupil dilates, the eye abducts, and the lid is ptotic; congenital, persists through life; more common in female patients; and usually unilateral.
- *Inverse Marcus-Gunn phenomenon*: ptotic lid elevates with opening of mouth (very rare).

Cause

Congenital miswiring of levator muscle by branch of trigeminal nerve usually directed to the external pterygoid muscle; acquired cases have been described.

Epidemiology

- Rarely, may have autosomal dominant inheritance
- No race or gender predilection.

Pathology

Aberrant innervation of the levator with branch of trigeminal nerve usually destined for the external pterygoid muscle; other possibilities have been suggested when other jaw muscles are involved.

TREATMENT

Diet and Lifestyle

No special precautions are necessary.

Pharmacologic Treatment

No pharmacologic treatment is recommended.

Nonpharmacologic Treatment

Mild cases can be treated with levator aponeurotic-muscle resection. Patients with large-amplitude winking may require ablation of the levator, followed by frontalis suspension.

Treatment Aims

Achieving symmetric lid positions and no synkinesis.

Prognosis

• The condition tends to improve slightly with age
• Typically, good results are obtained through current surgical techniques, but lagophthalmos on downgaze is still often present.

Follow-up and Management

Corneal protection after sling procedures is necessary.

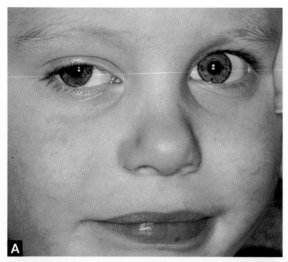

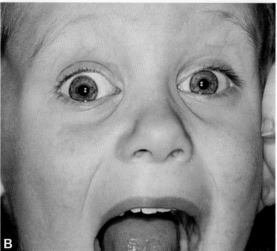

Figs 1A and B: Marcus-Gunn jaw-winking syndrome. (A) In primary gaze with the mouth closed, there is right upper eyelid ptosis; (B) With the jaw opened the right upper eyelid elevates due to synkinesis.

GENERAL REFERENCES

Beard C. Ptosis, 3rd edition. St Louis: Mosby; 1980.

Betharia SM, Kumar S. Levator sling for Marcus-Gunn ptosis. Br J Ophthalmol. 1987;71(9):685-9.

Blaydon SM. (2006). Marcus-Gunn jaw winking syndrome [online]. Available from www.emedicine.com.

Callahan A. Surgical correction of the blepharophimosis syndrome. Trans Am Acad Ophthalmol Otolaryngol. 1973;77: 687-90.

Doucet TW, Crawford JS. The quantification, natural course, and surgical results in 57 eyes with Marcus Gunn (jaw-winking) syndrome. Am J Ophthalmol. 1981;92:702-7.

Mosavy SH, Horiat M. Marcus-Gunn phenomenon associated with synkinetic oculopalpebral movements. Br Med J. 1976;2(6037):675-6.

DIAGNOSIS

Definition

Ocular motility disorder caused by mechanical forces preventing extraocular muscle function.

Synonyms

None

Symptoms

- Diplopia in strabismic positions
- Head postures and ptosis in some patients.

Signs (Figs 1 to 3)

Brown Syndrome

Limitation of elevation in adduction: possible depression in adduction, Y-pattern exotropia, head turn away from involved eye, head tilt to same side as affected eye.

Fibrosis Syndrome

Limitation of ductions with chin-up head posture: may be generalized with fixed globe, or limited to certain muscle groups, usually including inferior recti.

"Heavy Eye" Syndrome

Hypotropia and esotropia: in a myopic eye: may adopt head tilt toward side of affected eye.

Investigations

- Family history
- *Complete motility examination in all gaze positions*: patients who have mechanical strabismus will have ductions as limited as versions in pathologic gaze positions
- *Dilated fundus examination*: in patients who have "heavy eye" syndrome to look for staphyloma
- *Magnetic resonance imaging*: in patients with difficult motility patterns
- *Forced-duction testing*: will disclose tightness to elevation in adduction in patients who have Brown syndrome, tightness to elevation in patients who have "heavy eye" syndrome, and generalized tightness in patients who have fibrosis syndromes.

Differential Diagnosis

Brown syndrome

- *Inferior oblique palsy*: usually associated with A-pattern and superior oblique overaction, positive head tilt test; duction "up and in" better than version.
- *Blowout orbital fracture*: history of trauma, enophthalmos

Fibrosis syndromes

- *Partial third-nerve palsy*: not inherited; usually unilateral; may involve pupillary sphincter
- Blowout fracture.

"Heavy eye" syndrome

Esotropia and hypotropia from fusion break.

Causes

Brown syndrome

- *Congenital*: short superior oblique tendon
- *Acquired*: superior oblique tuck encircling element for retinal detachment repair, trauma, or inflammation of trochlea.

Fibrosis syndromes

Congenital: inherited as autosomal dominant in many families.

"Heavy eye" syndrome

Inferior misdirection of lateral rectus around equator of enlarged globe: with resultant limitation of elevation and abduction.

Epidemiology

Brown Syndrome

Predominantly females and occurs in the left eye.

Fibrosis Syndrome

- Often autosomal dominant without race or gender predilection
- Asymmetric but usually bilateral.

"Heavy Eye" Syndrome

No recognized patterns, typically associated with high myopia.

Diagnosis continued on p. 284

TREATMENT

Diet and Lifestyle

- Many patients will adopt a head posture to maintain comfortable single binocular vision
- Patients with fibrosis syndromes must adopt head posture to view straight ahead.

Pharmacologic Treatment

No pharmacologic treatment is recommended.

Nonpharmacologic Treatment

Brown Syndrome

Strabismus surgery is indicated in approximately 40% of patients who will adopt a head posture to view straight ahead with comfortable single binocular vision. Procedures include tenotomy (sparing intermuscular septum) and lengthening superior oblique tendon with plastic strips.

Fibrosis Syndromes

Strabismus surgery is indicated to permit patients to view in primary position without adopting a head posture. Large recessions are performed, using adjustable suture techniques when possible.

"Heavy Eye" Syndrome

Strabismus surgery is indicated to align the eyes and recover comfortable single inocular vision. Procedures include many different techniques, but information limited on most effective approach. Some surgeons advocate recession of inferior and medial recti, using adjustable suture techniques when possible.

Treatment Aims

Brown Syndrome
- To achieve straight eyes in primary position without the adoption of a head posture
- To achieve full elevation in adduction.

Fibrosis Syndromes
To achieve straight eyes in primary position without the adoption of a head posture; full ductions and versions are rarely obtainable.

"Heavy Eye" Syndrome
To achieve straight eyes in primary position with comfortable single binocular vision.

Prognosis

Brown Syndrome
Modern surgical techniques permit attainment of postoperative alignment without head posture in most patients.

Fibrosis Syndromes
Most patients can attain improved ductions and versions after strabismus surgery.

"Heavy Eye" Syndrome
Surgical experience is too limited to predict final outcomes.

Follow-up and Management
Individualized

Treatment continued on p. 285

DIAGNOSIS—cont'd

Complications

Neck deformities and amblyopia

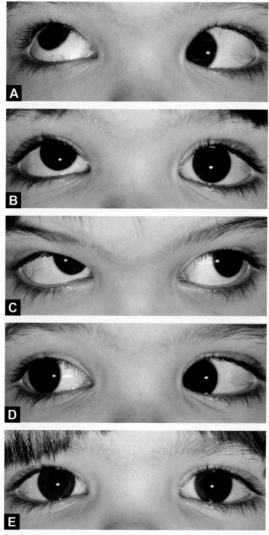

Figs 1A to E: Brown's syndrome. Elevation of the left eye is impaired most in right gaze. The differential diagnosis is one of inferior rectus paresis. Brown's syndrome is characterized by a positive traction test for elevation in adduction, but muscle paresis is not. (A) Gaze to right and up. Note limitation of elevation of adducted left eye; (B) Gazing upward shows mild limitation of elevation of left eye; (C) Gazing left and up shows no restrictions; (D) Gazing to the right shows no vertical deviation in this case, but one may be present; (E) Primary position shows no deviation.

Diagnosis continued on p. 286

TREATMENT—cont'd

Classification

- Brown syndrome (378.61)
- Fibrosis syndromes (378.60)
- "Heavy eye" syndrome (378.60).

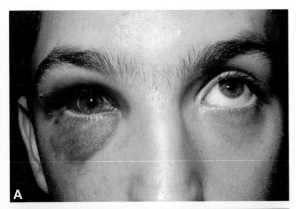

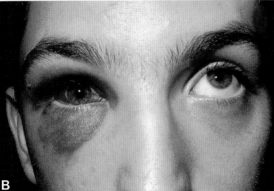

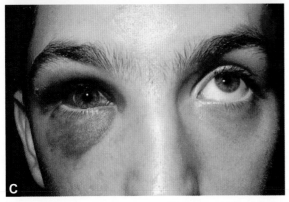

Figs 2A to C: Inferior Rectus Entrapment The inferior rectus muscle is entrapped within the blowout fracture. When the patient tries to look upward, the affected eye has limited upward gaze. The patient experiences diplopia with this maneuver.

Treatment continued on p. 287

DIAGNOSIS—cont'd

Pearls and Considerations

Vary depending on specific etiology

Commonly Associated Conditions

- *Brown syndrome*: as above; also, widening of lid fissure with attempted globe elevation in adduction; may have positive head-tilt test, but usually suggests ipsilateral palsy of inferior rectus not consistent with ductions and versions.
- *Fibrosis syndromes*: often associated with pseudoptosis and true ptosis and chin-up head posture
- *"Heavy eye" syndrome*: associated with unilateral high myopia, often with staphyloma.

Referral Information

Refer to appropriate specialist based on etiology (e.g. orthopedics, endocrinology, etc.).

TREATMENT—cont'd

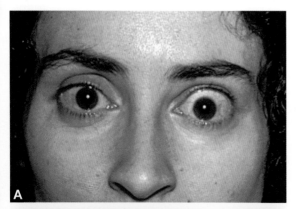

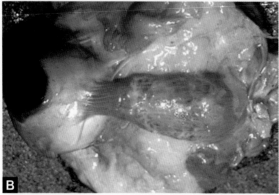

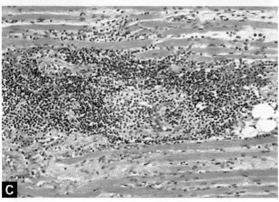

Figs 3A to C: A. Thyroid exophthalmos, greater right eye, causing mechanical strabismus; B. Autopsy of another patient shows marked enlargement of rectus muscles; C. Histopathology show chronic inflammation and edema of rectus muscle.

GENERAL REFERENCES

Andrews CV, Hunter DG, Engle EC. Congenital Fibrosis of the Extraocular Muscles. In: Pagon RA, Bird TD, Dolan CR, Stephens K, Adam MP (Eds). GeneReviews™ [Internet]. Seattle (WA): University of Washington, Seattle; 1993-2004.

Brown HW. True and simulated superior oblique tendon sheath syndromes. Doc Ophthalmol. 1973;34:123-8.

Hansen E. Congenital fibrosis of the extraocular muscles. Acta Ophthalmol. 1968;46:469-79.

Harley RD, Rodrigues MM, Crawford JS. Congenital fibrosis of the extraocular muscles, Trans Am Ophthalmol Soc. 1978;76:197-201.

Krzizok TH, Kaufmann H, Traupe H. Elucidation of restrictive motility in high myopia by magnetic resonance imaging. Arch Ophthalmol. 1997;115:1019-26.

Rutar T, Demer JL. "Heavy Eye" syndrome in the absence of high myopia: A connective tissue degeneration in elderly strabismic patients. J AAPOS. 2009;13(1):36-44. Epub 2008 Oct 18.

Wang FM, Wertenbaker C, Behrens MM, et al. Acquired Brown's syndrome in children with juvenile rheumatoid arthritis. Ophthalmology. 1984;91:23-31.

Wright KW. Brown's syndrome: diagnosis and management. Trans Am Ophthalmol Soc. 1999;97:1023-109.

Mechanical Strabismus (378.63), Blowout Fracture (802.6) and Graves' Dysthyroid Orbitopathy (242)

DIAGNOSIS

Definition

- A deficit in ocular motility secondary to mechanical forces limiting extraocular muscle function
- Blowout fracture refers to break in the bony orbital floor without involvement of the bony rim.

Synonyms

None

Symptoms

- *Diplopia and visual confusion*: in strabismic gaze positions
- *Dyscosmetic head postures (head tilts or turns)*: in some patients
- *Loss of visual field, visual acuity and color vision discrimination*: in some patients with Graves' dysthyroid orbitopathy (GDO)
- *Pain from ulcers related to corneal exposure*: in some patients with GDO.

Signs

Blowout Fracture

Enophthalmos, limitation of ductions (usually elevation with floor fracture, abduction with medial orbital wall fracture; *see* Figure 1), infraorbital hypesthesia.

Graves' Dysthyroid Orbitopathy

Lid retraction (Fig. 2), lid or conjunctival swelling and chemosis, duction limitations (usually elevation or abduction), exophthalmos, lagophthalmos, corneal exposure (with resultant scarring, infection or erosion).

Investigations

Blowout Fracture

- History, visual acuity test, alignment in all gaze positions, ductions and versions, measurement of enophthalmos
- *Magnetic resonance imaging or computed tomography*: to document location and extent of fracture, entrapment of orbital tissue in maxillary or ethmoid sinuses, and sinus opacity from inflammation or infection
- *Dilated anterior-segment and fundus examination*: to rule out retinal, vitreous damage or intraocular foreign body
- Clinical photographs.

Graves' Dysthyroid Orbitopathy

- History of thyroid disease, visual acuity and visual field tests, color vision evaluation, ductions and versions, measurement of exophthalmos and lid retraction
- *Magnetic resonance imaging*: to document enlargement of extraocular muscles (EOMs) and encroachment of muscles around optic nerve
- *Dilated fundus examination*: to evaluate optic nerve, retinal vasculature
- *Measurement of serum thyroid hormone*: total or free thyroxine (T_4), total or free triiodothyronine (T_3)
- Serum thyroid-stimulating hormone (TSH)
- *Autoantibody tests*: antithyroid peroxidase, antithyroglobulin antibodies, anti-TSH receptor antibodies.

Differential Diagnosis

Blowout Fracture

Brown syndrome, fibrosis syndromes, enophthalmos (caused by breast carcinoma metastatic to the orbit).

Graves' Dysthyroid Orbitopathy

Proptosis: caused by orbital masses, craniofacial anomalies, neurofibromatosis Type 1 (pulsatile).
Lid retraction: congenital, or caused by overcorrection during ptosis surgery, aberrant regeneration of third cranial nerve, or topical α-adrenergic drugs.
Enlarged EOMs: caused by orbital myositis, orbital cellulitis; rarely a primary anomaly.

Cause

Blowout Fracture

Usually caused by axial blunt trauma.

Graves' Dysthyroid Orbitopathy

Presumably an autoimmune disease.

Epidemiology

Blowout Fracture

Common in sports with small, hard projectiles (e.g. squash, tennis, baseball).

Graves' Dysthyroid Orbitopathy

Twenty percent of patients with GDO will be clinically euthyroid, and all laboratory tests will be negative; ~40% of this population will eventually become hyperthyroid.

Classification

- Blowout fracture (378.62)
- Graves' dysthyroid orbitopathy (378.63).

Associated Features

Blowout Fracture

Hyphema, ruptured globe, vitreous hemorrhage, retinal break or detachment, iris or retinal dialysis, uveitis, retinal hemorrhage, macular edema or hole.

Graves' Dysthyroid Orbitopathy

Hyperthyroidism or hypothyroidism, Cogan lid-twitch sign (retraction of lid after rapid downward eye movement), bruit over eye or eyelid, upper-lid lag on downgaze, increased intraocular pressure on attempted upgaze, resistance to globe retropulsion, pretibial myxedema, diffuse goiter.

Diagnosis continued on p. 290

TREATMENT

Diet and Lifestyle

Blowout Fracture

Protective eyewear during racquet sports and baseball will decrease incidence.

Graves' Dysthyroid Orbitopathy

- Treatment of hyperthyroidism may exacerbate GDO signs and symptoms
- Cigarette smoking significantly increases the risk of ophthalmopathy in Graves' disease.

Pharmacologic Treatment

For Blowout Fracture

- Oral antibiotics to prevent or treat sinus infection, orbital cellulitis
- Nasal antihistamines, decongestants
- As required for uveitis, ocular complications.

For Graves' Dysthyroid Orbitopathy

- Judicious treatment of hypothyroidism or hyperthyroidism
- Systemic prednisone may decrease orbital, lid and muscle swelling in acute cases
- Topical lubricants for exposed cornea.

Nonpharmacologic Treatment

For Blowout Fracture

Surgical reduction of fracture with placement of rigid substance to bridge bony defect; release of entrapped orbital contents; strabismus surgery for residual strabismus; procedures include recession of tight muscles, using adjustable sutures when possible.

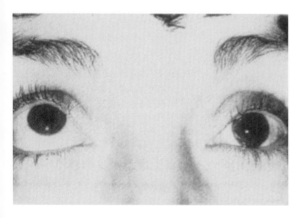

Fig. 1: Limitation of upgaze in left eye after blowout fracture.

Treatment continued on p. 291

DIAGNOSIS—cont'd

Complications

Blowout Fracture

- *Permanent duction limitation*: with head posture, strabismus in primary position
- Infraorbital hypesthesia, enophthalmos.

Graves' Dysthyroid Orbitopathy

- *Corneal exposure*: with resultant melting, scarring or infection
- *Optic nerve compression*: with loss of visual acuity, visual field, and color perception and discrimination
- *Head posture, diplopia*: in primary position and reading position
- Dyscosmetic lid retraction, exophthalmos, and chemosis of lids or conjunctivae.

Pearls and Considerations

Trapdoor entrapment of the EOMs refers to entrapment of the orbital contents in which the broken bone has snapped back into place after initial injury. This condition compromises blood supply to the affected structures and requires surgical intervention within 24 hours.

Referral Information

Refer to appropriate subspecialist based on etiology of disease (e.g. endocrinologist, head and neck surgeon).

TREATMENT—cont'd

For Graves' Dysthyroid Orbitopathy

Orbital decompression for optic nerve compression, profound exorbitism with corneal exposure, limited globe movement; lateral, medial tarsorrhapies for corneal protection; strabismus surgery for residual strabismus, limitation of ductions; procedures include recessions on tight muscles, using adjustable sutures when possible; resections are avoided; levator muscle and lower-lid retractor lengthening for lid retraction.

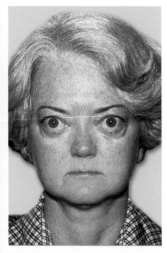

Fig. 2: Lid retraction and exorbitism in patient with Graves' disease.

GENERAL REFERENCE

Fells P. Thyroid-associated eye disease: clinical management. Lancet. 1991;338: 29-32.

Microhyphema (364.41)

DIAGNOSIS

Definition

Blood in the anterior chamber which is typically too small to settle or layer.

Synonyms

None

Symptoms

Blurry vision

Signs

- Hyphema
- Intraocular pressure (IOP) elevations.

Investigations

- History including type of injury, onset, and hematologic predispositions for bleeding
- Pupillary examination for afferent defects
- Ruling out a ruptured globe.

Complications

- Elevated IOPs
- Rebleeding with corneal blood staining
- Optic neuropathy depending on the etiology of trauma.

Pearls and Considerations

- Even microhyphemas can mask significant trauma
- Uncomplicated cases typically resolved within 1 week.

Commonly Associated Conditions

Angle recession from inciting injury.

Referral Information

Occasionally, patients will require inpatient hospitalization and follow-up.

Differential Diagnosis

Must rule out intraocular foreign bodies related to trauma.

Cause

- Typically a result of blunt trauma
- May occur spontaneously in patient with neovascularization of the iris, blood dyscrasias, and juvenile xanthogranuloma
- Chafing of the intraocular lens against the iris or ciliary body.

Epidemiology

Commonly associated with blunt trauma and intraocular lens dislocations.

Associated Features

Angle recession and other injuries to angle structures.

TREATMENT

Diet and Lifestyle

Protective eyewear while in contact sports or operating machinery is always recommended.

Pharmacologic Treatment

- Most can be treated as outpatient with cycloplegia and topical steroids for inflammation
- Atropine 1%, 2–3 times daily
- Prednisolone acetate 1%, every 2–6 hours for inflammation
- No aspirin
- Avoid acetazolamide in patients with sickle cell disease
- Antiglaucoma medications in instances of increased IOP.

Nonpharmacologic Treatment

- Eye shield and head up position at 30°
- Anterior chamber washout if microhyphema becomes larger or other complications arise including increased IOP and corneal blood staining.

Treatment Aims

- Control IOP
- Preventing rebleeding
- Preventing corneal blood staining.

Prognosis

Typically good if no rebleeding occurs.

Follow-up and Management

- Daily follow-up for the first 4–5 days checking IOP and visual acuity
- Eye shields for protection during first 2 weeks post injury
- One month post injury and resolution for gonioscopic examination and scleral depression.

GENERAL REFERENCES

Albert DM, Jakobiec FA. Principles and Practice of Ophthalmology, vol I. Philadelphia: Saunders; 1994.

American Academy of Ophthalmology. Basic and Clinical Science, section 8. San Francisco: The Academy; 1994-1995.

Foroozan R, Tabas JG, Moster ML. Recurrent microhyphema despite intracapsular fixation of a posterior chamber intraocular lens. J Cataract Refract Surg. 2003;29(8):1632-5.

Grieshaber MC, Schoetzau A, Flammer J, et al. Postoperative microhyphema as a positive prognostic indicator in canaloplasty. Acta Ophthalmol. 2011. doi: 10.1111/j.1755-3768.2011.02293.

Recchia FM, Saluja RK, Hammel K, et al. Outpatient management of traumatic microhyphema. Ophthalmology. 2002;109 (8):1465-70; discussion 1470-1.

Shepard J, Williams PB. (2005). Hyphema. [online] Available from www.emedicine.com.

Wilson FM. Traumatic hyphema: pathogenesis and management. Ophthalmology. 1980;687:910-9.

Wright K. Textbook of Ophthalmology. Baltimore: Lippincott Williams & Wilkins; 1997.

Monofixation Syndrome (378.34)

DIAGNOSIS

Definition

A sensory state that comprises features of both normal retinal correspondence and abnormal retinal correspondence (ARC) associated with binocular patients who have a small or absent tropia and possible superimposed phoria.

Synonyms

- Monofixation phoria
- Microtropia
- Microstrabismus
- Esotropic flick strabismus
- Small angle strabismus.

Symptoms

- Typically asymptomatic unless they have a large phoria
- Asthenopia.

Signs

- Up to 8 prism (Δ) esotropia or exotropia and 2Δ vertically up or down
- Most have strabismus which is not easily noticeable
- Absolute, facultative, central scotoma that usually measures 2.5–3° in diameter.

Investigations (Figs 1 and 2)

- The diagnosis is usually confirmed by sensory testing, demonstrating peripheral fusion without central fusion
- Normal fusional vergence amplitudes
- Stereopsis from nil to 67 arc seconds
- Facultative central scotoma of about 3° under binocular viewing conditions
- *Positive 4 Δ diopter base-out test*: holding the prism before the nonfixing eye will not lead to eye movement because the image is merely moved within the foveal scotoma
- *Cover test* may show larger deviation on alternate cover test than on cover-uncover test; monofixation syndrome (MFS) is the only form of strabismus in which this occurs.

Differential Diagnosis

Some authors separate MFS from "microtropia," "monofixational phoria," etc. These terms represent emphasis on one part of the presentation of some patients with MFS.

Cause

- Occurs spontaneously, often in patients who have anisometropia
- After strabismus surgery for early-onset esotropia or exotropia
- After strabismus surgery for intermittent exotropia (risk, 1%)
- After reversal of amblyopia in patients with aligned eyes
- After reversal of constant, acquired strabismus
- Organic foveal lesions (e.g. toxoplasmosis) in one eye.

Epidemiology

- The syndrome may develop spontaneously by unknown means
- It may be caused by anisometropia
- It is the best-expected sensory state in almost all patients who have "congenital" strabismus after successful surgical alignment.

Associated Features

Sensory status does not fit strict definitions of "normal" or "abnormal" retinal correspondence. Sensory testing is more consistent with normal because patients with MFS have normal fusional version amplitudes and some stereoptic ability.

Diagnosis continued on p. 296

TREATMENT

Diet and Lifestyle

No dietary precautions are necessary.

Pharmacologic Treatment

No pharmacologic treatment is recommended.

Treatment Aims
To prevent symptomatic phorias
Prognosis
- Esotropic patients tend to remain stable
- Exotropic patients tend to develop larger exotropia with time.
Follow-up and Management
Individualized per each instance

Monofixation Syndrome With No Tropia

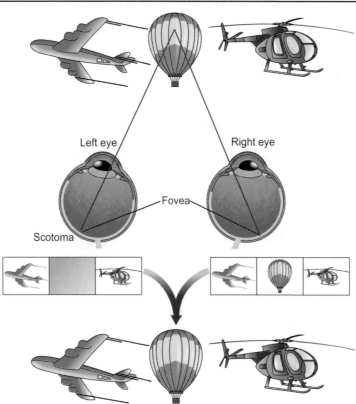

Fig. 1: Monofixation syndrome with no tropia. Note the central scotoma that envelops the area seen by the left fovea and fusion of peripheral information.

Treatment continued on p. 297

DIAGNOSIS—cont'd

Complications

Patients who have MFS are at risk for the development of amblyopia if they do not alternate fixation between the eyes. Age of onset is less than 5 years.

Sixty-six percent of patients with MFS are amblyopic, including:

- 33% of patients with early-onset strabismus and postoperative MFS
- 66% of patients with acquired esotropia and MFS
- 75% of patients with MFS with no known cause
- 90% of patients with strabismus and anisometropia with MFS
- 100% of patients with no history of strabismus but anisometropia and MFS.

Some MFS patients will decompensate and develop a larger tropia with suppression and anomalous retinal correspondence; seems to occur more frequently in those with exotropia than esotropia.

Pearls and Considerations

Adults with mild amblyopia, subnormal stereovision, or subtle differences in binocular visual acuity may have undiagnosed MFS.

Referral Information

No referral is required.

TREATMENT—cont'd

Nonpharmacologic Treatment

- Amblyopia should be treated
- Indicated only when patient develops larger angle strabismus or symptoms from a large phoria.

Monofixation Syndrome With Esotropia

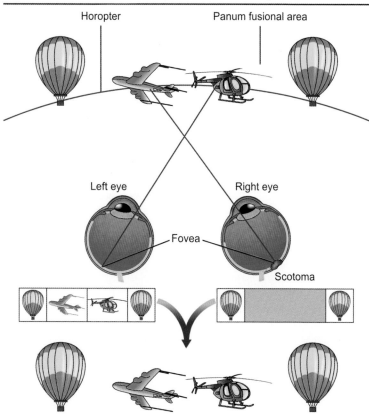

Fig. 2: Monofixation syndrome with 4Δ right esotropia. Note the right central scotoma that prevents perception of the plane and helicopter under binocular viewing conditions and fusion of peripheral information (balloons). The horopter is an infinitely thin surface in space that contains all the object points that project to corresponding retinal points. It is surrounded by the Panum fusional area, within which objects in space can be fused even though they project onto noncorresponding retinal points.

GENERAL REFERENCES

Arthur BW, Smith JT, Scott WE. Long-term stability of alignment in the mono-fixation syndrome. J Pediatr Ophthalmol Strabismus. 1989; 26:224-9.

Fawcett SL, Birch EE. Motion VEPs, stereopsis, and bifoveal fusion in children with strabismus. Invest Ophthalmol Vis Sci. 2000;41(2):411-6.

Gupta BK. (2005). Monofixation syndrome. [online] Available from www.emedicine.com.

Jampolsky A. Characteristics of suppression in strabismus. Arch Ophthalmol. 1955;54:683-6.

Parks MM. Stereoacuity as an indicator of bifixation. In: Knapp P (Ed). Strabismus Symposium. New York: Karger; 1968.

Parks MM. The monofixation syndrome. In: Dabezies O (Ed). Strabismus. St Louis: Mosby; 1971. pp. 131-5.

Parks MM. The monofixation syndrome. Trans Am Ophthalmol Soc. 1969;67: 609-57.

Siatkowski RM. The decompensated monofixation syndrome (an American Ophthalmological Society thesis). Trans Am Ophthalmol Soc. 2011;109:232-50.

Myasthenia Gravis, Ocular (358.0)

DIAGNOSIS

Definition

A disorder of the neuromuscular junction caused by an autoimmune attack on the acetylcholine (ACh) receptors at the neuromuscular junction.

Synonyms

None; myasthenia gravis (MG) also known as Erb-Goldflam disease.

Symptoms

Diplopia, ptosis, "flattened smile" (lips elevate but fail to retract), nasal speech, respiration weakness.

Signs

Medial rectus weakness, gaze nystagmus, convergence insufficiency, pupil-sparing pseudo-third-nerve palsy, pseudo-fourth-nerve palsy, pseudo-sixth-nerve palsy, pseudo-gaze palsy, isolated extraocular muscle (EOM) weakness, double-elevator palsy, hypermetric saccades (if gaze restricted), hypometric saccades (if gaze unrestricted), fatigue (on rapid following, in sustained lateral gaze, on optokinetic nystagmus), ptosis (alternating, unilateral or bilateral), diurnal eyelid fatigue, ptosis that worsens in bright sunlight, eyelid opposite ptotic lid is retracted, post-tetanic facilitation (may cause eyelid to be elevated), peek sign on attempted eyelid closure, weakness of orbicularis oculi, Cogan's eyelid twitch (in ~10% of patients) (Fig. 1).

Investigations

- *Ice pack test*: examination includes applying an ice pack to the ptotic eyelid for 2 minutes to assess ptosis improvement. Observe whether patients appear to be involuntarily "peeking" out of their eyelids when they close their eyes. Assess for weakness of orbicularis oculi muscle. Observe whether the eyelid overshoots the eye as the patient looks from a downgaze to the primary position (lid twitch). Ask the patient to look upward and suppress blinking (one eyelid is mechanically held while observing whether the fellow eyelid curtains).
- Appraise improvement of the ptosis or diplopia after sleep
- *Serum ACh receptor antibody*: positive in ~50% of patients with ocular myasthenia; 87% with generalized myasthenia. False negatives very uncommon; positive values generally considered diagnostic.
- *Edrophonium (tensilon) test*: false negatives and positives occur; false negatives occur 18% of the time in ocular myasthenic and 29% in generalized myasthenic patients. Also, there is a small risk of cardiorespiratory collapse.
- Neostigmine (prostigmin) test.
- Repetitive nerve stimulation [increased decrement (>10%) of the evoked compound muscle action potential in response to repetitive supramaximum nerve stimulation at 3 Hz].

Differential Diagnosis

- Graves' orbitopathy
- Other causes of ptosis (e.g. contact-lens syndrome)
- Cranial nerve palsies
- Generalized myasthenia
- Juvenile MG, neonatal MG or congenital MG
- Bulbar myasthenia (e.g. brainstem stroke, pseudobulbar palsy)
- Lambert-Eaton myasthenic syndrome
- Botulism
- Chronic progressive external ophthalmoplegia
- Oculopharyngeal dystrophy
- Miller-Fisher variant of Guillain-Barré syndrome
- Myotonic dystrophy
- Cavernous sinus syndrome
- Decompensated phoria
- Progressive supranuclear gaze palsy.

Cause

Reduction of available nicotinic ACh receptors at neuromuscular junctions; caused by autoimmune attack with destruction (distortion of postsynaptic membrane geometry) and antagonism (blockade) at the available receptor sites.

Epidemiology

- Incidence rate is 1:20,000 to 0.4:1 million per year
- Prevalence rate is 1:8,000-200,000
- Disease occurs from infancy to the senium
- Peak incidence is in second and third decades of life, affecting mostly women. Another peak in incidence occurs in sixth and seventh decades, affecting mostly men.
- There is no racial or geographic predilection.

Classification

Ocular myasthenia gravis (OMG) is a nonprogressive form involving only ocular motility problems and eyelid weakness.

Associated Features

- *Bulbar signs:* include chewing, eating, swallowing and breathing
- *Flaccid dysarthria*: characterized by hypernasality, decreased articulation, dysphonia, and decreased loudness
- *Associated immunologic disorder:* diabetes mellitus, thyroid disease, systemic lupus erythematosus, rheumatoid arthritis; increased incidence of malignancies; occur in 23% of patients
- *Thymomas:* in 10% of patients, particularly older men; 50% of patients with thymomas have MG.

Diagnosis continued on p. 300

TREATMENT

Diet and Lifestyle

- Thirty-three percent of patients with myasthenia experience the first symptoms after an emotional upset
- Sixty-six percent of myasthenic patients note aggravation of established symptoms by psychologic factors.

Pharmacologic Treatment

- *Corticosteroids* (e.g. prednisone): often considered first-line therapy, though still controversial; may prevent progression of OMG to generalized myasthenia
- *Anticholinesterases:* pyridostigmine, neostigmine, ambenonium. Used in conjunction with immunosuppressives, or as an alternative first-line therapy, particularly for patients with contraindications to corticosteroid therapy
- *Propantheline:* for adverse gastrointestinal side effects of anticholinesterase medication
- *Immunosuppressives:* azathioprine, cyclosporine
- *Intravenous immunoglobulin:* rarely required for OMG
- Avoidance of medications that can exacerbate symptoms (*see* Complications: e.g. muscle relaxants, antimalarials, β-blockers, verapamil and aminoglycosides).

Treatment Aims

- To minimize diplopia and ptosis
- To improve systemic weakness in generalized cases.

Other Treatments

- *Prisms and glasses for diplopia*: rarely successful
- Patches
- *Eyelid tape*: for ptosis
- *Ptosis crutch*: if available
- *Strabismus and ptosis surgery*: may be relatively contraindicated. Generally performed only when the ocular deviation appears to be stable over a period of at least 6 months.

Prognosis

- Eighty-five of patients who present with OMG convert to generalized myasthenia
- Approximately 90% of ocular myasthenic patients who convert to generalized myasthenia do so within 12 months
- Diplopia and ptosis are often resistant to systemic therapy.

Treatment continued on p. 301

Myasthenia Gravis, Ocular (358.0)

DIAGNOSIS—cont'd

- *Single-fiber electromyography*: if necessary; abnormal in 67% of patients with ocular myasthenia when examining the extensor digitorum brevis muscle; abnormal in 86% of patients when the facial muscle was also studied.
- Computed tomography of the mediastinum (exclude an associated thymoma)
- Pulmonary function studies
- Antinuclear antibody, rheumatoid factor, thyroid function tests, antithyroid antibodies, postprandial blood glucose, complete blood count.

Complications

- *Myasthenic crisis*: acute respiratory distress or bulbar symptoms. May be precipitated by steroid dosing titration, which should be done cautiously
- *Cholinergic crisis*: overmedication with cholinesterase inhibitor leading to increased ACh accounting for increased salivation, lacrimation, sweating, vomiting, diarrhea, abdominal cramps, urgent or frequent urination, bronchial asthma and pupillary miosis
- *Hypoadrenergic crisis*: may be precipitated by sudden corticosteroid withdrawal
- Thymoma
- The following may exacerbate MG: hyperthyroidism, hypothyroidism, occult infection, aminoglycoside and macrolide antibiotics, ciprofloxacin, D-penicillamine, intravenous contrast dye, procaine/lidocaine, lithium, phenothiazines, β-blockers (including topical ophthalmic medications, such as timolol and betaxolol), quinine and antiarrhythmic agents.

Pearls and Considerations

- Ptosis and diplopia will eventually be present in 90% of MG patients
- Pupils react normally in ocular myasthenia patients
- Weakness may be first noticed in subclinical patients after undergoing general anesthesia.

Referral Information

If previously undiagnosed, refer to primary care physician for additional workup and treatment as indicated.

TREATMENT—cont'd

Nonpharmacologic Treatment

- *Plasmapheresis* (plasma exchange): rarely required for OMG.
- *Thymectomy:* not usually required in OMG without thymoma.

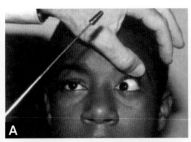
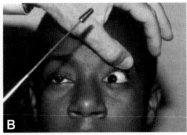
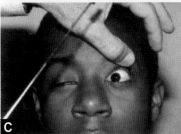

Figs 1A to C: (A) This child, age 10 years, presented with a right ptosis. His left eyelid is elevated by the examiner while he stares up without blinking; (B) Twenty seconds later, the right eyelid begins to "curtain"; (C) His eyelid position at 40 seconds demonstrates the eyelid fatigue consistent with myasthenia gravis.

GENERAL REFERENCES

Barton JJ, Fouladvand M. Ocular aspects of myasthenia gravis. Semin Neurol. 2000;20(1):7-20.

Elrod RD, Weinberg DA. Ocular myasthenia gravis. Ophthalmol Clin North Am. 2004;17(3):275-309.

Freidman DI. Disorders of the neuromuscular junction. In: Yanoff M, Duker JS (Eds). Ophthalmology. St Louis: Elsevier; 2006.

Gilbert ME, Savino PJ. Ocular myasthenia gravis. Int Ophthalmol Clin. 2007;47(4):93-103.

Haines SR, Thurtell MJ. Treatment of ocular myasthenia gravis. Curr Treat Options Neurol. 2012;14(1):103-12.

Mittal MK, Barohn RJ, Pasnoor M, et al. Ocular myasthenia gravis in an academic neuro-ophthalmology clinic: clinical features and therapeutic response. J Clin Neuromuscul Dis. 2011;13(1)46-52.

Vincent A, Palace J, Hilton-Jones D. Myasthenia gravis. Lancet. 2001;357 (9274):2122-8.

DIAGNOSIS

Definition

A blockage of the lacrimal drainage system due to a defect present at birth.

Synonyms

None

Symptoms

- Epiphora (Fig. 1)
- Decreased visual acuity
- Skin excoriation below the eyes.

Signs

- Elevated tear meniscus
- Epiphora
- Conjunctival injection
- Mucus and pus coming from the palpebral fissures.

Investigations

- *Dye-disappearance test*: instill fluorescein in conjunctivae, investigate with cobalt-blue light; fluorescein should clear tear film 2–5 minutes after instillation
- *Jones test 1*: retrieval of dye from the nose after above; proves system is open
- *Jones test 2*: irrigate dye from conjunctiva, anesthetize cornea; cannulate sac and irrigate; retrieval of dye from nose proves dye reached lacrimal sac; difficult in children
- *Sinus radiography*: shows bony abnormalities
- *Microscintigraphy*: ^{99}Tc instilled in conjunctiva; serial photographs made with microcollimator over time; useful for evaluating efficiency of lacrimal pump
- Diagnostic probing: discloses areas of obstruction and narrowing
- Dacryocystography: water-soluble contrast material (Renografin-C) irrigated into canaliculi and films taken; both tear drainage systems can be simultaneously evaluated (Figs 2 and 3)
- Nuclear magnetic resonance scanning: reserved for unusual cases (e.g. post-traumatic obstruction, craniofacial anomalies).

Differential Diagnosis

- *Congenital glaucoma*: typically with enlarged corneas and Haab Striae
- Bacterial/viral conjunctivitis
- Corneal abrasion.

Causes

- Imperforate membrane of Hasner
- Canalicular atresia
- Compression by nasal hemangioma
- In adults, can be caused by canaliculitis (*Actinomyces sp.*) and punctal stenosis.

Epidemiology

- Six to twenty percent of neonates are born with symptoms of nasolacrimal duct obstruction
- Ninety percent have spontaneous resolution by 1 year of age.

Associated Features

- Trauma to the nasal canthus
- Craniofacial anomalies
- Nasal hemangiomas.

Pathology

Pathology depends on cause of obstruction. Most children will have membrane at lower end of lacrimal duct or atresia of part of the tear drainage system. Most adults will have traumatic destruction of part of system, tumor infiltration, or bacterial inflammations of sac or duct.

Diagnosis continued on p. 304

TREATMENT

Diet and Lifestyle

No special precautions are necessary.

Pharmacologic Treatment

Broad-spectrum antibiotics help control the bacterial load, but do not affect opening of the system.

Treatment Aims

- To prevent infection
- To achieve a patent nasolacrimal drainage system.

Prognosis

Typically good, once system is patent

Follow-up and Management

- Probing is typically deferred until 1 year of age unless symptoms significant
- Occasionally, the system may have scarring and fibrosis requiring further intervention.

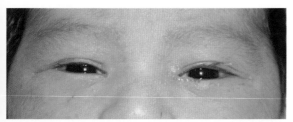

Fig. 1: Epiphora secondary to obstruction of nasolacrimal duct. (*Source*: http://newborns.stanford.edu/images/dacro2.jpg).

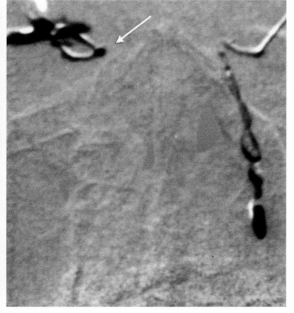

Fig. 2: Dacryocystogram. Complete obstruction of the lacrimal drainage pathways at the medial common canalicular level on the right side.

303

Treatment continued on p. 305

DIAGNOSIS—cont'd

Complications

- Dacrocystitis (Fig. 4)
- Orbital cellulitis
- Permanent strictures
- Facial fistulae
- Recurrent conjunctivitis.

Pearls and Considerations

- Ninety percent resolve spontaneously by 1 year of age
- Probing cures 95% of nasolacrimal duct obstructions.

Commonly Associated Conditions

- Craniofacial anomalies
- Nasal hemangioma
- Previous trauma to the nasal canthal area.

Referral Information

- Pediatric ophthalmologist for assessment
- Probing and surgical intervention as needed.

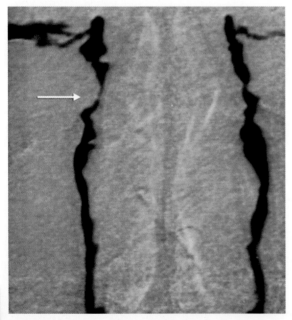

Fig. 3: Dacryocystogram. Medial deflection of contrast material within the right sac indicates sac stones.

TREATMENT—cont'd

Nonpharmacologic Treatment

- Lacrimal sac massage, following with topical antibiotic, can help control bacterial load
- Balloon dilation of the nasolacrimal system has shown promise in children who have difficult probing history; some surgeons perform as a first procedure
- Irrigation and probing of tearing children at approximately 1 year of age, or sooner if recurrent conjunctivitis, orbital cellulitis, or dacryocystitis occurs; perform twice, with infracturing of the inferior nasal turbinate if repeated; usually performed in an operating room, may be performed in an office
- *Intubation of system*: with silastic tube stents that remain for 6 months to 1 year
- *Dacryocystorhinostomy*: if silastic intubation fails
- *Conjunctivodacryocystorhinostomy*: in patients without patent canaliculi.

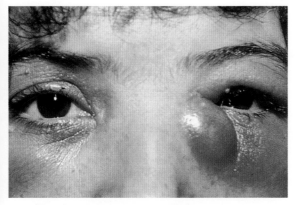

Fig. 4: Swelling, redness, and pain secondary to acute dacrocystitis.

GENERAL REFERENCES

Bashour M. (2005) Nasolacrimal duct, congenital anomalies. [online] Available from www.emedicine.com.

Druse F, Hand SI, Ellis FD, et al. Silicone intubation in children with nasolacrimal obstruction. J Pediatr Ophthalmol Strabismus. 1982;17:389-93.

Hornblass A, Ingis TM. Lacrimal function tests. Arch Ophthalmol. 1979;97: 1654-8.

Kushner BJ. Congenital nasolacrimal system obstruction. Arch Ophthalmol. 1982;100:597-601.

MacEwen CJ, Young JD. The fluorescein disappearance test: an evaluation of its use in infants. J Pediatr Ophthalmol Strabismus. 1991;28:302-28.

Massaro BM, Gonnering RS, Harris GJ. Endonasal lacrimal dacryostorhinostomy: a new approach to nasolacrmial duct obstruction. Arch Ophthalmol. 1990; 108:1172-6.

Pediatric Eye Disease Investigator Group, Repka MX, Chandler DL, et al. Repeat probing for treatment of persistent nasolacrimal duct obstruction. J AAPOS. 2009;13(3):306-7.

Pediatric Eye Disease Investigator Group, Repka MX, Melia BM, et al. Primary treatment of nasolacrimal duct obstruction with balloon catheter dilation in children younger than 4 years of age. J AAPOS. 2008;12(5):451-5.

Repka MX, Chandler DL, Holmes JM, et al. Balloon catheter dilation and nasolacrimal duct intubation for treatment of nasolacrimal duct obstruction after failed probing. Arch Ophthalmol. 2009;127(5):633-9.

Nystagmus, Congenital (379.51)

DIAGNOSIS

Definition

- Rhythmic oscillation of one or both eyes that are usually involuntary and either sensory or motor in etiology
- It is a high-frequency, horizontal nystagmus that begins in the first few months of life.

Symptoms

- Photophobia
- Decreased vision
- Unsteady eye movements or head posturing.

Signs

- Rhythmic eye movements that maintain the same plane in all gaze positions
- Strabismus and head positions.

Investigations (Fig. 1)

- Age of onset
- Family history
- Medication or illicit drug use by mother
- Systemic and neurologic evaluation for anomalies, developmental delay, and hypotony
- Evaluation looking for media opacities, strabismus, and head positions
- Urine catecholamines
- Brain magnetic resonance imaging (MRI), electroretinography (ERG), and eye movement recording
- *Complete eye examination*: with special attention to iris transillumination, optic nerve hypoplasia or atrophy, perimacular depigmentation, aniridia, foveal aplasia, decreased skin or choroidal pigmentation, severely decreased or absent color vision discrimination.

Complications

- In Aniridia, 40% of patients develop glaucoma
- In congenital cone dystrophy—photophobia
- In optic nerve hypoplasia—hypopituitarism and cerebral deformity
- Decreased binocular visual acuity of 20/200 at distance and 20/30 at near.

Pearls and Considerations

- Time of onset is usually 2–3 months and before 6 months of age
- Often associated with ocular albinism
- Sensory defect nystagmus refers to visual disorders.

Commonly Associated Conditions

Congenital cone dystrophy, optic nerve hypoplasia, aniridia, albinism, bilateral macular lesions, kernicterus, achromatopsia, midline anomalies of central nervous system, cerebellar or brainstem hypoplasia.

Referral Information

No referral is necessary.

Differential Diagnosis

- Congenital/infantile nystagmus
- If due to vision deprivation before 2 years of age, consider:
  - Corneal opacity, cataract, glaucoma
  - Retinal diseases
  - Optic nerve diseases
- *Latent nystagmus*: usually associated with strabismus and affected by monocular occlusion
- *Spasmus nutans*: onset in first year of life in healthy children. Typically a high frequency nystagmus confused with chiasmal, suprachiasmal, or third ventricle glioma.
- Gaze-evoked nystagmus
- Vestibular diseases
- Toxins and drugs such as alcohol, lithium, and antiseizure medications.

Causes

- The cause is not truly understood when the globes are anatomically normal; may represent inaccuracy in the eye's positional feedback loop ("leaky integrator"). Most patients who have congenital nystagmus have decreased visual acuity at distance.
- Patients who have aniridia have increased chiasmal decussation, which may contribute to unsteady eye movements.

Epidemiology

- Congenital is the most common form, comprising nearly 80% of all nystagmus
- Incidence: 1 in 2850 live births
- Prevalence: 0.5% including those associated with strabismus and other diseases
- No race or gender predilection.

Pathology

- *Congenital cone dystrophy*: aberrant retinal cone receptors
- *Optic nerve hypoplasia*: missing ganglion cell fibers in all amounts
- *Achromatopsia*: aberrant retinal cone receptors
- *Aniridia*: remnant of iris root usually detectable on gonioscopy; optic nerve hypoplasia typically found; often a large vessel crosses the usual macular location, absent foveal depression.

TREATMENT

Diet and Lifestyle

- Many patients who have congenital nystagmus have photophobia and benefit from sunglasses and wide-brimmed hats
- Patients with albinism have increased incidence of skin cancer and must wear ultraviolet-ray protective lotion when outdoors.

Pharmacologic Treatment

Baclofen and tegretol benefit some patients with periodic alternating nystagmus.

Nonpharmacologic Treatment

- Surgery is the mainstay of treatment for patients who have significant reproducible head postures caused by eccentric null points
- *Kestenbaum procedure*: generally requires surgery on muscles in both eyes; may be used for patients with horizontal, vertical, or oblique null points; often improves visual acuity
- Creation of exotropia with medial rectus recessions in both eyes: stimulation of convergence may dampen nystagmus
- Recession of four horizontal rectus muscles in patients who have horizontal null point: usually does not improve visual acuity, but patients find viewing target easier; perhaps eyes spend more time in primary position.

Treatment Aims

- Improve visual acuity
- Decreased asthenopia
- Remove head postures.

Prognosis

Visual acuity does not improve with age, although amplitude and frequency of the nystagmus do improve.

Follow-up and Management

- Patients who have suspected spasmus nutans must have intracranial scanning to rule out chiasmatic and hypothalamic gliomas
- Patients who have sporadic aniridia must have abdominal scanning and examination to rule out Wilms tumor. They should be examined every few months to rule out filtration-angle obstruction and glaucoma.

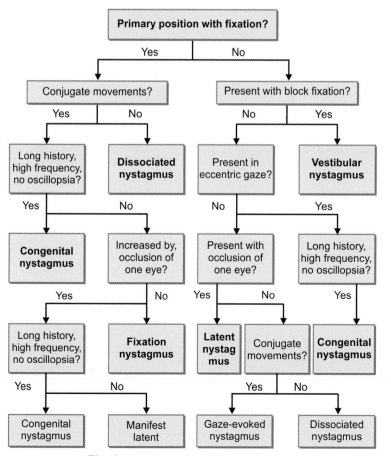

Fig. 1: Identification of types of nystagmus.

GENERAL REFERENCES

Abadi RV, Whittle J. The nature of head postures in congenital nystagmus. Arch Ophthalmol. 1991;109:216-20.

Abadi RV, Whittle JP, Worfolk R. Oscillopsia and tolerance to retinal image movement in congenital nystagmus. Invest Ophthalmol Vis Sci. 1999; 40(2): 339-45.

Dell'Osso LF, Flynn JT. Congenital nystagmus surgery: a quantitative evaluation of the effects. Arch Ophthalmol. 1979;97: 462-8.

Roussi M, Dalens H, Marcellier JJ, et al. Congenital nystagmus and negative electroretinography. Clin Ophthalmol. 2011; 5:429-34. Epub 2011.

Weiss AH, Kelly JP. Acuity development in infantile nystagmus. Invest Ophthalmol Vis Sci. 2007;48(9): 4093-9.

Yee RD. Nystagmus and saccadic intrusions and oscillations. In: Yanoff M, Duker JS (Eds). Ophthalmology. St Louis: Elsevier; 2006.

Zubcov AA, Stark N, Weber A, et al. Improvement of visual acuity after surgery for nystagmus. Ophthalmology. 1993;100:1488.

Oblique Muscle Dysfunctions and Dissociated Vertical Deviation (378.31)

DIAGNOSIS

Definition

Dysfunction of the inferior or superior oblique muscle is enough to cause measurable deviation.

Epidemiology

- *Inferior oblique overaction*: noted in 72% of patients who have early-onset esotropia, 35% of those who have accommodative esotropia and intermittent exotropia
- *Dissociated vertical deviation (DVD)*: noted in 75% of patients who have early-onset esotropia, 15% of those who have accommodative esotropia, and 10% of those who have intermittent exotropia.

Synonyms

None

Symptoms

- *Oblique muscle dysfunction*: diplopia and blurry vision
- *Dissociated vertical deviation*: typically asymptomatic due to limited binocular vision during DVD movement.

Signs (Figs 1 to 3)

Oblique Muscle Dysfunctions

- Inferior oblique overaction (overelevation in adduction)
- Inferior oblique underaction (underelevation in adduction)
- Superior oblique overaction (overdepression in adduction)
- Superior oblique underaction (underelevation in adduction).

Dissociated Vertical Deviation

- Elevation, abduction, and extorsion in nonfixing eye
- Present in primary position
- Not associated with V-Pattern.

Investigations

Oblique Muscle Deviations

- Gaze measurements in all positions
- Measurements of ocular torsion
- Evaluation of any cyclovertical palsy.

Dissociated Vertical Deviation

Gaze measurements in all positions.

Differential Diagnosis

- Congenital esotropia
- Monofixational syndrome
- Amblyopia.

Causes

Oblique Muscle Dysfunction

Primary: Unknown
Secondary:
- *Inferior oblique overaction*: ipsilateral superior oblique or contralateral superior rectus palsy
- *Superior oblique overaction*: ipsilateral inferior oblique or contralateral inferior rectus palsy.

Dissociated vertical deviation: Unknown

Epidemiology

- Congenital is the most common form, comprising nearly 80% of all nystagmus
- *Incidence*: 1 in 2850 live births
- *Prevalence*: 0.5% including those associated with strabismus and other diseases
- No race or gender predilection.

Diagnosis continued on p. 310

TREATMENT

Diet and Lifestyle

No special precautions necessary.

Pharmacologic Treatment

No pharmacologic treatment is recommended.

Treatment Aims
- Achieve straight primary gaze positions
- Decrease the degree of strabismus and improved appearance.

Prognosis
Strabismus surgery is typically very successful.

Follow-up and Management
Specific to each clinical situation.

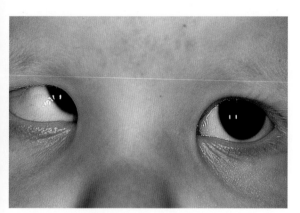

Fig. 1: Right eye inferior oblique overaction and overelevation in adduction.

Treatment continued on p. 311

Oblique Muscle Dysfunctions and Dissociated Vertical Deviation (378.31)

DIAGNOSIS—cont'd

Complications

- Inability to achieve single binocular vision
- Amblyopia
- Development of head postures/torticollis and neck contracture.

Pearls and Considerations

- Dissociated vertical deviation is present in all gaze positions
- Dissociated vertical deviation is not associated with an A- or V-pattern.

Commonly Associated Conditions

Oblique Muscle Deviations

- Oblique overaction results in abduction movement in extreme elevation or depression
- Underacting oblique results in deficiency of eye movements in extreme elevation or depression
- A-pattern in superior oblique overaction or inferior oblique underaction.

Dissociated vertical deviation

Very few patients have globe depression with loss of fusion.

Referral Information

Surgical evaluation is suggested.

TREATMENT—cont'd

Nonpharmacologic Treatment

- *Inferior oblique overaction*: inferior oblique recession, myectomy
- *Inferior oblique underaction*: superior oblique tuck
- *Superior oblique overaction*: superior oblique tendon recession, lengthening or tenotomy
- *Superior oblique underaction*: superior oblique tendon tuck, Harada-Ito procedure.

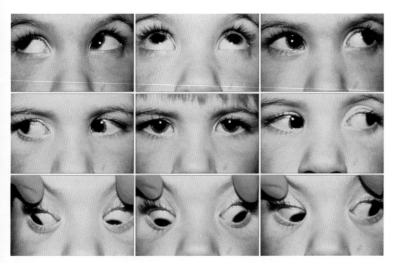

Fig. 2: Child who has bilateral superior oblique overaction, overdepression in adduction, and an A-pattern exotropia.

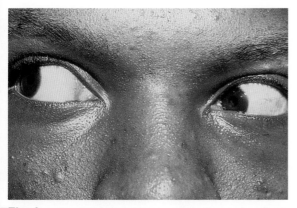

Fig. 3: Left eye inferior oblique underaction and underelevation in adduction. This must be differentiated from the more common Brown's vertical retraction syndrome.

GENERAL REFERENCES

Boylan C, Clement RA, Howrie A. Normal visual pathway routing in dissociated vertical deviation. Invest Ophthalmol Vis Sci. 1988;29(7):1165-7.

Diamond GR. Esotropia. In: Yanoff M, Duker JS (Eds). Ophthalmology. St Louis: Elsevier; 2006.

Gobin MH. Sagitallization of the oblique muscles as a possible cause for the "A", "V", and "X" phenomena. Br J Ophthalmol. 1968;52:13.

Kushner BJ. Effect of ocular torsion on A and V patterns and apparent oblique muscle overaction. Arch Ophthalmol. 2010;128(6):712-8.

Kushner BJ. Incomitant strabismus: does extraocular muscle form denote function? Arch Ophthalmol. 2010;128(12):1604-9.

MacDonald AL, Pratt-Johnson JA. The suppression patterns and sensory adaptations to dissociated vertical divergent strabismus. Can J Ophthalmol. 1974;9:113.

Sprague JB, Moore S, Eggers HM, et al. Dissociated vertical deviation: with the Faden operation of Cuppers. Arch Ophthalmol. 1980;98:465.

Wilson ME, Parks MM. Primary inferior oblique overaction in congenital esotropia, accommodative esotropia, and intermittent exotropia. Ophthalmology. 1989;96:7.

Oculosympathetic Paresis (Horner's Syndrome) (337.9)

DIAGNOSIS

Definition

A condition arising from interruption of sympathetic innervation to the eye and presenting with miosis, partial ptosis, and loss of hemifacial sweating.

Synonyms

Horner-Bernard syndrome; Horner's ptosis; oculosympathetic paresis usually abbreviated OSP.

Symptoms

- *Ptosis of 2–3 mm*: can be variable
- *Inverse ptosis of 1–2 mm*: creating the illusion of enophthalmos
- Miosis
- *Anhidrosis*: occasionally helpful when the patient is questioned about perspiration or skin temperature during exercise
- Horner's syndrome refers to the triad of ptosis, miosis and anhidrosis
- Oculosympathetic paresis can be applied to ptosis and miosis
- Neck pain (history of neck trauma or manipulation, e.g. by chiropractor).

Signs (Fig. 1)

- *Subtle ptosis*: without the loss of the eyelid crease
- *Miosis creating an anisocoria*: greater in dim than bright illumination
- Less helpful signs include an increased amplitude of accommodation, transient decrease in intraocular pressure, and change in tear viscosity.

Investigations

In darkness, a paretic dilator will dilate the pupil at a slower rate than a normal pupil, called "dilation lag". Therefore, look for an anisocoria that is greater at 4–5 sec than at 10–12 sec into darkness.

Apraclonidine Ophthalmic Solution: Current Test of Choice

- Apraclonidine ophthalmic solution of 0.5% (weak alpha1-agonist and a strong alpha 2-agonist) is used as a supersensitivity test. The denervation supersensitivity in Horner's syndrome results in pupillary dilatation and lid elevation on the abnormal side, but no response or mild miosis on the normal side from alpha2-activity following apraclonidine.
- Readily available, and good sensitivity of about 87%. Mydriatic effect on abnormal pupil easier to interpret than other tests
- Upregulation of alpha1-receptors may take 5–8 days; in acute cases, a negative apraclonidine test does not exclude Horner's, and a cocaine test should be considered.

Cocaine Ophthalmic Solution

- Cocaine ophthalmic solution of 4–10% (indirect sympathomimetic agent) is also used as a supersensitivity test. (This test is less effective in darkly pigmented patients. The cocaine solution must be instilled onto untouched corneas.) After instilling equal drops into both eyes, an OSP pupil will not dilate to cocaine, whereas a normal eye will enlarge. A postcocaine anisocoria of 0.5 mm suggests that the odds of an OSP are 77:1; less than 0.8 mm of anisocoria translates to a 1054:1 chance of OSP; and 1 mm of anisocoria means a 5990:1 chance of OSP.
- *Disadvantages*: availability, controlled substance, metabolites detectable in urine (should warn patient of this prior to instilling).

Differential Diagnosis

- Congenital ptosis with physiologic anisocoria
- Dermatochalasis with physiologic anisocoria
- History of chest, neck, and otolaryngologic procedures (e.g. chest tube; botox injections for glabellar lines)
- Tonic pupil
- Argyll-Robertson pupil
- Cluster headache.

Cause

- In adults, 40% of OSP is idiopathic, whereas 8% is neoplastic. Neoplasm is the presenting sign in only 3%
- Eighteen percent of children with neuroblastoma manifest OSP. It is the presenting sign in only 2%. Other causes include benign tumors (e.g. neurofibromas), iatrogenic, idiopathic and congenital.

Specific Causes According to the "Three-Neuron Chain"

Central (First-Order Neuron)
- Brainstem glioma
- Syringomyelia
- Tumor (hypothalamus, brainstem, cervicothoracic spinal cord)
- Wallenberg's syndrome
- Stroke (hypothalamus, brainstem)
- Arteriovenous malformation.

Preganglionic (Second-Order Neuron)
- Cervical trauma
- Cervical arthritis
- Poliomyelitis
- Neural crest tumors
- Pneumothorax
- Lung tumor (typically, apical "Pancoast" tumor)
- Cervical rib
- Intrathoracic aneurysm
- Neoplasm of thyroid gland or other neck structures.

Postganglionic (Third-Order Neuron)
- Cluster headache
- Tumor (nasopharyngeal carcinoma, lymphoma)
- Otitis media
- Internal carotid artery disease (thrombosis, aneurysm, trauma, dissection)
- Cavernous sinus syndrome.

Diagnosis continued on p. 314

TREATMENT

Diet and Lifestyle

No special precautions are necessary.

Pharmacologic Treatment

2.5% phenylephrine, or apraclonidine (iopidine) 0.5%, three times daily.

Nonpharmacologic Treatment

No nonpharmacologic treatment is recommended.

Complications

- Heterochromia iridis in children younger than age 2 (iris pigmentation is under sympathetic control during early childhood development), straighter hair on side of OSP, or lower brachial plexus palsy (Klumpke's paralysis) all support a congenital cause.
- Oculosympathetic paresis may be component of telodiencephalic, Foville's or Wallenberg's syndrome. OSP with a contralateral fourth-nerve paresis suggest a brainstem lesion. Hoarseness and hiccupping in a woman with OSP suggest involvement of the phrenic nerve and recurrent laryngeal nerve from breast cancer at sixth cervical level.

Treatment Aims

- Ptosis repair
- Exclusion of life-threatening causes of OSP.

Prognosis

Variable

313

Treatment continued on p. 315

Oculosympathetic Paresis (Horner's Syndrome) (337.9)

DIAGNOSIS—cont'd

Paredrine Ophthalmic Solution

Warning! Do not instill paredrine until 48 hours after instilling cocaine.

- Paredrine ophthalmic solution 1% (hydroxyamphetamine) offers anatomic localization either above or below the level of the mandible (head or chest)
- If the OSP miotic pupil does not dilate to paredrine, the lesion is "third order", or postganglionic, and above the level of the mandible
- If the OSP miotic pupil does dilate to paredrine, the lesion is preganglionic, or "first and second order", and below the level of the mandible
- Other pupils that do not dilate well to paredrine include an iris affected by trans-synaptic dysgenesis, those of darkly-pigmented patients, and dark irides. The diagnostic specificity of paredrine is 84% for third-order OSP and 97% for first- and second-order OSP. If the postparedrine anisocoria is 1 mm, there is an 85% probability for third-order OSP. If there is 2 mm of postparedrine anisocoria, there is a 99% probability of OSP.
- Anhidrosis has been employed for anatomic localization of the lesion. If the forehead is hypohidrotic, the lesion is in the head. If the face and cheek are hypohidrotic, the lesion is in the chest. (If the lesion is in the spinal cord, the face and upper half of body become hypohidrotic. If the lesion causing the OSP is in the brainstem, there is anhidrosis over half the face and body).

Other

- Always review old photographs for long-standing ptosis and anisocoria
- A computed tomography (CT) scan of the head and neck is indicated
- Also, in children, obtain 24-hour vanillylmandelic acid levels. *Every child with a "congenital Horner's" should be screened for a neuroblastoma*
- Depending on symptoms and signs, may need magnetic resonance imaging (MRI), with and without gadolinium contrast, of brain, neck, upper part of chest, C- and T-spine, and lung or a mammogram
- Angiography (catheter digital subtraction versus magnetic resonance angiography with fat suppression) of carotid artery, particularly in painful Horner's.

Pearls and Considerations

- Facial flushing may be present with preganglionic lesions, whereas ipsilateral orbital pain or migraine-like headache may be present in postganglionic lesions
- Most patients presenting with Horner's syndrome in isolation without additional clinical features will have a postganglionic lesion or idiopathic etiology.

Referral Information

Refer for imaging studies to help elucidate organic cause.

TREATMENT—cont'd

- *Painful OSP* is seen in carotid artery dissection, otitis media, cavernous sinus syndrome, and cluster headache. OSP with an earache suggests carotid artery dissection or otitis media. A neck ache and dysgeusia imply a carotid dissection. OSP that occurs with a headache, red eye and stuffy nose could be a cluster headache.
- Oculosympathetic paresis and ipsilateral shoulder, arm and chest pain suggest an apical pulmonary sulcus tumor (Pancoast's syndrome)
- Hoarseness and hiccuping suggest Vernet's syndrome or phrenic nerve syndrome
- Diplopia and an OSP suggest a cavernous sinus syndrome.

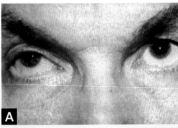
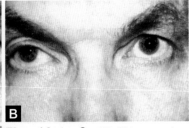
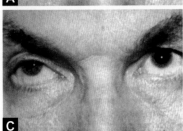

Figs 1A to C: (A) This man has Horner's syndrome in his right eye; (B) Anisocoria is more conspicuous in dark illumination; (C) Anisocoria 45 minutes after cocaine drop instillation; notice how the normal left pupil has dilated to cocaine, whereas the right pupil is unchanged, creating a greater postcocaine anisocoria.

GENERAL REFERENCES

Jeret JS, Bluth M. Stroke following chiropractic manipulation: report of 3 cases and review of the literature. Cerebrovasc Dis. 2002; 13(3):210-3.

George A, Haydar AA, Adams WM. Imaging of Horner's syndrome. Clin Radiol. 2008;63(5):499-505.

Orssaud C, Roche O, Renard G, et al. Carotid artery dissection revealed by an oculosympathetic spasm. J Emerg Med. 2010;39(5):586-8.

Parmar MS. (2012). Horner syndrome. [Online] Available from www.emedicine.com.

Patel S, Ilsen PF. Acquired Horner's syndrome: clinical review. Optometry. 2003;74(4):245-56.

Robertson WC, Pettigrew LC. "Congenital" Horner's syndrome and carotid dissection. J Neuroimaging. 2003;13(4): 367-70.

Walton KA, Buono LM. Horner's syndrome. Curr Opin Ophthalmol. 2003;14(6): 357-63.

Ophthalmia Neonatorum (771.6)

DIAGNOSIS

Definition

Conjunctivitis of the newborn is defined as any conjunctivitis that occurs within the first 4 weeks of life.

Synonyms

Neonatal conjunctivitis

Symptoms

Irritability

Signs (Figs 1 and 3)

* *Neisserial*: purulent discharge, injection, possible corneal ulcer (*Neisseria gonorrheae*)
* *Chlamydial*: watery or purulent discharge, injection, pseudomembranes
* *Herpes*: watery discharge, injection, lid vesicles
* *Chemical*: watery discharge, injection.

Investigations

* History of sexually transmitted infections in parents
* Tissue stains and cultures (Fig. 2)
* *Neisseria*: pneumonia, meningitis, sepsis
* *Chlamydial*: pneumonia, rhinitis, nasopharyngitis, tracheitis, otitis media
* *Herpes*: chorioretinitis, encephalitis.

Complications

* *Neisseria*: possible penetration of intact corneal epithelium
* *Chlamydial*: self-limited, but may result in peripheral pannus and scarring
* *Herpes*: corneal scarring and vascularization
* *Chemical*: self-limited, no sequelae.

Differential Diagnosis

* Nasolacrimal duct obstruction
* Neonatal blepharitis/blepharoconjunctivitis
* Diffuse retinoblastoma
* Neonatal leukemia with ocular involvement
* Uveitis due to prenatal infection
* Epiphora due to glaucoma.

Cause

* *Neisseria*: lids are very puffy and occurs between 3 and 6 days
* *Chlamydial*: occurs between 5 and 10 days
* *Herpes*: unilateral and occurs at 7–10 days or later
* *Chemical*: from 1% silver nitrate and generally from birth to 3 days.

Epidemiology

* *Gonococcal*: 0.3/1000 births
* *Chlamydial*: 8.2/1,000 births
* *Developing countries*: 15–60% of live births.

Pathology

* Inoculated by maternal or iatrogenic routes
* Due to deficient infant immune defense mechanism.

Diagnosis continued on p. 318

TREATMENT

Diet and Lifestyle

Prenatal care and treatment of maternal infections can prevent newborn infection.

Pharmacologic Treatment

- *Bacterial*: Penicillin G 50,000 U/Kg IM or IV every 12 hours
- *Chlamydial*: Erythromycin 40 mg/kg/day PO for 2–3 weeks
- *Herpes*: Topical vidaribine 9x daily.

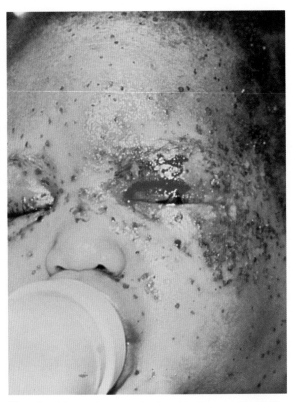

Fig. 1: Primary herpes simplex blepharoconjunctivitis. Note the bilateral vesicular eruptions in this child who has a primary herpes simplex infection.

Treatment continued on p. 319

Ophthalmia Neonatorum (771.6)

DIAGNOSIS—cont'd

Pearls and Considerations

- Length of exposure is an important factor in developing conjunctivitis from the infectious organisms present in the birth canal
- Most common cause in the US is *Chlamydial trachomatis.*

Commonly Associated Conditions

- Maternal infections
- Premature or prolonged rupture of placental membranes
- *Gentamicin toxicity*: lid skin erosions.

Referral Information

Cornea consult if perforation or impending perforation.

TREATMENT—cont'd

Nonpharmacologic Treatment

Neisseria: Admit to Hospital

- Lavage secretions hourly
- Work-up for other concomitant sexually transmitted diseases
- Referral for parental treatment of subsequent conditions.

Chlamydia: Outpatient Management

Consider presence of other sexually transmitted diseases.

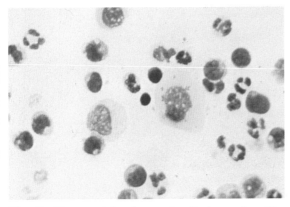

Fig. 2: Giemsa stain of a conjunctival scraping. The epithelial cells show basophilic cytoplasmic inclusions typical of a chlamydial infection.

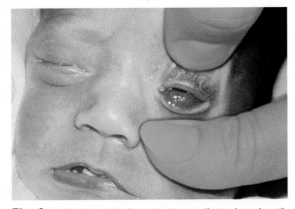

Fig. 3: A 10-day-old infant who has unilateral conjunctivitis. The mother had an untreated chlamydial infection of the birth canal.

GENERAL REFERENCES

Dinsmoor MJ. Ophthalmia neonatorum. Contemp Obstet Gynecol. 1992;37: 112-8.

Prentice MJ, Hitchinson GR, Taylor-Robinson D. A microbiological study of neonatal conjunctivae and conjunctivitis. Br J Ophthalmol. 1977;61:601-12.

Rubenstein JB, Jick SL. Disorders of the conjunctiva and limbus. In: Yanoff M, Duker JS (Eds). Ophthalmology. St. Louis: Elsevier; 2006.

Rudd P. Diagnosis of ophthalmia neonatorum. Br Med J (Clin Res Ed). 1988; 296(6616):212.

Sandstrom I, Kallings I, Melen B. Neonatal chlamydial conjunctivitis. Acta Pediatr Scand. 1988;77:207-12.

Simon JW. Povidone-iodine prophylaxis of ophthalmia neonatorum. Br J Ophthalmol. 2003;87(12):1437.

Thygesen. Historical review of oculogenital disease. Am J Ophthalmol. 1971; 71:975-81.

Vedanta V. Prophylaxis of ophthalmia neonatorum. Br J Ophthalmol. 2004;88 (10):1352.

Optic Neuritis (377.3)

DIAGNOSIS

Definition

Demyelinating inflammation of the optic nerve of unknown etiology.

Synonyms

None; typically abbreviated ON (optic neuritis).

Symptoms

- *Blurred, painful vision*: in 92.2% of patients
- *Pain on eye movement*: before, during and after visual loss
- *Positive visual phenomenon*: photopsias on eye movement or auditory-induced
- Photophobia
- *Depth perception difficulties*: Pulfrich stereo phenomenon
- Uhtoff's phenomenon.

Signs (Fig. 1)

- Relative afferent pupillary defect
- *Reduced Snellen acuity*: the initial median of ON patients is 20/50; ~10% of ON patients have Snellen acuity of 20/20; ~15% have acuity of finger counting or worse
- *Visual field loss*: can be diffuse (50%) or local (50%); local defects include altitudinal (29.2%), three-quadrant involvement (14.6%), quadrant (13.2%), hemianopic (11.1%), centrocecal (8.3%), arcuate (6.3%), and other (17.3%); 48% of fellow eyes have an abnormal visual field.
- Decreased contrast sensitivity (may be more sensitive measure of residual functional damage than automated perimetry)
- Dyschromatopsia
- Reduced brightness sense
- Nerve fiber bundle defects
- *Retrobulbar ON*: 65% of patients
- *Papillitis*: 35% of patients
- *Peripapillary hemorrhage*: infrequent; 6% of patients
- *Multiple sclerosis (MS)*: associated with anterior uveitis and pars planitis
- Systemic neurologic abnormality.

Differential Diagnosis

- *Idiopathic*: most common
- Ischemic optic neuropathy
- Multiple sclerosis (demyelinating disease)
- Sarcoid
- Systemic lupus erythematosus
- Wegener's syndrome
- Syphilis
- Sjögren's syndrome
- Dysthyroid optic neuropathy
- Cytomegalovirus
- Leber's mitochondrial optic neuropathy
- Lyme disease
- Leprosy
- Cat-scratch disease (*Bartonella henselae*)
- Acute zonal occult outer retinopathy
- Mucocele
- Toxins associated with optic neuropathy (e.g. carbon monoxide, ethylene glycol, perchloroethylene, methanol and tobacco)
- Drugs associated with optic neuropathy (e.g. ethambutol, clioquinol, isoniazid, amiodarone, linezolid, methotrexate, sildenafil, oxymetazoline, infliximab, chemotherapeutic agents, such as vincristine, cisplatin, carboplatin and paclitaxel).
- Nutritional deficiencies associated with optic neuropathy (e.g. vitamin B_{12} deficiency).

Cause

- Forme fruste of MS
- Optic neuritis demyelination.

Epidemiology

- Female/male ratio is 2:1
- Whites more affected than blacks
- Age of onset is 15–40 years (average, 30 years)
- Rapid decrease in visual acuity, with maximal visual deficit in ~5 days
- Incidence is 1–4:100,000 per year
- Environmental influence against background of genetic susceptibility.

Immunology

An autoimmune inflammatory cascade is believed to mediate myelin destruction in MS.

Diagnosis continued on p. 322

TREATMENT

Diet and Lifestyle

No special precautions are necessary.

Pharmacologic Treatment

Corticosteroids

- High-dose IV corticosteroids followed by a quick oral corticosteroid taper quickens visual recovery but has no effect on final visual outcome. A recent Cochrane meta-analysis and systematic review of six randomized controlled trials examining the use of corticosteroid therapy in ON also found no conclusive benefit in terms of final visual outcome. IV corticosteroid treatment does seem to reduce the risk of developing MS at 2 years.
- However, treatment of ON with oral prednisone more than doubles the risk of a new attack of ON (30%) in either the affected or the fellow eye. Thus, oral prednisone is relatively contraindicated in the treatment of ON.
- Treatment with IV methylprednisolone followed by oral prednisone halves the risk of developing a clinical attack of MS at 2 years in patients with a critical number of white-matter lesions.

Prognosis

Visual Recovery

- In most ON patients, as per the Optic Neuritis Treatment Trial, visual recovery begins rapidly within 3 weeks after the onset of symptoms with or without treatment. Visual recovery seems to plateau at 6 weeks but may continue to improve up to 1 year. At 5 years, 87% will have visual acuity of 20/25 or better, and 94% will have an acuity of 20/40 or better. Visual recovery is less evident in patients with finger-counting vision or worse. These patients have 20/40 acuity or better at 6 months. Although Snellen acuity may return to normal, many patients have subtle symptomatic visual deficits.
- The probability of experiencing a repeat attack of ON in the same eye or fellow eye is ~20% in 5 years.

Probability of Developing Clinically Definite Multiple Sclerosis

- Thirty percent chance of developing clinically definite MS at 5 years. Fifty percent chance at 15 years; the risk of developing MS is greatest within the first 5 years.
- Clinical features of ON associated with a low 5-year risk of developing clinically definite MS are absence of brain lesions on MRI; absence of pain; mild visual loss; and presence of optic disk edema, hemorrhage or exudate.
- High-signal abnormalities on brain MRI are the strongest predictor of developing MS. At 5 years the absence of lesions indicates a 16% chance of developing MS (which should not be misinterpreted to mean that MS will not develop). The presence of one or two lesions indicates a 37% risk (double the risk of those with no lesions); three or more lesions, a 51% risk.

Treatment continued on p. 323

Optic Neuritis (377.3)

DIAGNOSIS—cont'd

Investigations

- *Magnetic resonance imaging (MRI) of brain*: to detect high-signal white-matter abnormalities
- *Magnetic resonance imaging of orbit*: to rule out orbital lesions
- *Optical coherence tomography (OCT) of optic nerve*: retinal nerve fiber layer (RFNL) thickness reflects both disease activity and visual prognosis
- *Visual evoked potentials (VEPs)*: may be more sensitive than OCT in the early detection of ON
- *Lumbar puncture (LP)*: to detect oligoclonal bands.

Pearls and Considerations

- In all ON patients, MS must be considered
- About a third of ON patients will have papillitis presenting as diffuse edema of the optic nerve head
- Loss of vision from ON may be permanent.

Referral Information

Refer to neurologist for imaging and evaluation of possible MS or neuromyelitis optica (NMO).

TREATMENT—cont'd

Immunomodulators

Disease modifying drugs (DMDs) such as interferon-1a (Avonex®), interferon-1b (Betaseron®) and glatirimer acetate (Copaxone®) in patients at high risk of developing MS.

Others

Intravenous immunoglobulins (IVIG), plasmapharesis.

Nonpharmacologic Treatment

No nonpharmacologic treatment is recommended.

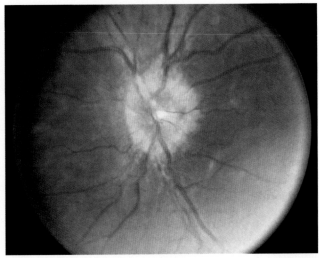

Fig. 1: Left eye of a woman aged 42 years who presented with painful visual loss, afferent pupillary defect, dyschromatopsia, and central and arcuate scotoma. Her disk edema is consistent with papillitis. This is distinguished from early papilledema by abnormal optic nerve function.

GENERAL REFERENCES

Arnold AC. Evolving management of optic neuritis and multiple sclerosis. Am J Ophthalmol. 2005;139(6):1101-8.

Balcer LJ, Calabresi PA, Frohman EM. Can retinal imaging accurately detect optic neuritis? Nat Rev Neurol. 2010;6(3):125.

Balcer LJ, Galetta SL. Treatment of acute demyelinating optic neuritis. Semin Ophthalmol. 2002;17(1):4-10.

Beck RW, Cleary PA, Anderson MM, et al. A randomized, controlled trial of corticosteroids in the treatment of optic neuritis. N Engl J Med. 1992;326:581-8.

Beck RW, Kupersmith MJ, Cleary PA, et al. Fellow eye abnormalities in acute unilateral optic neuritis. Ophthalmology. 1993;100:691-8.

Burton EV, Greenberg BM, Frohman EM. Optic neuritis: a mechanistic view. Pathophysiology. 2011;18(1):81-92.

Ergene E. (2004). Adult optic neuritis. [Online] Available from www.emedicine.com.

Gal RL, Vedula SS, Beck R. Corticosteroids for treating optic neuritis. Cochrane Database Syst Rev. 2012;4:CD001430.

Hoorbakht H, Bagherkashi F. Optic neuritis, its differential diagnosis and management. Open Ophthalmol J. 2012;6:65-72.

Levin A, Arnold A. Neuro-ophthalmology. New York: Thieme Medical; 2005.

Martinelli V, Bianchi Marzoli S. Non-demyelinating optic neuropathy: clinical entities. Neurol Sci. 2001;22(suppl 2):S55-9.

Optic Neuritis Study Group. Visual function 5 year after optic neuritis. Arch Ophthalmol. 1997;115:1545-52.

Petzold A, de Boer JF, Schippling S, et al. Optical coherence tomography in multiple sclerosis: a systematic review and meta-analysis. Lancet Neurol. 2010;9(9):921-32.

The Optic Neuritis Study Group. Multiple sclerosis risk after optic neuritis: final optic neuritis treatment trial follow-up. Arch Neurol. 2008;65(6):727-32.

Orbital Inflammation, Acute (376.0)

DIAGNOSIS

Definition

Acute inflammation of the anterior preseptal and/or posterior orbit.

Synonym

Preseptal cellulitis, orbital cellulitis.

Symptoms

Decreased vision: generally, mildly decreased vision is caused by abnormalities of the tear film secondary to the inflammation; rarely, a rapid loss of vision results from spread of the inflammation to the optic nerve.

Pain and redness: the area of cellulitis tends to be red, warm and painful (Fig. 1). *Swelling/pressure*: the swelling may be so severe as to cause complete closure of the eyelids; also, the swelling often crosses over to involve secondarily the eyelids on the uninvolved side.

Tearing

Blurred vision: the uninvolved contralateral eye may show blurred vision caused by secondary tearing and eyelid swelling.

Diplopia (double vision): decreased ocular motility results in strabismus and thus double vision.

Signs

- Redness of lids
- *Chemosis of conjunctiva*: may be so severe that the chemotic conjunctiva protrudes through the semiclosed eyelids
- *Lid swelling*: the patient may present with swelling to such a degree that complete closure of the eyelids occurs (Figs 2A and B)
- *Exophthalmos (ocular proptosis)*: inflammation posterior to the septum orbitale (i.e. postseptal extension) may cause exophthalmos, except in children less than 5 years of age, in whom exophthalmos does not occur
- *Ocular motility problems*: the orbital swelling and direct inflammation of the extraocular muscles may limit the mobility of the muscles resulting in strabismus and diplopia
- Appearance of acute systemic illness.

Investigations

History: especially of sinusitis, orbital trauma and systemic complaints.
Ocular examination:

- Complete ocular examination (if eyelids are swollen shut completely, local anesthesia may be necessary to examine the eyes adequately), exophthalmometry (measurement of exophthalmos by an exophthalmometer), intraocular pressure, undilated and dilated slit-lamp examinations, and dilated fundus examination.
- A dilated pupil, marked ophthalmoplegia, loss of vision and afferent pupillary defect are all warning signs of serious orbital cellulitis. Also, phycomycosis (usually *Mucor*) can present as an acute fulminating infection of the sinuses and orbit, generally in an acidotic or immunosuppressed patient.

Differential Diagnosis

Graves' disease, allergic reaction (angioneurotic edema), pseudotumor of orbit (*see* Orbital inflammation, chronic), Parinaud's oculoglandular syndrome (granulomatous conjunctivitis and ipsilateral enlargement of the preauricular lymph nodes), Wegener's granulomatosis, orbital mucocele, carotid cavernous fistula, orbital neoplasms.

Cause

- Most cases (> 60%) arise from infection of contiguous sinuses, especially ethmoiditis and especially in children
- The most common cause of infectious orbital cellulitis in children is *Haemophilus influenzae*. In adults, the most common causes are *Staphylococcus* and *Streptococcus* spp.; it can be secondary to trauma, upper respiratory infection, dental abscess and many other systemic infections.

Epidemiology

Acute orbital inflammation is rare but extremely important because it is potentially life threatening.

Classification

Preseptal inflammation [orbital cellulitis (376.1)]: inflammation contained anterior to the septum orbitale, mainly limited to lids and superficial tissue.
Postseptal extension: inflammation extends posterior to the septum orbitale into orbital tissues.

Associated Features

- Fever, leukocytosis
- With posterior spread, signs and symptoms of orbital apex syndrome, cavernous sinus thrombosis, or meningitis may develop.

Pathology

- An acute inflammatory reaction characterized by neutrophils, and necrosis is seen
- Special stains may show a bacterial cause, most often *Staphylococcus aureus* and *Streptococcus* spp.

Diagnosis continued on p. 326

TREATMENT

Diet and Lifestyle

In general, patients who have acute orbital inflammation (most prevalent in children) tend to be acutely ill. Bed rest, warm compresses and a light diet generally supplement the parenteral antibiotics.

Pharmacologic Treatment

Antibiotic Therapy

- Any purulent material should be cultured
- Most children need systemic antibiotic therapy. The type of antibiotic used depends on such factors as the Gram-stained appearance of the organism, physician protocol for orbital cellulitis and results of culture.
- In adults, Gram-stained sections of any purulent material are the best guide to antibiotic therapy. Most physicians start with a broad-spectrum antibiotic while they await the results of culture and sensitivity.
- If cavernous sinus thrombosis is imminent or present, prompt systemic antibiotic therapy can be life saving.

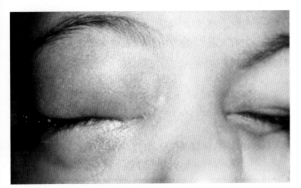

Fig. 1: This child has swollen red eyelids (cellulitis) of her right eye caused by acute ethmoiditis.

Treatment Aims

- *To preserve vision and ocular function*: the key to visual and ocular rehabilitation is prompt therapy; other specialists (e.g. pediatricians, otolaryngologists, oral surgeons, internists) may need to be consulted.
- *To prevent posterior spread of infection to avoid complications such as orbital apex syndrome, cavernous sinus thrombosis, or meningitis*: in the case of posterior spread of the inflammation toward the orbital apex, prompt antibiotic therapy can be life saving.
- *To identify and treat any underlying systemic disease*: particularly important in phycomycosis, which is often accompanied by systemic acidosis; the acidosis can be caused by diabetes mellitus, chronic diarrhea and conditions that cause immunosuppression.

Other Treatments

- Any systemic infection (e.g. sinusitis, dental abscess) should be treated accordingly
- Sinus drainage will have to be performed, generally by an otolaryngologist, in a significant percentage of patients (especially children) who have acute orbital inflammation.

Prognosis

With prompt antibiotic therapy and drainage of any sites where purulent material has formed, the prognosis for visual and ocular rehabilitation is excellent.

Follow-up and Management

Close initial follow-up is crucial to determine the effectiveness of therapy and if surgical drainage of any pockets of purulent material is necessary. Also, any systemic problems need to be followed and dealt with appropriately.

Treatment continued on p. 327

Orbital Inflammation, Acute (376.0)

DIAGNOSIS—cont'd

General examination: general physical examination, white blood count and differential, culture of any ocular purulent material.

Special examination: computed tomography, magnetic resonance imaging or orbital ultrasound may be indicated, especially if swelling precludes an adequate ocular examination or if an intraocular or orbital foreign body is suspected.

Complications

- Visual loss, ocular motility problems, orbital apex syndrome
- *Cavernous sinus thrombosis*: with cavernous sinus involvement, headache, nausea, vomiting and varying levels of consciousness may occur
- *Meningitis*: extension of the orbital inflammation posteriorly in the orbit can result in subdural empyema, intracranial abscess or meningitis.

Pearls and Considerations

Because phycomycosis (*Mucor*) may present initially in the orbit, and because it may be lethal, early recognition by the ophthalmologist may be life saving.

Referral Information

Consider referral to otolaryngologist if spread of infection from adjacent sinuses is suspected.

TREATMENT—cont'd

Phycomycosis (*Mucor*)

Phycomycosis usually can be recognized easily in hematoxylin-eosin-stained sections by the hyphae, which are large, branching, and contain septa. The fungus tends to invade, causing thrombosis and an immediate threat to both vision and life. Because the acute orbital inflammation may be the initial sign of systemic phycomycosis, proper recognition of this fungal disease can be life saving. Immediate IV administration of antifungal agents (generally by an infectious disease expert) is essential. At the same time, prompt attention must be paid to the underlying condition (e.g. diabetes mellitus).

Nonpharmacologic Treatment

- If sinusitis, otitis or dental abscess is suspected, consultation with an otolaryngologist or oral surgeon is indicated
- Any intraorbital purulent material should be drained surgically and cultured. In children, sinus drainage is needed in ~50% of patients. In adults, sinus and abscess drainage is necessary in ~90% of patients.
- Blood cultures are indicated if hematogenous spread is suspected.

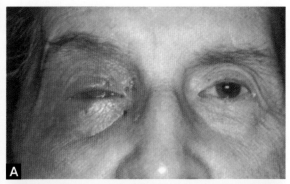

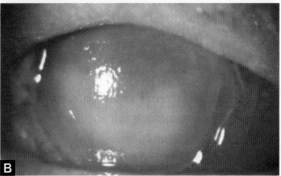

Figs 2A and B: (A) The red right eye is secondary to panophthalmitis with orbital spread; (B) On closer observation of the right eye, a hypopyon (pus) is seen behind the cornea in the anterior chamber.

GENERAL REFERENCES

Fairley C, Sullivan TJ, Bartley P, et al. Survival after rhino-orbital-cerebral mucormycosis in an immunocompetent patient. Ophthalmology. 2000;107(3): 555-8.

Hodges E, Tabbara KF. Orbital cellulitis: review of 23 cases from Saudi Arabia. Br J Ophthalmol. 1989;73:205-8.

Klapper SR, Patrinely JR, Kaplan SL, et al. Atypical mycobacterial infection of the orbit. Ophthalmology. 1995;102(10): 1536-41.

Read RW. Endophthalmitis. In: Yanoff M, Duker JS (Eds). Ophthalmology, 3rd Edition. St Louis: Elsevier; 2006.

Orbital Inflammation, Chronic (376.1)

DIAGNOSIS

Definition

An ongoing, low-grade inflammation of the anterior (preseptal) and/or posterior orbit.

Synonyms

None

Symptoms

- Exophthalmos (synonymous with ocular proptosis)
- *Red, painful eye*: if exophthalmos is excessive, exposure keratitis may cause redness and pain in the eye
- Swelling/pressure, tearing, blurred vision, diplopia.

Signs

- *Exophthalmos*: a lesion within the muscle cone causes more exophthalmos than a similar-sized lesion outside the muscle cone: paresis of the extraocular muscles as a result of inflammation (ophthalmoplegia) can cause 2.0 mm of ocular proptosis; in Graves' exophthalmos, extraocular and periorbital muscle involvement by edema, lymphocytic infiltration (mainly CD4+ and CD8+ T cells along with focal accumulations of B, plasma, and mast cells), and mucopolysaccharide deposition are responsible for the exophthalmos.
- Chemosis and injection of conjunctiva
- Periorbital and eyelid edema
- *Lid lag*: especially in Graves' disease
- Ocular motility problems.

Investigations

History

Especially of systemic complaints and presence of Graves' disease, sarcoidosis, lymphoma, leukemia, or immunosuppression (e.g. AIDS).

Ocular Examination

Visual acuity, ocular motility, complete external examination, exophthalmometry (measurement of exophthalmos by an exophthalmometer), intraocular pressure, undilated and dilated slit-lamp examination, dilated fundus examination; can perform computed tomography (CT) or magnetic resonance imaging (MRI) of the orbit, paying particular attention to the extraocular muscles (the best way to diagnose thyroid exophthalmos).

Sarcoidosis

Chest radiograph, "blind" conjunctival biopsy, and biopsy of lacrimal gland may be performed to diagnose sarcoidosis.

Differential Diagnosis

Graves' disease, acute orbital inflammation, orbital mucocele, carotid cavernous fistula, orbital neoplasms.

Causes

- *Secondary to bacteria*: Tuberculosis, syphilis, cat-scratch disease (*Bartonella henselae*)
- *Secondary to fungi*: phycomycosis (mucormycosis), sporotrichosis, aspergillosis
- *Secondary to parasites*: trichinosis, schistosomiasis, cysticercosis
- *Secondary to other entities*: sarcoidosis, Wegener's granulomatosis, Crohn's disease, midline lethal granuloma syndrome
- *Paranoids ocular glandular syndrome*: granulomatous conjunctivitis and ipsilateral enlargement of preauricular lymph nodes
- *Unknown cause*: e.g. pseudotumor, benign lymphoepithelial lesion of Godwin.

Epidemiology

- All forms of chronic inflammation of the orbit are rare
- Although granulomatous infectious orbital inflammation is rare, it is extremely important because it is potentially life threatening, especially phycomycosis (mucormycosis).

Classification

- Infectious granulomatous, e.g. phycomycosis (mucormycosis)
- Noninfectious granulomatous, e.g. sarcoidosis, Crohn's disease, cat-scratch disease
- Noninfectious nongranulomatous, e.g. pseudotumor.

Associated Features

Depend on course (e.g. sarcoidosis may have multisystem involvement).

Immunology

An immunologic course has been postulated for several noninfectious entities, but not with certainty.

Diagnosis continued on p. 330

TREATMENT

Diet and Lifestyle

No special precautions are necessary; however, if the patient is acutely ill (as often occurs with some infectious causes, e.g. phycomycosis), bed rest, warm compresses, and a light diet generally supplement other, more specific treatments.

Pharmacologic Treatment

- If an infectious agent is identified, appropriate therapy should be instituted as soon as possible
- If exposure keratitis is present, frequent lubrication (even every half an hour if needed) with either lubricating drops or ointment during the day and ointment at bedtime.

Phycomycosis (Mucormycosis) and Aspergillosis

Both phycomycosis and aspergillosis can be present as an acute orbital inflammation (often fulminating) or as a limited chronic form; both can be life-threatening. Usually, phycomycosis can be recognized easily in Gram-stained or eosin-hematoxylin-stained sections of purulent material by the hyphae, which are large, branching, and contain septa. The fungus tends to invade early into arterioles, causing thrombosis and therefore posing an immediate threat to both vision and life. Because the acute orbital inflammation may be the initial sign of systemic phycomycosis, proper recognition of this fungal disease can be lifesaving. Similarly, the fungus of aspergillosis can be recognized best (with Grocott or periodic acid-Schiff staining techniques) by its branching, septated hyphae, which are about one-fifth the size of *Mucor*. Immediate IV administration of antifungal agents, generally by an infectious disease expert, is essential. At the same time, prompt attention must be paid to the underlying condition (e.g. diabetes mellitus, AIDS, chronic renal disease).

Nonpharmacologic Treatment

- Orbital biopsy may be necessary to establish a diagnosis
- Often, noninfectious chronic orbital inflammation responds well to corticosteroid or low-dose orbital radiation therapy.

Exposure Keratitis

If conservative therapy (lubricating drops/ointment) is not successful, tarsorrhaphy (lateral or regular) can be performed. With extreme exophthalmos (e.g. advanced thyroid exophthalmopathy), more extreme measures, such as orbital decompression, may be needed.

Suspected Sarcoidosis

- If chest radiograph is not helpful, a "blind" conjunctival biopsy can be performed; "blind" refers to not seeing any nodule within the conjunctiva in the inferior cul-de-sac. Under topical anesthesia, the conjunctiva in the inferior cul-de-sac is tented up, and a strip of conjunctiva approximately 8 × 3 mm is removed with scissors. Suturing is usually not needed.
- If a conjunctival nodule (granuloma) is detected clinically, this should be included in the biopsy. It is extremely important to communicate with the pathologist that a strip of 4–6 sections should be placed on one glass slide and repeated at three different levels. This procedure yields 12–18 sections in which to search for the subconjunctival noncaseating granuloma characteristic of sarcoidosis.

Treatment Aims

- To preserve vision and ocular function
- *To identify and free of any underlying systemic disease*: particularly important in phycomycosis, which often is accompanied by systemic acidosis; the acidosis could result from diabetes mellitus, chronic diarrhea, and conditions that cause immunosuppression; if sarcoidosis presents initially with ocular involvement, the patient must be referred to a primary physician to check for systemic involvement and future monitoring.

Other Treatments

Any systemic infection or noninfectious condition (e.g. tuberculosis, AIDS, phycomycosis, sarcoidosis) should be treated accordingly.

Prognosis

- With prompt, appropriate therapy, the prognosis for visual and ocular rehabilitation is excellent for most of the conditions
- The key to visual and ocular rehabilitation is prompt therapy. Other specialists (e.g. pediatricians, otolaryngologist, oral surgeons, internists) may need to be consulted.

Follow-up and Management

- Close initial follow-up is essential to monitor the effectiveness of therapy
- Long-term follow-up is necessary to recognize any early recurrence. Also, any systemic problems need to be followed off and dealt with appropriately there.

Treatment continued on p. 331

Orbital Inflammation, Chronic (376.1)

DIAGNOSIS—cont'd

Infectious Agents

The main bacteria that cause chronic orbital inflammation are those that cause tuberculosis *(Mycobacterium tuberculosis)*, syphilis *(Treponema pallidum)*, and cat-scratch disease *(Bartonella henselae);* the main fungi that cause chronic orbital inflammation are those that cause phycomycosis *(Mucor, Rhizopus)*, aspergillosis *(Aspergillus fumigatus)*, and sporotrichosis *(Sporotrichum schenckii);* and the main parasites that cause chronic orbital inflammation are those that cause trichinosis *(Trichinella spiralis)*, schistosomiasis *(Schistosoma haematobium, S. japonicum)*, and cysticercosis *(Cysticercus cellulosae)*.

General Examination

Physical examination, white blood cell count and differential, any other laboratory test as indicated.

Special Examination

Computed tomography, MRI (Fig. 1), orbital ultrasound: these tests are extremely important in diagnosing Graves' disease, orbital mucocele, carotid cavernous fistula, and orbital neoplasms.

Complications

- Exposure keratitis, visual loss, uveitis, intraocular involvement
- Strabismus and diplopia (double vision)
- Systemic involvement and even death (e.g. from phycomycosis) (Fig. 2).

Pearls and Considerations

Topic is too broad to make specific recommendations.

Referral Information

Refer to appropriate subspecialist based on suspected etiology of inflammation (e.g. endocrinologist for Graves' disease).

TREATMENT—cont'd

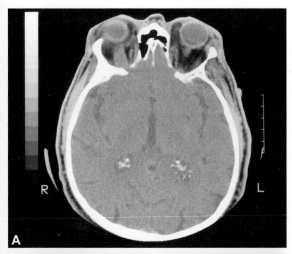

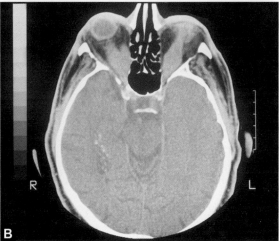

Figs 1A and B: Different CT views of thickened rectus muscles in a patient with Graves' ophthalmopathy.

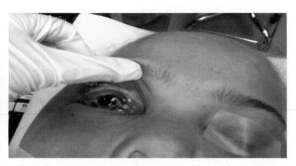

Fig. 2: Patient had phycomycosis (*Rhizopus oryzae*) of the orbit.

GENERAL REFERENCES

Parken B, Chew JB, White VA, et al. Lymphocytic infiltration and enlargement of the lacrimal glands: a new subtype of primary Sjögren's syndrome? Ophthalmology. 2005;112: 2040.

Santos GP, Blanco PP, Batuecas CA, et al. Rhino-orbito-cerebral mucormycosis, a retrospective study of 7 cases. Acta Otorrinolaringol Esp. 2010;61: 48-53. Epub 2009.

Yanoff M, Sassani JW. Ocular Pathology, 6th edition. St Louis: Mosby; 2009. pp. 532-4.

Pars Planitis (363.21)

DIAGNOSIS

Definition
Intraocular inflammation, primarily of the anterior vitreous.

Synonym
Intermediate uveitis (IU).

Symptoms
- Floaters
- Decreased vision
- Photophobia.

Signs
- Mild anterior-chamber inflammation
- Cells in the anterior vitreous
- Cellular aggregations in the predominantly inferior vitreous: "snowballs"
- "*Snowbanking*": white exudative material over the inferior ora serrata
- Peripheral retinal vascular sheathing
- Cystoid macular edema
- Posterior subcapsular cataract
- Secondary glaucoma
- Peripheral retinal neovascularization
- Vitreous hemorrhage
- Peripapillary edema.

Investigations
- *History and appropriate laboratory studies*: to rule out Lyme's disease, sarcoidosis, toxoplasmosis, tuberculosis, syphilis, multiple sclerosis
- *Complete ocular examination including peripheral depression*: to view the inferior ora serrata
- *Fluorescein angiography*: to rule out retinal vasculitis and/or cystoid macular edema
- *Optical coherence tomography*: to rule out cystoid macular edema.

Complications
- Cystoid macular edema
- Peripheral neovascularization
- Cataract
- Vitreous hemorrhage
- Secondary glaucoma
- Epiretinal membranes
- Traction or rhegmatogenous detachment.

Pearls and Considerations
- Pars planitis tends to follow a prolonged course of exacerbations and remissions
- Children tend to have worse visual outcomes with IU than adults.

Referral Information
Refer to retinal specialist for oral steroids, intravitreal steroids or even vitrectomy as appropriate.

Differential Diagnosis
- Tumor
- Anterior uveitis
- Rhegmatogenous retinal detachment
- Endophthalmitis.

Cause
Chronic inflammatory disorder of unknown cause.

Epidemiology
- Usually found in patients 14-40 years old
- Bilateral 80% of patients
- May remain active for years.

Pathology
- Peripheral lymphocyte cuffing of venules
- Loose fibrovascular membrane.

TREATMENT

Diet and Lifestyle

No special precautions are necessary.

Pharmacologic Treatment

- Steroid therapy is used in patients with cystoid macular edema. Treatment usually consists of intravitreal injection of steroid and often needs to be repeated
- Cytotoxic agents are reserved for intractable cases
- Oral therapy may be necessary if the vitreous infiltrate causes decreased vision.

Nonpharmacologic Treatment

- *Cryoablation*: of the pars plana membrane in severe cases
- *Peripheral laser or cryoablation*: to neovascularization
- *Vitrectomy*: for dense vitreous infiltrates with or without traction that cause significant visual loss.

Treatment Aims

To prevent secondary complications (e.g. chronic cystoid macular edema, vitreous hemorrhage).

Prognosis

- Clinical course is usually self-limited with gradual improvement of vision
- Cases can smolder with intermittent acute exacerbation, limiting the visual end result because of chronic cystoid macular edema.

Follow-up and Management

Patients are followed every few months, depending on the severity of disease, response to treatment, and rate of recurrence.

GENERAL REFERENCES

Henderly DE, Haymond RS, Rao NA, et al. The significance of the pars plana exudate in pars planitis. Am J Ophthalmol. 1987;103:669-71.

Read RW, Zamir E, Rao NA. Nongranulomatous inflammation: uveitis, endophthalmitis, panophthalmitis and sequelae. In: Tasman W, et al. (Eds). Duane's Clinical Ophthalmology (CD-ROM). Baltimore: Lippincott Williams & Wilkins; 2004.

Smith RE. Pars planitis. In: Ryan SJ (Ed). Retina, vol. 2. St Louis: Mosby; 1989. pp. 637-45.

Welsh RB, Maumenee AE, Wahler HE. Peripheral posterior segment inflammation, vitreous opacities and edema of the posterior pole: pars planitis. Arch Ophthalmol. 1960;64:540-9.

Phacoanaphylactic Endophthalmitis (360.19)

DIAGNOSIS

Definition
Inflammation of the ocular tissues secondary to rupture of the crystalline lens.

Synonyms
Phacoimmune endophthalmitis.

Symptoms
Phacoanaphylactic endophthalmitis always follows a penetrating ocular injury in which the lens is ruptured; characterized by a zonal granulomatous inflammatory reaction centered around the ruptured lens (Figs 1 and 2), with symptoms of:
- Photophobia
- Ocular irritation or pain
- Blurred vision.

Signs
- Red eye secondary to ciliary injection
- Evidence of previous penetrating ocular injury
- Mutton-fat keratic precipitates
- Corneal edema secondary to glaucoma.

Investigations (Fig. 3)
- *History*: penetrating ocular injury
- Visual acuity test
- *Complete ocular examination*: including undilated and dilated slit-lamp examination
- Dilated fundus examination.

Complications
- Decreased visual acuity
- Glaucoma
- Cataract
- Macular edema
- Retinal detachment
- *Phthisis bulbi*: the end stage of ocular disease—a shrunken, functionless eye.

Pearls and Considerations
As with other forms of endophthalmitis, this is a true medical emergency.

Referral Information
Refer immediately for surgical removal of remaining pieces of the lens.

Differential Diagnosis
- Anterior iridocyclitis
- Phacolytic glaucoma
- Sympathetic uveitis
- Vogt-Koyanagi-Harada syndrome.

Epidemiology
Phacoanaphylactic endophthalmitis only occurs when the lens capsule is traumatically ruptured and only rarely.

Immunology
Phacoanaphylactic endophthalmitis, an autoimmune condition, may result from the breakdown or reversal of central tolerance to the T-cell level. Small amounts of circulating lens proteins normally maintain T-cell tolerance, but it may be altered as a result of trauma, possibly through the adjuvant effects of wound contamination, bacterial products, or both. After the abrogation of tolerance to lens protein, antilens antibodies are produced and reach the lens remnants in the eye, where an antibody-antigen reaction takes place (phacoanaphylactic endophthalmitis).

Pathology
A zonal granulomatous inflammation surrounds lens remnants. Activated neutrophils surround and seem to dissolve or "eat away" lens material, probably releasing proteolytic enzymes, arachidonic acid metabolites, and oxygen-derived free radicals. Epithelioid cells and occasional (sometimes in abundance) multinucleated inflammatory giant cells are seen beyond the neutrophils. Lymphocytes, plasma cells, fibroblasts, and blood vessels (i.e. granulation tissue) surround the epithelioid cells. Usually the iris is encased in the inflammatory reaction and inseparable from it. The uveal tract generally shows a reactive, chronic nongranulomatous inflammatory reaction.

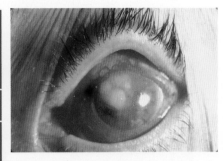

Fig. 1: Patient had a complicated extracapsular cataract extraction. Postoperatively, patient developed photophobia and endophthalmititis. Eye was enucleated.

TREATMENT

Diet and Lifestyle

No special precautions are necessary.

Pharmacologic Treatment

Phacoanaphylactic endophthalmitis basically is a surgical disease. However, the usual precautions (e.g. topical antiglaucoma drops for accompanying glaucoma, topical corticosteroids to reduce inflammation) are recommended before surgery.

Nonpharmacologic Treatment

Surgery: removing the remaining lens remnants may relieve the situation.

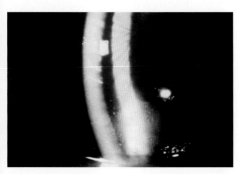

Fig. 2: Mutton-fat keratic precipitates present in another case.

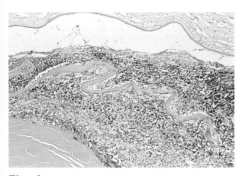

Fig. 3: Histology shows zonular granulomatous inflammatory reaction around lens remnant (lower right). The lens remnant is surrounded by polynuclear leukocytes, surrounded epithelioid and giant cells, surrounded by granulation tissue. The lens capsule is ruptured.

GENERAL REFERENCES

Chan CC. Relationship between sympathetic ophthalmia, phacoanaphylactic endophthalmitis, and Vogt–Koyanagi–Harada disease. Ophthalmology. 1988; 95:619.

Marak GE. Phacoanaphylactic endophthalmitis (major review). Surv Ophthalmol. 1992;36:325-39.

Yanoff M, Sassani JW. Ocular Pathology, 6th edition. St Louis: Mosby; 2009. pp. 75-6.

Phakomatoses

DIAGNOSIS

Definition

A group of different diseases characterized by multiple tumors (benign or malignant) developing in different organs of the body.

Synonyms

None; see terms used for specific tumors.

Symptoms

- Phakomatoses are a heredofamilial group of congenital tumors that have disseminated, benign (usually) hamartomas (tumors of tissue normally found in an area) in common
- *Neurofibromatosis*: Facial deformities (i.e. cosmetic problems), multiple skin tumors, ocular proptosis (exophthalmos), blurred vision
- *Sturge-Weber syndrome*: Facial blemish (i.e. cosmetic problems secondary to "port-wine stain"), blurred vision (Figs 1A and B)
- *Von Hippel's disease*: Blurred vision
- *Tuberous sclerosis*: Facial blemish (i.e. cosmetic problems secondary to adenoma sebaceum), mental impairment, blurred vision.

Signs

Neurofibromatosis (237.71)

Café au lait spots, cutaneous neurofibromas (Fig. 2), thickening of conjunctival and corneal nerves, Lisch iris nodules (characteristic of neurofibromatosis type 1 and present in approximately 90% of patients by age 6 years, Fig. 3), intraocular uveal and neural retinal hamartomas, orbital plexiform neurofibromas (Figs 4A and B) and neurilemmomas (orbital neurofibroma often presents with typical S-shaped deformity of upper lid), optic nerve glioma (approximately 25% of patients who have optic nerve gliomas have neurofibromatosis, almost exclusively in type 1), glaucoma (especially when upper eyelid involved).

Sturge-Weber Syndrome (Meningocutaneous Angiomatosis) (759.7)

Choroidal cavernous hemangioma (tends to involve choroid diffusely and blend into surrounding normal choroid), facial nevus flammeus or port-wine stain (usually along distribution of trigeminal nerve), glaucoma (approximately 30% of patients; especially when upper eyelid involved).

Von Hippel's Disease (Angiomatosis Retinae) (759.6)

Neural retinal capillary hemangioma (similar to cerebellar capillary hemangioma), neural retinal exudates (even when capillary hemangioma located in peripheral retina, exudates can appear in macula and cause blurred vision; in a child, any unexplained macular exudation may indicate von Hippel's disease or Coats' disease), glaucoma (usually angle-closure glaucoma secondary to iris neovascularization and peripheral anterior synechiae associated with long-standing retinal detachment).

Tuberous Sclerosis (Bourneville's Disease) (759.5)

Facial cutaneous adenoma sebaceum, glial hamartomas (giant drusen) of optic disc (these can be misdiagnosed as optic disc edema; however, the history and other clues, e.g. adenoma sebaceum and retinal glial hamartomas, should make the diagnosis obvious), glial (astrocytic) hamartomas of neural retina (approximately 53% of patients).

Differential Diagnosis

- Retinal hemangiomas, astrocytic hamartomas, choroidal hemangiomas, orbital neurofibromatoses and neurilemmomas, and giant drusen of the optic disc all can occur primarily without phakomatosis.
- Neuromas, café au lait spots, and prominent corneal nerves—old similar to findings in neurofibromatosis—may also be seen a multiple endocrine neoplasia, which is caused by an abnormality of chromosomes 11 q13 and 10q11.2.

Causes

- *Neurofibromatosis type 1*: irregular autosomal dominant; chromosome 17 (band 17 q11.2)
- *Neurofibromatosis type 2*: irregular autosomal dominant; chromosome 22 (band 22 q12)
- *Sturge-Weber syndrome*: irregular autosomal dominant
- *Von Hippel's disease*: congenital; autosomal dominant with incomplete penetrance; short arm of chromosome 3
- *Tuberous sclerosis*: irregular autosomal dominant; wall and arm of chromosome 39.

Epidemiology

- *Neurofibromatosis type 1*: prevalence 1:3000-4000
- *Neurofibromatosis type 2*: prevalence 1:50,000
- *Sturge-Weber syndrome*: Very rare
- *von Hippel's disease*: prevalence 1:40,000
- *Tuberous sclerosis*: Incident 0.56:100,000 person-years; prevalence 10.6:100,000.

Pathology

- *Neurofibromatosis type 1*: depends on the type of tumor (e.g. neurofibroma, optic nerve glioma)
- *Neurofibromatosis type 2*: depends on the type of tumor [e.g. eight-nerve tumor (neurilemmoma), meningioma]
- *Sturge-Weber syndrome*: choroidal cavernous hemangioma
- *Von Hippel disease*: retinal capillary hemangioma.

Diagnosis continued on p. 338

TREATMENT

Diet and Lifestyle

- If blindness is anticipated, the family should be informed of the many interventions available to blind patients
- Central nervous system lesions in von Hippel's disease, Sturge-Weber syndrome, and tuberous sclerosis may require considerable modification of lifestyle.

Pharmacologic Treatment

No pharmacologic treatment for phakomatoses is available; however, the secondary effects (e.g. glaucoma) can be treated.

Nonpharmacologic Treatment

- The phakomatoses should be treated surgically as indicated
- Generally, the optic nerve glioma found in neurofibromatosis should be treated conservatively. Because the tumor is essentially a benign hamartoma, the indications for removal depend on factors other than the tumor (e.g. exophthalmos may cause exposure keratitis). Deciding whether to remove only the orbital optic nerve glioma or both the globe and the glioma is based on clinical data.
- An orbital neurofibroma may cause severe ocular proptosis and exposure keratitis, and removal of the neurofibroma may be warranted
- Choroidal hemangiomas in Sturge-Weber syndrome tend to leak fluid, resulting in a secondary serous neural retinal detachment. This can be treated by laser photocoagulation, usually in a scatter form over the tumor
- In von Hippel's disease, if exudation has decreased vision, cryotherapy of the peripheral retinal lesion or laser photocoagulation of the lesion's feeder vessels may cause partial or complete resolution of the exudate
- Usually, no specific therapy is needed in tuberous sclerosis.

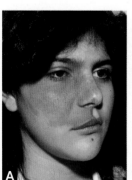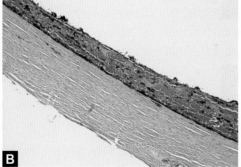

Figs 1A and B: (A) Sturge-Weber syndrome. Port-wine stain present along distribution of trigeminal nerve; (B) Sturge-Weber syndrome. Choroid thickened by cavernous hemangioma.

337

Treatment continued on p. 339

Phakomatoses

DIAGNOSIS—cont'd

Investigations

History (including family history), complete external examination, visual acuity testing, refraction, intraocular pressure, undilated and dilated slit-lamp examination, dilated fundus examination.

Pearls and Considerations

Varied and specific to the type of underlying disorder; topic too broad.

Referral Information

Refer to primary care physician and/or plastic surgeon for intervention as appropriate based on the specific condition.

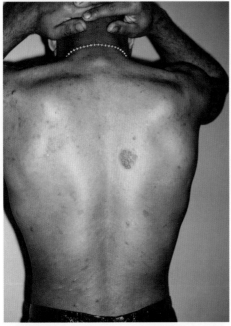

Fig. 2: Neurofibromatosis. Café au lait spots and cutaneous neurofibromas.

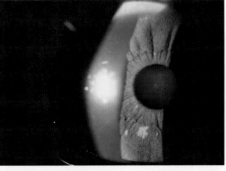

Fig. 3: Neurofibromatosis. Iris shows multiple tan, spider-like nevi (Lisch nodules).

TREATMENT—cont'd

Complications

- Neurofibromatosis, Sturge-Weber syndrome, and von Hippel's disease all can be associated with glaucoma, retinal exudation and detachment, and eventually blindness
- Neurofibromatosis of the orbit can cause exophthalmos, which can become marked and result in exposure keratitis
- Neurofibromatosis of the optic nerve can cause optic nerve glioma and subsequent blindness
- The neural retinal lesions of tuberous sclerosis disease generally remain stationary.

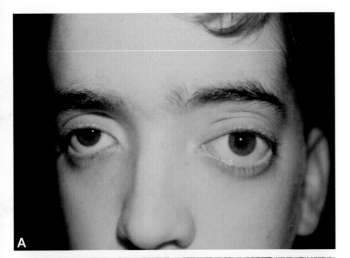

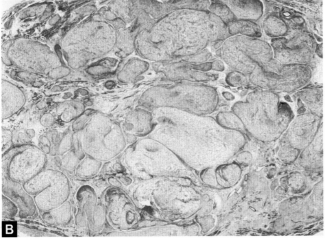

Figs 4A and B: (A) Neurofibromatosis. Left eye proptosis caused by retrobulbar tumor (plexiform neurofibroma); (B) Neurofibromatosis. Plexiform neurofibroma shows a tangle of enlarged nerves (left, H & E stain, right trichrome stain).

GENERAL REFERENCES

Bosch MM, Boltshauser E, Harpes P, et al. Ophthalmologic findings and long-term course in patients with neurofibromatosis type 2. Am J Ophthalmol. 2006;141:1068.

Khaier A, Nischal KK, Espinosa M, et al. Periocular port wine stain: the Great Ormand Street Hospital experience. Ophthalmology. 2011;118:2274.

Pinna A, Demontis S, Maltese G, et al. Absence of the greater sphenoid wing in neurofibromatosis 1. Arch Ophthalmol. 2005;123:1454.

Shields CL, Reichstein DA, Bianciotto C, et al. Retinal pigment epithelial depigmented lesions associated with tuberous sclerosis complex. Arch Ophthalmol. 2012;130:387.

Yanoff M, Sassani JW. Ocular Pathology, 6th edition. St Louis: Mosby; 2009. pp. 29-36.

Pseudoexfoliation of the Lens (366.11)

DIAGNOSIS

Definition
Accumulation of white flakes at the pupillary margin and on the anterior surface of the lens.

Synonyms
None; often abbreviated PEX.

Symptoms
Patients are usually asymptomatic, and PEX is discovered on routine examination. *See also* Glaucoma, pseudoexfoliative (365.52).

Signs
* Pseudoexfoliation is bilateral in slightly greater than 50% of cases. In following a patient for years, the clinician may note PEX in one eye. This usually prompts a careful examination of the other eye, which generally is normal. Continued examination of the uninvolved eye can result in normal findings until suddenly, years later, the second eye becomes involved.
* *Pseudoexfoliation material (PEXM)*: dandruff-like material on the pupillary margin of the undilated pupil, usually the earliest sign (Fig. 1)
* After dilation, the anterior surface of lens shows a characteristic thin, homogeneous, white deposit centrally located and surrounded by a relatively clear zone, which in turn is surrounded by a more peripheral, coarse, granular "hoarfrost" material that extends to the equator (Figs 2 to 4). In aphakic and pseudophakic eyes, PEXM may appear years after cataract surgery on the pupillary border, anterior and posterior surfaces of the lens implant, anterior hyaloid surface, and vitreous framework.
* *Corneal endothelial abnormalities*: may include powdery PEXM on the internal corneal surface and within its cytoplasm (seen as intraendothelial inclusions)
* *"Leathery" and poorly dilating iris*: PEXM collects on the posterior surface of the iris and acts as a strut. Also, atrophy of the iris dilator muscle fibers occurs, causing difficulty in dilating
* *Subtle iridodonesis and phacodonesis*: seen in many patients; caused by instability of the zonules supporting the lens
* Spontaneous subluxation (lens displaced but still in posterior chamber) and dislocation (lens displaced out of the posterior chamber into the anterior chamber or vitreous) of the lens: rare.

Differential Diagnosis
* Pigment dispersion syndrome
* Inflammatory deposits on lens surface.

Cause
The cause is unknown.

Epidemiology
* Pseudoexfoliation of the lens has a worldwide distribution but seems to be most common in Scandinavian people (especially those living in Norway and Finland) and is rare and African people
* Pseudoexfoliation probably is inherited (possibly autosomal dominant) with incomplete penetrance
* Pseudoexfoliation tends to involve an older population, mainly ages 60–80 years.

Classification
Generally, PEX of the lens is classified as unilateral or bilateral, with or without elevated intraocular pressure.

Associated Features
Pseudoexfoliation material has been found histologically in the following structures:
* *Ocular*: Iris, ciliary body, posterior ciliary vessels, palpebral and bulbar conjunctiva, eyelid comment orbital tissue
* *Nonocular*: Skin, lungs, heart, liver, gallbladder, kidney, cerebral meninges
* The significance of the systemic findings is not known.

Pathology
Pseudoexfoliation material appears eosinophilic in routine histology and is found prominently on the anterior surface of the lens, the posterior surface of the iris, and the internal surface of the ciliary body. The material stains positively with periodic acid-Schiff; it is probably a type of basement membrane.

Diagnosis continued on p. 342

TREATMENT

Diet and Lifestyle

No special precautions are necessary.

Pharmacologic Treatment

Pharmacologic treatment has no effect on PEX unless glaucoma develops.

Nonpharmacologic Treatment

Unless a cataract develops, no treatment is necessary for the lens. Any associated glaucoma should be treated appropriately.

Cataract Surgery in Pseudoexfoliation Eyes

- Complications occur more frequently in patients with PEX syndrome. The instability of the zonules supporting the lens often leads to a subtle iridodonesis and phacodonesis in many patients and, rarely, spontaneous lens subluxation (lens in posterior chamber but not in its normal location) and dislocation (lens not in posterior chamber but in vitreous or anterior chamber).
- The instability of the cataractous PEX lens during surgery can lead to capsular tears and vitreous loss. Some advocate nuclear-expression extracapsular cataract (ECC) surgery, and others recommend phacoemulsification ECC surgery; level of comfort and experience should guide the surgeon's choice of procedure.
- Another question is whether to put the intraocular lens (IOL) implant into the "lens bag" or on top of the bag into the ciliary sulcus. Initially, many surgeons thought that it was safer to put the IOL into the sulcus. Then the pendulum swung strongly to in-the-bag insertions. However, many surgeons now prefer in-the-sulcus insertions because of the recent findings of subluxated and dislocated IOLs years after in-the-bag insertions.

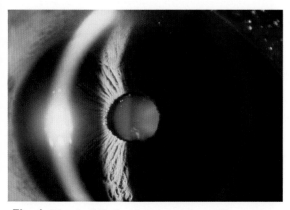

Fig. 1: "Dandruff-like" material seen in papillary region, an early sign of PEX.

Treatment Aims

To control any associated glaucoma.

Other Treatments

- Because of the increased risk associated with cataract surgery in PEX patients, appropriate care must be taken if a cataract develops.
- Informed consent is extremely important, especially considering the increased risk of cataract surgery in PEX patients (see Nonpharmacologic treatment). Also, the patient must be informed that careful postoperative follow-up (including long-term follow-up) is essential because of the increased risk of developing glaucoma.

Prognosis

If no other vision-threatening ocular conditions are present, cataract extraction and lens implantation result in greater than 90% visual improvement to an acuity of greater than or equal to 20/40.

Follow-up and Management

- The cumulative probability of PEX eyes developing abnormally high intraocular pressure (IOP) is approximately 5% in 5 years and approximately 15% in 10 years. Long-term follow-up, therefore, is mandatory.
- Patients with PEX of the lens should be considered glaucoma suspect and followed yearly if IOP is normal. The IOP is elevated, appropriate testing [e.g. visual fields, ocular computerized tonometry (OCT), optic nerve photos] should be performed on follow-up visits tailored to do the individual patient.

Treatment continued on p. 343

Pseudoexfoliation of the Lens (366.11)

DIAGNOSIS—cont'd

- *Glaucoma*: will develop in approximately 8% of patients, and an additional 12% will be glaucoma suspects (ocular hypertension); the cumulative probability for PEX eyes to develop abnormally high intraocular pressure is approximately 5% in 5 years and 15% in 10 years; the cause of the glaucoma is not known; both mechanical (PEXM "clogging" the trabecular meshwork) and genetic theories have been proposed.
- *Findings similar to those of pigment dispersion syndrome*: the iris pigment epithelium undergoes degeneration, liberating melanin pigment. This pigment can deposit on the posterior surface of the cornea (pseudo-Krukenberg spindle) in the anterior-chamber angle and within the trabecular meshwork, mimicking the pigment dispersion syndrome; an early sign is a pigmented linear deposit lying on the corneal side of Schwalbe's line, called Sampaolesi's line.

Investigations

- Visual acuity testing
- Refraction
- Intraocular pressure
- Undilated and dilated slit-lamp examination
- Gonioscopy
- Dilated fundus examination.

Complications

- Secondary open-angle glaucoma
- Increased chance of complications during cataract surgery.

Pearls and Considerations

- Can lead to pseudoexfoliative glaucoma, the most common secondary open-angle glaucoma worldwide
- True exfoliation syndrome only occurs with heat or infrared changes in the anterior lens capsule.

Referral Information

Refer to glaucoma specialist for argon laser or selective laser trabeculoplasty.

TREATMENT—cont'd

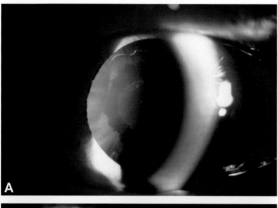

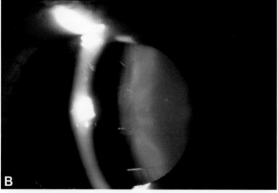

Figs 2A and B: The central disc and peripheral granular "hoarfrost" material are seen in the slit beam.

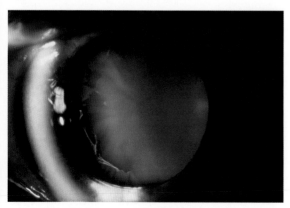

Fig. 3: The peripheral granular "hoarfrost" material is seen easily.

GENERAL REFERENCES

Kang JH, Loomis S, Wiggs JL, et al. Demographic and geographic features of exfoliation glaucaoma in 2 United States-based prospective cohorts. Ophthalmol. 2012;119:27.

Rautenbach RM, Bardien S, Harvey J, et al. An investigation into LOXL1 variants in Black African individuals with exfoliation syndrome. Arch Ophthalmol. 2011;129:206.

Thorleifsson G, Magnusson KP, Sulem P, et al. Common sequence variants in the LOXL1 gene confer susceptibility to exfoliation glaucoma. Science. 2007;317:1397.

Yanoff M, Sassani JW. Ocular Pathology, 6th edition. St Louis: Mosby; 2009. pp. 368-73.

Yilmaz A, Ayaz L, Tamer L. Selenium and pseudoexfoliation syndrome. Am J Ophthalmolol. 2011;151:272.

Pseudotumor Cerebri (Idiopathic Intracranial Hypertension) (348.2)

DIAGNOSIS

Definition

Papilledema associated with idiopathic intracranial hypertension.

Synonyms

Idiopathic intracranial hypertension; benign intracranial hypertension.

Symptoms

- Five to ten percent of patients are asymptomatic, and papilledema is detected on routine eye examination
- *Headache*: 90% of patients
- *Transient visual obscuration*: 54% of patients
- *Diplopia*: 36% of patients
- *Painful neck stiffness*: 31% of patients
- *Pulsatile tinnitus (usually on right side)*: 27% of patients.

Signs

- Normal visual acuity; no afferent pupillary defect unless chronic atrophic papilledema
- *Papilledema*: can be acute, chronic or chronic atrophic (Fig. 1)
- *Visual field loss*: includes arcuate nerve fiber bundle loss, enlarged blind spot, constricted visual fields, inferior nasal field depression, decreased color vision (by Ishihara color plates), and cecocentral and central scotomas
- Modified Dandy's diagnostic criteria
  - Patient is awake and alert.
  - Signs and symptoms of increased intracranial pressure (ICP)
  - Absence of localized neurologic signs except for sixth-nerve palsy
  - Opening pressure of cerebrospinal fluid (CSF) on lumbar puncture (LP) is greater than 25 cm H_2O (caution: opening pressure may be higher in some normal patients, particularly in children) and is of normal composition
  - Normal ventricles and normal study on computed tomography (CT) and magnetic resonance imaging (MRI)
- Relative afferent pupillary defects may occur if there is asymmetric visual field loss or chronic atrophic papilledema in one eye.

Differential Diagnosis

- Lateral sinus or superior sagittal sinus thrombosis
- Combination of anomalous disks, obesity and migraine
- Papilledema from an intracranial mass
- Bilateral perioptic neuritis
- Spinal cord tumor.

Cause

Idiopathic

- Decreased rate of CSF absorption, increased rate of CSF formation, increased venous ICP, and increased brain interstitial fluid (edema)
- *Secondary causes*: vitamin A, tetracycline, nalidixic acid, anabolic steroids, oral contraceptives, lithium
- Obstructive sleep apnea.

Epidemiology

- Incidence is 13:100,000 in women ages 20–40 years who are 10% above their ideal body weight. Incidence increases to 19:100,000 if they are 20% above their ideal body weight
- There is no racial predilection, though black patients are associated with a worse visual outcome
- Ninety-two percent of patients are women
- In children, the gender ratio is equal, and obesity is not as important. The child may become irritable, apathetic, and somnolent instead of suffering headache. Children have a higher prevalence of sixth-nerve palsy than adults. They may develop a third- or fourth-nerve palsy and a unilateral lower-motor-neuron facial palsy or skew deviation. Dandy's criteria do not apply to children (*see* Signs).
- In men, pseudotumor cerebri may be a different disease. Dural arteriovenous malformations may be causative.
- Although familial pseudotumor cerebri has many causes, no genetic linkage studies have been done.

Pathology

Unknown

Diagnosis continued on p. 346

TREATMENT

Diet and Lifestyle

- Weight loss: the one proven treatment for pseudotumor cerebri. Typically, only modest weight loss is required
- Behavior modification.

Pharmacologic Treatment

Standard dosage: Carbonic anhydrase inhibitor: acetazolamide (diamox), 500 mg–1 g BID

Furosemide, 20–80 mg, maximum 600 mg/day

Digoxin, 0.25 mg/day

Oral corticosteroids (occasionally used as "bridge therapy" in rapidly-progressive visual loss pending more definitive treatment)

Topiramate, octreotide (investigational).

There is no role for long-term use of steroids in pseudotumor cerebri.

Nonpharmacologic Treatment

- Optic nerve fenestration
- Serial LPs
- Cerebrospinal fluid diversion procedure (e.g. ventriculoperitoneal or lumbo-peritoneal shunt)
- Endovascular stenting of transverse venous sinus stenoses (can have serious complications)
- Subtemporal decompression
- Gastric reduction surgery (e.g. "lap band" bariatric surgery).

Associated Features

Association Criteria

- Associated feature satisfies the Dandy criteria (*see* Signs)
- Underlying condition should be proved to increase ICP
- Treatment of the association should improve it
- Properly controlled studies should show an association.

Proven associations (meet all four criteria for association): obesity.

Likely associations (meet three criteria but lacks case-control studies): chlordecone (kepone), hypervitaminosis A.

Probable associations (meet two criteria): steroid withdrawal in children, hypothyroid children receiving replacement therapy, ketoprofen and indomethacin in Bartter's syndrome, hypoparathyroidism, Addison's disease, uremia, iron deficiency anemia, tetracycline, nalidixic acid, danazol, lithium, amiodarone, phenytoin, nitrofurantoin, ciprofloxacin, nitroglycerin.

Treatment Aims

To prevent or reverse vision loss.

Prognosis

- Severe, permanent visual impairment occurs in 25% of patients in months to years
- Eighty percent improve visual function in 8 months with treatment
- Recurrence rate is 10–40%.

Follow-up and Management

- Patients should have serial visual function evaluation
- Monitor visual function with visual fields, color vision, contrast sensitivity, Snellen acuity, and optic disk OCT and photos.

Treatment continued on p. 347

Pseudotumor Cerebri (Idiopathic Intracranial Hypertension) (348.2)

DIAGNOSIS—cont'd

Investigations

- To avoid brainstem herniation, CT of head before LP to rule out intracranial lesion
- Threshold visual fields, Goldmann visual field, contrast sensitivity, CT or MRI (may see flattening of the posterior pole of both eyes, possibly empty sella turcica, and/or stenosis of one or both transverse cerebral venous sinuses), magnetic resonance arteriography and venography, LP [cell count, glucose, protein, opening-pressure cytology, venereal disease research laboratory (VDRL)], optical coherence tomography (OCT), erythrocyte sedimentation rate, complete blood count, rapid plasma reagin test, fluorescent treponemal antibody absorption test, calcium (Ca++), phosphorus, thyroxine, blood urea nitrogen, electrolytes, overnight polysomnography.

Complications

- Progressive loss of vision, secondary vein occlusion from papilledema
- Factors that may influence visual loss: hypertension, older age, myopia, anemia, chronic disk edema of more than 4 diopters, optochoroidal shunts, subretinal hemorrhage
- Disk infarction, choroidal folds, vein occlusion.

Pearls and Considerations

Associated optic atrophy may lead to permanent vision loss and is the only permanent morbidity associated with idiopathic intracranial hypertension.

Referral Information

Refer to neurologist or neuro-ophthalmologist for complete workup and imaging; consider referral to nutritionist for assistance with weight reduction therapy.

TREATMENT—cont'd

Possible associations (meet one criterion): menstrual irregularity, oral contraceptive use, Cushing's syndrome, vitamin A deficiency, minor head trauma, Behçet's syndrome.

Unlikely (no criteria met): hyperthyroidism, steroid ingestion, immunization.

Unsupported: pregnancy, menarche.

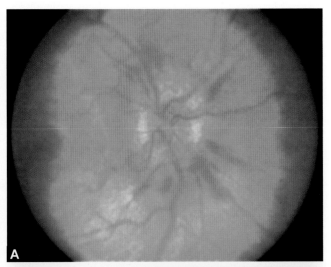

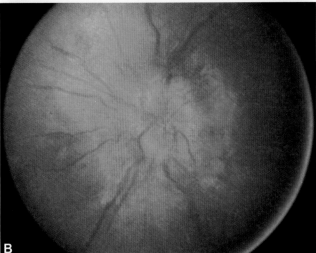

Figs 1A and B: Acute papilledema in a woman (height 5 ft, 2 in; weight 300 lb) who had an opening pressure of 450 mm H$_2$O. Note elevation of optic disk with flame-shaped hemorrhages.

GENERAL REFERENCES

Ball AK, Howman A, Wheatley K, et al. A randomised controlled trial of treatment for idiopathic intracranial hypertension. J Neurol. 2011;258(5):874-81.

Biousse V, Bruce BB, Newman NJ. Review: update on the pathophysiology and management of idiopathic intracranial hypertension. J Neurol Neurosurg Psychiatry. 2012;83(5):488-94.

Friedman DI. Papilledema and pseudotumor cerebri. Ophthalmol Clin North Am. 2001;14(1):129-47.

Goodwin J. (2006). Pseudotumor cerebri. [Online] Available from www.emedicine.com.

Mathews MK, Sergott RC, Savino PJ. Pseudotumor cerebri. Curr Opin Ophthalmol. 2003;14(6):364-70.

Movsas TZ, Liu GT, Galetta SL, et al. Current neuro-ophthalmic therapies. Neurol Clin. 2001;19(1):145-72.

Newman SA. Interventional neuro-ophthalmology: not an oxymoron. J Neuro-ophthalmol. 2012;32(2):177-84.

Scott CJ, Kardon RH, Lee AG, et al. Diagnosis and grading of papilledema in patients with raised intracranial pressure using optical coherence tomography vs clinical expert assessment using a clinical staging scale. Arch Ophthalmol. 2010;128(6):705-11.

Wall M, George D. Idiopathic intracranial hypertension (pseudotumor cerebri): a prospective study of 50 patients. Brain. 1991;114:155-80.

Refraction and Accommodation Disorders (367.0)

DIAGNOSIS

Definition

- Conditions occur when parallel light rays from a distant object do not come to focus on the retina
- *Accommodation disorder*: an abnormality with focusing near objects.

Synonyms

- None
- Associated terms include: myopia (near-sighted), hyperopia (far-sighted), astigmatism, presbyopia, accommodative insufficiency, convergence insufficiency.

Symptoms

- Decreased visual acuity
- Asthenopia.

Signs

- Squinting
- Holding objects too close or far from the eyes.

Investigations

- Evaluating near point of convergence
- Proper cycloplegic refraction.

Complications

- *Amblyopia*: associated with uncorrected anisometropia, keratoconus
- *High hyperopia*: risk for developing accommodative esotropia, narrow angle glaucoma
- *Progressive myopia*: associated with uncorrected astigmatism, retinal detachment, myopic degeneration with choroidal neovascular membrane.

Pearls and Considerations

Contact lenses greatly reduce minification and magnification which allows large anisometropic corrections.

Commonly Associated Conditions

- *Hyperopia*: microphthalmos, cornea plana
- *Myopia*: Stickler's syndrome, Ehler-Danlos syndrome, retinopathy of prematurity, Marfan's syndrome, Weill-Marchesani syndrome.

Referral Information

None

Differential Diagnosis

- Decreased visual acuity from any pathologic ocular condition
- Nanophthalmos
- Macular hyperplasia and thickened sclera.

Causes

- Unknown, but may run in families
- Mismatches between axial length and focusing power of the eye (primarily the cornea and lens).

Pathology

- *Hyperopia*: at risk for angle-closure glaucoma
- *Myopia*: oblique optic disc with exposed sclera viewed as a white crescent.

Epidemiology

- Varies, but up to 20% of patients are myopic and 75% require prescriptions between -0.50 and $+8.00$ D
- Sixty-five percent of all refractive prescriptions are for presbyopes
- Many children have bilateral symmetric astigmatism that resolves by age 3
- Typically, young children have hyperopia that decreases with age
- A small group are myopic in childhood which continues to increase as the child grows.

TREATMENT

Diet and Lifestyle

No particular diet/lifestyle modifications have been proven to attribute to refractive error.

Pharmacologic Treatment

No pharmacologic management has been proven to prevent refractive errors.

Nonpharmacologic Treatment

- Glasses and contact lenses
- Refractive surgery when indicated.

Treatment Aims

Improve visual acuity

Prognosis

Children typically accept new prescriptions without difficulty.

Follow-up and Management

- Children with refractive errors are followed annually
- Adults can be examined biannually.

GENERAL REFERENCES

Davidson S, Quinn GE. The impact of pediatric vision disorders in adulthood. Pediatrics. 2011;127(2):334-9. Epub 2011.

Monga S, Kekunnaya R, Gupta A, et al. Accommodative esotropia. Ophthalmology. 2012;119(3):655-6; author reply 656.

Dusek WA, Pierscionek BK, McClelland JF. An evaluation of clinical treatment of convergence insufficiency for children with reading difficulties. BMC Ophthalmol. 2011;11:21.

Goss DA. Attempts to reduce the rate of increase of myopia in young people: a critical literature review. Am J Optom Physiol Opt. 1982;59:828-41.

McBrien N, Moghaddam HO, Reeder AP. Atropine reduces experimental myopia and eye enlargement via a nonaccommodative mechanism. Invest Ophthalmol Vis Sci. 1993;34:205-15.

O'Leary DJ, Millodot M. Eyelid closure causes myopia in humans. Experientia. 1979;35:1478-9.

Wallman J, Turkel J, Trachtman J. Extreme myopia produced by modest changes in early visual experience. Science. 1978;201:1249-51.

Retinal Artery Occlusion (362.31)

DIAGNOSIS

Definition

Blockage of an artery supplying the retina (can be the central artery or an arterial branch).

Synonyms

None; common abbreviations include BRAO (branch retinal artery occlusion) and CRAO (central retinal artery occlusion).

Symptoms

- Acute
- Severe
- Painless loss of vision.

Signs

Branch Retinal Artery Occlusion (Fig. 1)

- May see one or more emboli in a branch arteriole
- Cotton-wool spots
- Arteriolar narrowing
- Retinal whitening: in distribution of the blocked arteriole.

Central Retinal Artery Occlusion (Fig. 2)

- Retinal whitening
- Cherry-red spot in the fovea (xanthophyllic pigment of fovea stands out in an otherwise white macula)
- Narrowing or segmentation of retinal arterioles
- Optic nerve pallor: can be seen in the late stages.

Investigations

Branch Retinal Artery Occlusion

- *Fluorescein angiography*: will help map out the area of retinal involvement
- Noninvasive carotid artery blood flow studies
- Echocardiography.

Central Retinal Artery Occlusion

- *Fluorescein angiography*: demonstrates delayed or even complete lack of retinal arterial filling
- *Echoretinography (ERG)*: shows a reduction in the B-wave amplitude
- *Systemic workup*: carotid artery noninvasive testing, echocardiography, erythrocyte sedimentation rate if temporal arteritis suspected; further studies should be considered if sickle cell disease, intravenous drug use, or hyperviscosity syndromes are suspected.

Differential Diagnosis

Branch Retinal Artery Occlusion

- Transient retinal ischemia
- Transient visual disturbance
- Commotio retinae secondary to trauma.
- Arteriolar vasospasm.

Central Retinal Artery Occlusion

Ophthalmic artery occlusion

Causes

Branch Retinal Artery Occlusion

- Embolization of a branch retinal arteriole from atherosclerotic plaque in the carotid artery or a calcific heart valve: most common cause
- Atrial myxoma in younger patients
- Talc emboli associated with IV drug use
- Intranasal cocaine causing arteriolar spasm
- Fat emboli after long-bone fractures.

Central Retinal Artery Occlusion

Thrombosis or embolic blockage to the central retinal artery; the most common source of emboli comes from the carotid arteries.

Epidemiology

Branch Retinal Artery Occlusion

- Most patients will resume a vision of 20/40 or better, although the paracentral scotoma can be visually disabling in some patients
- Most patients will have a permanent visual field defect in the area of retinal distribution supplied by that arteriole.

Central Retinal Artery Occlusion

- Ninety percent of patients will have vision less than finger-counting range
- Up to 25% of patients will describe a preceding episode of transient visual loss
- Five-year mortality results from myocardial infarction in approximately 40% of patients.

Pathology

Branch Retinal Artery Occlusion

Similar to that seen with CRAO, although the area of retinal necrosis confined to the inner layers of the retina is small; the outer layers are well preserved; late in the healing phase, the inner layer of the retina becomes acellular.

Central Retinal Artery Occlusion

Initially, ischemic necrosis is seen, followed by acellular scarring of the inner retinal layers.

Diagnosis continued on p. 352

TREATMENT

Diet and Lifestyle

Diet that promotes cardiovascular health, including decreased fat and salt intake, is indicated.

Pharmacologic Treatment

- An aspirin a day may help prevent future episodes of BRAO and is recommended for CRAO patients with a negative workup who are in the atherosclerotic age range.
- In selected patients (e.g. monocular patients presenting within 180 minutes), the risks and benefits need to be discussed thoroughly before considering administration of intravenous tissue plasminogen activator. This may lead to reperfusion and restoration of vision in some patients.

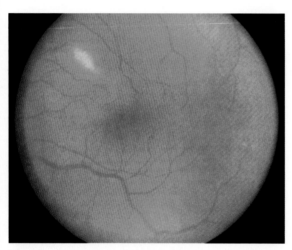

Fig. 1: Supratemporal branch occlusion (BRAO) with intraretinal whitening in the superior macula and a prominent cotton-wool spot.

Treatment Aims

Branch Retinal Artery Occlusion
Prompt workup to rule out any treatable causes that would decrease future morbidity.

Central Retinal Artery Occlusion
To lower intraocular pressure and vasodilate the arterioles to dislodge the emboli into a smaller branch arteriole.

Other Treatments

Central Retinal Artery Occlusion
Panretinal photocoagulation should be instituted for evidence of iris, angle, or retinal neovascularization and for associated secondary glaucoma.

Prognosis

Branch Retinal Artery Occlusion
- Most patients see an improvement in vision as the retinal edema resolves
- Patients will have a relative scotoma in the distribution of the occlusion that may be permanent.

Central Retinal Artery Occlusion
- Prognosis for normal vision is poor; however, central vision may be spared if a patent cilioretinal artery is present
- If suspected, temporal arteritis must be ruled out in an attempt to preserve vision in the fellow eye.

Follow-up and Management

Branch Retinal Artery Occlusion
Patients should be followed closely for the first 6 months to look for signs of neovascularization.

Central Retinal Artery Occlusion
Patients should be followed every 4 weeks to look for signs of neovascular glaucoma, which has been reported in up to 10% of patients.

351

Treatment continued on p. 353

Retinal Artery Occlusion (362.31)

DIAGNOSIS—cont'd

Complications

Branch Retinal Artery Occlusion

Neovascularization of the retina: from ischemia.

Central Retinal Artery Occlusion

- Neovascularization of the retina, iris, or angle
- Neovascular glaucoma.

Pearls and Considerations

- Central retinal artery occlusion is a true ocular emergency requiring immediate intervention
- Afferent pupillary defect will be present in CRAO
- Less than 10% of eyes with CRAO will eventually develop rubeosis iridis in the affected eye
- Ninety percent of BRAO events involve the temporal vessels
- Patients with CRAO have a high 5-year mortality rate because of cardiovascular disease and stroke
- If no cholesterol plaque is seen and the patient is in the appropriate age group, a sedimentation rate needs to be done to rule out temporal arteritis.

Referral Information

Refer to a retinal specialist for further evaluation and treatment immediately.

TREATMENT—cont'd

Nonpharmacologic Treatment

For Branch Retinal Artery Occlusion

If there is evidence of retinal neovascularization, sector laser photocoagulation in the distribution of the ischemia is recommended.

For Central Retinal Artery Occlusion

- Prompt evaluation within 180 minutes of the occlusion of the central retinal artery is optimal before irreparable damage to the retina occurs
- If the patient is seen within this time frame, a paracentesis should be performed in an attempt to lower the intraocular pressure
- Digital ocular massage may be able to dislodge the clot and improve vision; although rarely successful it should be attempted, since there are minimal side effects to the maneuver, the most common being bradycardia from the oculocardiac reflex.

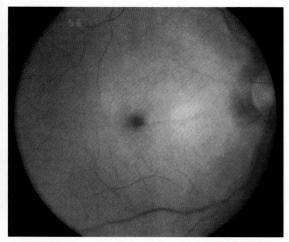

Fig. 2: Central occlusion (CRAO) with diffuse whitening of the posterior pole, cherry-red spot in the fovea, and telangiectasia of the optic nerve vessels.

GENERAL REFERENCES

Biousse V. Thrombolysis for acute central retinal artery occlusion: is it time? Am J Ophthalmol. 2008;146:631-4.

Brown GC, Magargal LE, Simeone FA, et al. Arterial obstruction and ocular neovascularization. Ophthalmology. 1982; 89:139-46.

Brown GC, Magargal LE. Central retinal artery obstruction and visual acuity, Ophthalmology. 1982;89:14-9.

Heyreh SS, Kolder HE, Weingeist TA. Central retinal artery occlusion and retinal tolerance time. Ophthalmology. 1980;87:75-8.

Sharma S, Brown GC. Retinal artery obstruction. Retina, 4th edition. St Louis: Elsevier; 2006.

Retinal Degeneration, Peripheral Cystoid (362.62)

DIAGNOSIS

Definition
Cyst like spaces associated with focal thinning of the peripheral retina.

Synonyms
None

Symptoms
Patients are asymptomatic.

Signs
Small, stippled areas of the inner retinal surface just posterior to the ora serrata: often aligned with the dentate processes; more frequently found inferotemporally and supratemporally.

Investigations
- Visual acuity testing
- Slit-lamp biomicroscopic examination
- Dilated fundus examination.

Complications
The cystoid spaces may coalesce into retinoschisis cavities that over time may cause peripheral visual loss.

Pearls and Considerations
Often detected with careful inspection of retina on routine examination.

Referral Information
No referral is necessary.

Differential Diagnosis
- Lattice degeneration
- Bullous retinoschisis.

Cause
Peripheral degeneration.

Epidemiology
- Most adults will have evidence of typical cystoid degeneration by age 20 or older. Over time, the cysts may coalesce to form typical retinoschisis.
- Eighteen percent of adults will have reticular cystoid degeneration, 41% of whom will have bilateral involvement. This can develop into reticular retinoschisis over time.

Classification
Classification is based on pathologic findings:
- *Typical cystoid degeneration*
- *Reticular cystiod degeneration*: often found posterior to areas of typical cystoid degeneration; more common inferotemporally.

Pathology
- *Reticular cystoid degeneration*: cysts are found in the nerve fiber layer
- *Typical cystoid degeneration*: cysts are found between the outer plexiform layer and the inner nuclear layer.

TREATMENT

Diet and Lifestyle

No special precautions are necessary.

Pharmacologic Treatment

No pharmacologic treatment is recommended.

Nonpharmacologic Treatment

No nonpharmacologic treatment is recommended.

Treatment Aims

None

Prognosis

Excellent

Follow-up and Management

Follow-up with annual dilated eye examinations.

GENERAL REFERENCE

Byer NE. Cystic retinal tuft and miscellaneous peripheral retinal findings. In: Albert DM, Jakobiec FA (Eds). Principles and Practice of Ophthalmology, vol. 2. Philadelphia: Saunders; 1994. pp. 1067-8.

Retinal Detachment (361)

DIAGNOSIS

Definition
- Separation of the sensory retina from the retinal pigment epithelium (RPE)
- *Rhegmatogenous retinal detachment*: a retinal detachment caused by one or more full-thickness breaks in the retina
- *Nonrhegmatogenous tractional retinal detachment*: a retinal detachment caused by mechanical force from vitreoretinal adhesions
- *Nonrhegmatogenous serous retinal detachment*: a retinal detachment that results from an accumulation of subretinal fluid.

Synonyms
None; often abbreviated as RD (retinal detachment).

Symptoms

Rhegmatogenous Retinal Detachment
- Flashes; floaters
- Veil- or curtain-like loss of vision: starting in the peripheral visual field and progressing toward the center.

Nonrhegmatogenous Retinal Detachment (Serous and Tractional)
Progressive loss of vision, floaters, pain.

Signs (Figs 1 to 4)

Rhegmatogenous Retinal Detachment
Decreased central and peripheral vision, pigment in the anterior vitreous, detached retina with or without identifiable breaks in the retina.

Nonrhegmatogenous Serous Retinal Detachment
Serous detachment of the retina is secondary to fluid building up in the subretinal space without evidence of a retinal break. These detachments take on a typical bullous, convex appearance and have a characteristic "shifting of fluid" when the patient changes from an erect to a supine position.

Nonrhegmatogenous Tractional Retinal Detachment
Tractional detachment is caused by vitreoretinal fibroproliferative membranes that form on the surface of the retina; with contraction, the retinal surface takes on a concave appearance. These RDs occasionally advance to the ora serrata.

Investigations

Rhegmatogenous Retinal Detachment
- *Careful history*: ask if the patient is nearsighted; if history of trauma or history of recent eye surgery or laser, check visual acuity and visual fields by confrontation
- *Slit-lamp evaluation*: of the anterior vitreous looking for pigment dispersion.
- *Dilated fundus examination*: with peripheral depression to look for retinal breaks
- *Examination of the posterior vitreous*: look for a vitreous detachment.

Nonrhegmatogenous Serous Retinal Detachment
- *Slit-lamp and indirect ophthalmoscopic examination*: of peripheral retina to rule out a break; a contact lens may improve peripheral view; scleral depression should be performed to view adequately the retinal-ora serrata junction
- Serous detachment lacks corrugated appearance and pigmented demarcation line.

Differential Diagnosis
- White without pressure
- Choroidal effusion or choroidal hemorrhage
- Posterior vitreous detachment, hemorrhage or vitritis with vitreous opacities limiting the view of attached retina
- Uveal melanoma.

Cause
- Rhegmatogenous detachment is caused by peripheral vitreoretinal adhesions causing a break in the retina through which vitreous fluid moves into the subretinal space.
- Serous retinal detachment is usually caused by inflammatory conditions in which fluid leaks out of the vasculature and accumulates in the subretinal space.
- Tractional retinal detachment is most commonly caused by diabetes, but can also be caused by any chronic condition such as uveitis in which the posterior vitreous becomes fibrotic and adherent to the retina.

Immunology/Epidemiology (Whatever applies)
- Risk factors for rhegmatogenous detachment include family history of RD, high myopia, lattice degeneration and pseudophakia.
- Serous detachments are usually a result of an immunologic condition causing posterior uveitis such as Harada's disease. They are the least frequent type of detachment.
- Traction detachments are usually seen in longstanding poorly controlled diabetic patients.

Pathology
- Rhegmatogenous detachments will initially display an area of vitreous which is attached to the retina, but if the vitreous separates from the break then no adherence will be seen on microscopic pathologic analysis of the tear.
- Depending upon the underlying cause of the serous detachment the subretinal fluid will contain inflammatory cells and cytokines within the serous fluid.
- Traction detachments demonstrate areas of vitreous and retinal fibroblastic proliferation with particular adherence to the intraretinal vessels and varying amounts of blood within and overlying these areas.

Diagnosis continued on p. 358

TREATMENT

Diet and Lifestyle

Rhegmatogenous Retinal Detachment

- Safety glasses should be worn by individuals with high-risk characteristics (e.g. high myopia, increased axial length, large patches of lattice)
- Avoid contact sports if the individual has high-risk characteristics.

Nonpharmacologic Treatment

For Rhegmatogenous Retinal Detachment

- *Laser*: to wall off the detached area if it is peripheral and if only a small area is detached
- *Pneumatic retinopexy with cryotherapy*: if the break is above the 4 and 8 o'clock positions
- *Scleral buckle and cryotherapy*: with or without drainage of subretinal fluid
- *Vitrectomy, laser, gas or silicone-oil tamponade*: most commonly done in pseudophakic patients.

For Nonrhegmatogenous Retinal Detachment (Serous and Tractional)

Pars plana vitrectomy with membrane delamination: indicated for tractional RDs that threaten the fovea.

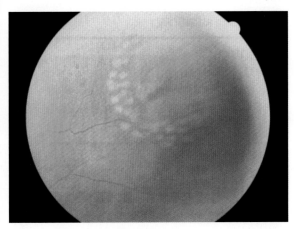

Fig. 1: Peripheral horseshoe-shaped retinal break with surrounding laser photocoagulation.

Treatment Aims

Rhegmatogenous Retinal Detachment

- To prevent extension of the RD into the macular region
- To reattach the retina.

Nonrhegmatogenous Retinal Detachment

To preserve vision.

Prognosis

Rhegmatogenous Retinal Detachment

The prognosis depends on the involvement of the macula, size of the break, and duration of the detachment. If the macula is off, the longer the retina is detached, the more permanent the damage to the retina. Larger breaks are more difficult to repair due to the formation of proliferative vitreoretinopathy.

Nonrhegmatogenous Retinal Detachment

The overall prognosis depends on the underlying condition causing the detachment.

Follow-up and Management

Rhegmatogenous Retinal Detachment

- Careful education for patients with high-risk characteristics
- Yearly dilated eye examination for patients with lattice degeneration.

Nonrhegmatogenous Retinal Detachment

Varies for each cause.

357

Treatment continued on p. 359

DIAGNOSIS—cont'd

Complications

Rhegmatogenous Retinal Detachment

- *Decreased intraocular pressure (IOP)*: common; IOP can be elevated rarely
- Cataract formation
- *Proliferative vitreoretinopathy*: contraction and folding of the retina secondary to membrane formation on the retinal surface
- Peripheral neovascularization, permanent visual loss, inflammation in the vitreous, iris neovascularization.

Nonrhegmatogenous Serous Retinal Detachment

Permanent visual loss: from disruption of the RPE layer.

Nonrhegmatogenous Tractional Retinal Detachment

- *Retinal break*: from advancing vitreoretinal traction; creates a combined tractional-rhegmatogenous RD
- *Visual loss*: will occur if the traction advances to involve the macula.

Pearls and Considerations

- All patients with predisposing peripheral degenerations (e.g. lattice degeneration) should be advised of the signs and symptoms of RD
- Three factors must be present for a rhegmatogenous RD to occur:
  - Liquefaction of the vitreous (factors that contribute to liquefaction include cataract extraction, trauma, high myopia, and intraocular inflammation)
  - Tractional force
  - Presence of a retinal break
- Rhegmatogenous RD has a familial component; siblings of an RD patient are three times more likely to experience a rhegmatogenous RD.

Referral Information

Immediate referral to a retinal specialist for surgical repair is indicated.

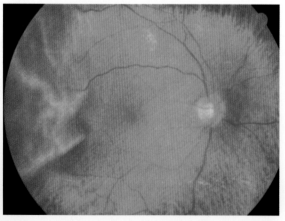

Fig. 2: Rhegmatogenous retinal detachment with elevation and corrugation of the retina temporal to the fovea.

TREATMENT—cont'd

Other Treatments

For Rhegmatogenous Retinal Detachment

- Laser prophylaxis to symptomatic retinal breaks (breaks associated with flashes and floaters)
- Laser prophylaxis to areas of lattice degeneration, atrophic holes, or asymptomatic horseshoe-shaped tears in the fellow eye, in patients with a history of RD (remains controversial).

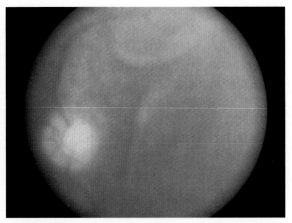

Fig. 3: Serous retinal detachment in patient with recurrent Harada's disease involving the macula.

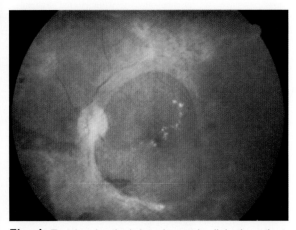

Fig. 4: Tractional retinal detachment in diabetic patient. Note the concave appearance of the retinal elevation caused by contraction of fibrovascular tissue emanating from the optic nerve and arcade vessels.

GENERAL REFERENCES

Benson WE, Morse PH. The prognosis of retina detachment due to lattice degeneration. Ann Ophthalmol. 1978;10:1197-200.

Bouldry EE. Risk of retinal tears in patients with vitreous floaters. Am Ophthalmol. 1983;96:783-7.

Oh KT, Hartnett MT, Landers MB. Pathogenetic mechanisms of retinal detachment. Retina, 4th edition. St Louis: Elsevier; 2006.

Tasman WS. Posterior vitreous detachment and peripheral retinal breaks. Trans Am Acad Ophthalmol Otolaryngol. 1968;72:217-24.

Weichel ED, Martidis A, Fineman MS, et al. Pars plana vitrectomy versus combined pars plana vitrectomy-scleral buckle for primary repair of pseudophakic retinal detachment. Ophthalmol. 2006; 113:2033-40.

Young LHY, D'Amico DJ. Retinal detachments. In: Albert DM, Jakobiec FA (Eds). Principles and Practice of Ophthalmology, vol. 2. Philadelphia: Saunders; 1994. pp. 1084-92.

Retinal Dystrophies (362.70)

DIAGNOSIS

Definition
A family of inherited degenerative disorders of the retinal structure.

Synonyms
See diseases below.

Symptoms

Best's Disease (Vitelliform Macular Dystrophy, 362.76) (Fig. 1)
- Blurry vision
- Metamorphopsia
- Decreased vision.

Stargardt's Disease (Fundus Flavimaculatus, 362.75) (Fig. 2)
- Gradual decrease in central vision: by teenage years
- Decreased color vision: red-green dyschromatopsia.

Signs

Best's Disease
Based on the stage of the disease: see Classification.

Stargardt's Disease
- Decreased vision: in the 20/100 range
- Absolute central scotoma
- Acquired red-green dyschromatopsia
- *Yellow-white irregular flecks*: at level of retinal pigment epithelium (RPE)
- Beaten-metal or bull's-eye appearance of the macula.

Investigations

Best's Disease
- Careful family history
- *Electrooculogram*: abnormal ratio of <1.5 (normal >1.8)
- *Full electroretinograms (ERGs)*: normal
- *Fluorescein angiography*: shows areas of blockage by the vitelliform lesion.

Stargardt's Disease
- Dark adaptation is normal
- *Fluorescein angiography*: shows a classic silent choroid with window-defect changes caused by alteration of RPE
- *Full ERGs*: normal.

Complications

Best's Disease
Secondary choroidal neovascularization.

Stargardt's Disease
- *Decreased vision to legal blindness*: by the 20s
- Secondary choroidal neovascularization.

Pearls and Considerations
Topic is too broad for specific recommendations.

Referral Information
Refer for genetic counseling as appropriate.

Differential Diagnosis

Stargardt's Disease
- Toxic maculopathy
- Cone-rod degeneration.

Cause

Best's Disease
- Autosomal dominance seen in individuals of European, Hispanic, and African ancestry
- A disease-specific mutation in a retina-specific protein, bestrophin, has been found to be the cause of the disease.

Stargardt's Disease
- Autosomal recessive inheritance with variable penetrance
- Mutations in the ABCA4 gene, which encodes an ATP-binding cassette transporter, have been found to be the cause of the disease.

Epidemiology

Stargardt's Disease
- Eighty percent of patients will have greater than 20/40 vision
- Only 4% of patients will have less than 20/200 vision.

Classification

Best's Disease
Stage 1: Previtelliform: normal fundus appearance with normal vision.
Stage 2: Vitelliform: occurs in early childhood; patients are asymptomatic, and disease often goes undetected; a yellow lesion 0.5–2.0 disc diameters in size is often seen in the macula under the RPE, resembling yolk of an egg.
Stage 3: Pseudohypopyon: usually occurs in teenage years; the lipofuscin breaks through the RPE and settles inferiorly in the subretinal space.
Stage 4: "Scrambled egg": yellow deposits scattered throughout the posterior pole; varying amounts of RPE atrophy and hypertrophy.

A variant of Best's disease occurs at an older age. Multiple vitelliform lesions throughout the posterior pole can be seen.

Pathology

Best's Disease
Excessive lipofuscin-like material in the RPE cells throughout the posterior pole, particularly in the fovea

Stargardt's Disease
Accumulation of a lipofuscin material at the apical level of the RPE cells

TREATMENT

Diet and Lifestyle

No special precautions are necessary.

Pharmacologic Treatment

No pharmacologic treatment is recommended.

Nonpharmacologic Treatment

Patients with either disease should receive genetic counseling.

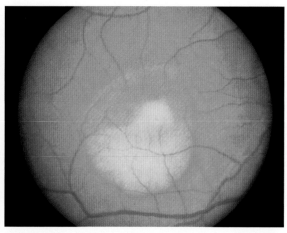

Fig. 1: Stage 3 Best's disease. Note the layered pseudo-hypopyon. The lipofuscin has broken through the retinal pigment epithelium and settled inferiorly in the subretinal space.

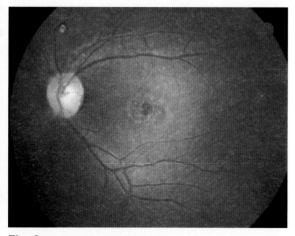

Fig. 2: Stargardt's disease. Note the yellow-white irregular flecks at the level of the retinal pigment epithelium and the beaten-metal appearance of the macula.

Treatment Aims

None

Prognosis

Best's Disease
Good, with vision in the 20/40–20/60 range.
Stargardt's Disease
Legal blindness

Follow-up and Management

Best's Disease
• Educate the patient on the signs of secondary choroidal neovascularization
• Annual eye examinations
• Because it is a dominant inheritance pattern, all family members should be examined.

Stargardt's Disease
Education on the symptoms of secondary choroidal neovascularization.

GENERAL REFERENCES

Deutman AF, Hoyng CB, van-Lith Verhoeven JJC. Macular dystrophies. Retina, 4th edition. St Louis: Elsevier; 2006.

Eagle RC, Lucier AC, Bernadino VB, et al. Retinal pigment epithelial abnormalities in fundus flavimaculatus: a light and electron microscope study. Ophthalmology. 1980;87:1189-200.

Frangieh GT, Green WR, Fine SL. A histopathologic study of Best's vitelliform dystrophy. Arch Ophthalmol. 1982;100:1115-21.

MacDonald IM, Tran M, Musarella MA. Ocular genetics: current understanding, Survey Ophthalmol. 2004;49:159-96.

Website for Genetic Testing Information. www.genetests.org.

DIAGNOSIS

Definition

Obstruction of a vein draining the retina (can be the central vein or a branch retinal vein).

Synonyms

None; common abbreviations are CRVO (central retinal vein occlusion) and BRVO (branch retinal vein occlusion).

Symptoms

Branch Retinal Vein Occlusion

- Decreased vision
- *Floaters*: indicates vitreous hemorrhage.

Central Retinal Vein Occlusion

- *Loss of vision, decreased vision*: related to degree of obstruction, ischemia
- *Eye pain*: if associated elevation in intraocular pressure (IOP)
- *Floaters*: indicates a vitreous hemorrhage.

Signs

Branch Retinal Vein Occlusion (Fig. 1)

- *Intraretinal hemorrhages*: distributed in one quadrant of the retina
- Cotton-wool spots
- Retinal edema
- Intraretinal lipid
- Vitreous hemorrhage
- *Neovascularization*: of the disc or elsewhere.

Central Retinal Vein Occlusion (Fig. 2)

- *Intraretinal hemorrhages*: in all four quadrants
- Cotton-wool spots
- Lipid exudates
- Retinal edema
- Vitreous hemorrhage
- *Neovascularization*: of the retina, iris, or angle
- Elevated IOP
- Collateral vessels on the optic nerve head imply a resolved occlusion.

Differential Diagnosis

Trauma, vasculitis, severe anemia, ocular ischemic syndrome.

Cause

Hypertension, chronic open-angle glaucoma, atherosclerosis, history of cardiovascular disease, oral contraceptives, chronic elevated systemic hypertension, glaucoma, diabetes mellitus, syphilis, antiphospholipid antibody syndrome, blood dyscrasias, collagen vascular diseases.

Epidemiology

Branch Retinal Vein Occlusion

- Two-thirds involve the supratemporal retinal vein; occurs at the crossing of the artery and vein that share a common adventitial sheath
- Fifty percent have associated decreased vision secondary to macular edema
- Occurs in the fifth and sixth decades of life.

Central Retinal Vein Occlusion

- Peak incidence in those more than 60 years of age; more common in men
- Thirty percent are ischemic
- Sixty percent with more than 10 disc areas of ischemia will develop neovascular glaucoma within 90 days
- Seventy percent are nonischemic; may convert to ischemic within first 3–6 months.

Classification

Ischemic versus Nonischemic BRVO/CVRO

- In patients with ischemic BRVO, if more than 5 disc diameters of capillary nonperfusion on fluorescein angiography, they are at risk of developing neovascularization of the retina.
- Ischemic CRVOs have extensive hemorrhage in all four quadrants of the retina, more cotton-wool spots, marked macular edema, and a presenting vision of less than 20/200. Fluorescein angiography usually shows 10 disc areas of capillary nonperfusion.
- Nonischemic CRVOs have mild disc edema, mild dilation of retinal veins, and intraretinal hemorrhages in all four quadrants of the retina. Macular edema may develop gradually. Presenting visual acuity implies prognosis.

Diagnosis continued on p. 364

TREATMENT

Diet and Lifestyle

No precautions are necessary.

Pharmacologic Treatment

Branch Retinal Vein Occlusion

- Lower IOP if elevated
- Discontinue oral contraceptives if applicable
- Intravitreal steroid such as Triesence (triamcinolone), Avastin (bevacizumab), or Lucentis (ranibizumab) for macular edema.

Central Retinal Vein Occlusion

- Intravitreal steroid, bevacizumab or ranibizumab for macular edema. Bevacizumab and ranibizumab can also be used to decrease the neovascular drive if vessels still growing after panretinal layer
- Lower IOP if there is evidence of glaucoma.

Standard Dosage

- Nonselective beta-blocker (timolol, metipranolol, or levobunolol), one drop twice daily
- Selective beta-blocker (betaxolol 0.5%), one drop twice daily
- Topical carbonic anhydrase inhibitor, one drop three times daily
- Oral carbonic anhydrase inhibitor (acetazolamide), 250 mg four times daily or 500 mg twice daily
- If there is evidence of iris neovascularization, administer atropine sulfate 1%. One drop twice daily is recommended to maintain long-term pupillary dilation.

Treatment Aims

- To maintain IOP within the normal range
- To resolve intraretinal hemorrhage and macular edema.

Prognosis

Branch Retinal Vein Occlusion

Often depends on presenting visual acuity; better in patients without macular ischemia.

Central Retinal Vein Occlusion

Often depends on visual acuity, level of ischemia.

Follow-up and Management

Branch Retinal Vein Occlusion

Every 4–6 weeks to look for evidence of edema or neovascularization.

Central Retinal Vein Occlusion

- Every 4 weeks for at least 6 months; gonioscopy at all visits to look for evidence of angle neovascularization
- Fundus photographs to document changes and allow future comparison
- Fluorescein angiography for patients suspected of ischemic CRVO or if evidence of macular edema; often this needs to be repeated within the first 6 months if clinical signs of progression.

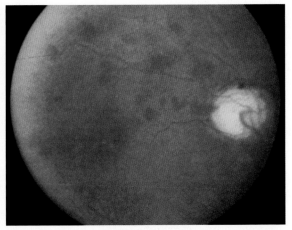

Fig. 1: Branch retinal vein occlusion involving the supratemporal vein. The intraretinal blot hemorrhages extend into the macula and respect the horizontal midline.

Treatment continued on p. 365

Retinal Vein Occlusion (362.35)

DIAGNOSIS—cont'd

Investigations

Branch Retinal Vein Occlusion

- *Fluorescein angiography*: to assess retinal capillary perfusion and ischemia, retinal leakage, and extent of occlusion
- *Optical coherence tomography*: to assess degree of macular edema and response to treatment.

Central Retinal Vein Occlusion

- *Intraocular pressure*: to rule out glaucoma
- *Gonioscopy*: to rule out angle neovascularization
- *Fluorescein angiography*: used to determine if there is retinal ischemia, edema, or neovascularization
- *Optical coherence tomography*: to gauge level of macular edema and response to treatment
- Systemic blood pressure
- *Laboratory studies*: complete blood count with differential, rapid plasma reagin, antinuclear antibodies, anticardiolipin antibodies, serum protein electrophoresis, cholesterol, carotid ultrasound, sedimentation rate
- *Electroretinogram*: depressed B/A-wave amplitude indicates retinal ischemia. This test is rarely ordered, because fluorescein can usually be done to detect ischemia.

Complications

Branch Retinal Vein Occlusion

Vitreous hemorrhage, neovascularization of the disc and elsewhere, retinal macular edema.

Central Retinal Vein Occlusion

- Retinal macular edema, optic nerve and retinal neovascularization, neovascular glaucoma
- *Vitreous hemorrhage*: from optic nerve or peripheral retinal neovascularization.

Pearls and Considerations

- The earlier CRVO is treated, the lower the risk of developing ocular neovascularization
- Branch retinal vein occlusion almost always occurs at arteriovenous crossings.

Referral Information

Refer to a retinal specialist for laser photocoagulation and/or intravitreal injections as indicated.

Pathology

Branch Retinal Vein Occlusion

Contraction of the sheath, increased rigidity of the crossing artery, atherosclerosis, and thrombotic occlusion of the corresponding vein.

Central Retinal Vein Occlusion

Occlusion of the central retinal vein occurs behind the lamina cribrosa in the substance of the optic nerve or where the vein enters the subarachnoid space; can see blood throughout all layers of the retina.

TREATMENT—cont'd

Nonpharmacologic Treatment

Branch Retinal Vein Occlusion

- *Grid laser photocoagulation*: for macular edema and vision greater than 20/40 without evidence of macular ischemia
- *Sector panretinal photocoagulation*: for ischemic BRVO for evidence of retinal or optic nerve neovascularization.

Central Retinal Vein Occlusion

- Panretinal photocoagulation for ischemic CRVOs is recommended when there is evidence of iris or angle neovascularization with or without elevated IOP. It is also recommended when severe ischemia as documented by fluorescein angiography is present.
- Focal grid laser therapy for macular edema has not shown significant benefit in the older population.

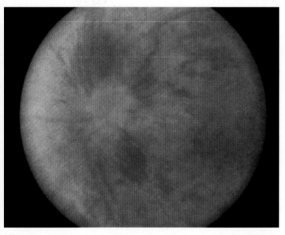

Fig. 2: Central retinal vein occlusion. The hemorrhages involve all four quadrants of the posterior pole and dilated venous system.

GENERAL REFERENCES

Branch Retinal Vein Occlusion Study Group. Argon laser photocoagulation for macular edema and branch vein occlusion. Am J Ophthalmol. 1984;98: 271-82.

Branch Retinal Vein Occlusion Study Group. Argon laser scatter photocoagulation for prevention of neovascularization and vitreous hemorrhage in branch retinal vein occlusion. Arch Ophthalmol. 1986;104:34-41.

Brown DM, Campochiaro PA, Singh RP, et al. Ranibizumab for macular edema following central retinal vein occlusion: six month primary end point results of a phase III study. Ophthalmology. 2010; 117:1124-33.

Central Retinal Vein Occlusion Study Group. A randomized clinical trial of early panretinal photocoagulation for ischemic central retinal vein occlusion. Ophthalmology. 1995;102:1434-43.

Central Retinal Vein Occlusion Study Group. Evaluation of grid pattern photocoagulation for macular edema in central retinal vein occlusion. Ophthalmology. 1995;102:1425-33.

Ip MS, Scott IU, VanVeldhuisen PC, et al. A randomized trial comparing the efficacy and safety of intravitreal triamcinolone with observation to treat vision loss associated with macular edema secondary to central retinal vein occlusion: the Standard Care vs Corticosteroid for Retinal Vein Occlusion (SCORE) study report 5. Arch Ophthalmol. 2009;127:1101-14.

Mruthyunjaya P, Fekrat S. Central retinal vein occlusion. Retina, 4th edition. St Louis: Elsevier; 2006.

Phillips S, Fekrat S, Finkelstein D. Branch retinal vein occlusion. Retina, 4th edition. St Louis: Elsevier; 2006.

Yanoff M, Fine BS. Neural (sensory) retina. Ocular Pathology, 4th edition. Barcelona, Spain: Mosby; 1996. p. 491.

Retinitis Pigmentosa (362.74)

DIAGNOSIS

Definition

A group of disorders characterized by progressive retinal dysfunction, cell loss and atrophy of the retinal tissue.

Synonym

"Night blindness"; commonly abbreviated RP.

Symptoms

- Decreased night vision (nyctalopia)
- Decreased color vision
- Loss of peripheral vision
- Blurry vision.

Signs

- *Pigment clumping or "bone spicule formation" in the peripheral retina*: see Figure 1
- Areas of retinal pigment atrophy
- Arteriolar attenuation
- Optic nerve "waxy" pallor
- Pigmented cells in the vitreous
- Stellate pattern to posterior lens capsule opacification
- Cystoid macular edema
- Epimacular membrane.

Investigations

- *Careful family history*: to detect any history of blindness
- *Careful drug history*: to rule out pseudo-RP as a possible cause
- Full-color examination
- *Goldmann visual field analysis*: to look for constriction and ring scotomas
- *Electroretinography*: results usually abnormal to nonrecordable
- Rule in or out possible systemic associations
- *Phytanic acid level*: rule out Refsum disease
- *Cardiology consult*: to rule out heart block
- *Peripheral blood smear*: to look for acanthocytosis
- Genetic counseling and workup
- Examine family members for possible subclinical levels of disease.

Complications

- Decreased vision
- Cataracts
- Cystoid macular edema
- Drusen in the optic nerve head.

Differential Diagnosis

Toxic retinopathy secondary to phenothiazines, congenital rubella, syphilis, resolution of previous retinal detachment (serous or rhegmatogenous), vitamin A deficiency, choroideremia, end-stage Stargardt's disease, gyrate atrophy, congenital stationary night blindness, diffuse unilateral neuroretinitis

Cause

Hereditary or Spontaneous Retinitis Pigmentosa

Autosomal dominant: late onset, less severe
Autosomal recessive: variable onset and severity.
X-linked recessive: least frequent, most severe, earliest onset.

Retinitis Pigmentosa Associated with Systemic Disease

Refsum disease: elevated phytanic acid levels.
Bassen-Kornzweig syndrome: deficiency in lipoproteins and malabsorption of vitamins A, D, E and K.
Kearns-Sayre syndrome: chronic progressive external ophthalmoplegia, limitation of ocular motility, ptosis and heart block before 20 years of age.
Usher's syndrome: hearing loss.
β-Lipoproteinemia: acanthocytosis of red blood cells.

Epidemiology

- Retinitis pigmentosa affects 1:5,000 individuals worldwide
- 44% are isolated
- 16% autosomal dominant
- 31% autosomal recessive
- 9% X-linked recessive.

Associated Features

See Cause section.

Pathology

- Photoreceptor loss
- Retinal pigment epithelium hyperplasia into the retina and surrounds retinal vessels
- Arteriolar thickening and hyalinization of vessel walls
- Diffuse or sectorial atrophy with late gliosis in the optic nerve.

Diagnosis continued on p. 368

TREATMENT

Diet and Lifestyle

- Genetic counseling
- Low-vision training and aids for activities of daily living
- Vocational rehabilitation
- Protective eyewear with ultraviolet-absorbing lenses.

Pharmacologic Treatment

- Treat underlying cause if associated with a systemic syndrome
- Supplement vitamins E and C, and carotene.

Treatment Aims

- To monitor vision
- To detect secondary side effects early.

Prognosis

Guarded, because of gradual progression of visual field loss and development of macular edema.

Follow-up and Management

Patients should have a baseline visual field examination and electroretinography performed annually; visual field examination should be performed annually until visual field is stable.

Treatment continued on p. 369

Retinitis Pigmentosa (362.74)

DIAGNOSIS—cont'd

Classification

- *Hereditary RP*: autosomal dominant most common; autosomal recessive; X-linked most severe
- Kearns-Sayre syndrome
- Usher's syndrome
- Refsum disease
- Vitamin A deficiency
- Congenital stationary night blindness.

Pearls and Considerations

- The term "retinitis" is misleading because it implies inflammation, which is not a part of the pathologic process of RP
- Night problems typically present within the first or second decade of life
- Night blindness is not diagnostic of RP; it can occur with other retinal disorders as well
- Color vision in RP usually remains good until vision is worse than 20/40
- Bone spicule formation results from the migration of pigment after retinal pigment epithelium (RPE) cells disintegrate.

Referral Information

Refer for genetic counseling or advanced diagnostic techniques as appropriate.

TREATMENT—cont'd

Nonpharmacologic Treatment

No nonpharmacologic treatment is recommended.

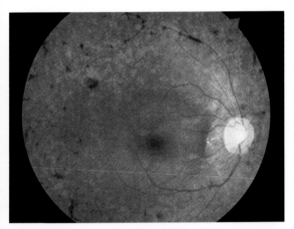

Fig. 1: Typical appearance of a patient with retinitis pigmentosa with bone spicule formation and retinal attenuation.

GENERAL REFERENCES

Kalloniatis M. Fletcher EL. Retinitis pigmentosa: understanding the clinical presentation, mechanisms and treatment options. Clin Exp Optom. 2004;87(2): 65-80.

Wang DY, Chan WM, Tam PO, et al. Gene mutations in retinitis pigmentosa and their clinical implications. Clin Chim Acta. 2005;351(1-2):5-16.

Weleber RG, Gregory-Evans K. Retinitis pigmentosa and allied disorders. In: Ryan SJ (Ed). Retina, 4th edition. St Louis: Elsevier; 2006.

Weleber RG, Kurz DE, Trzupek KM. Treatment of retinal and choroidal degenerations and dystrophies: current status and prospects for gene-based therapy. Ophthalmol Clin North Am. 2003;16(4): 583-93.

Retinopathy of Prematurity (362.21)

DIAGNOSIS

Definition

A proliferative retinopathy that develops in premature infants due to incomplete vasculogenesis of the retina at the time of birth.

Synonyms

- None
- Abbreviated as ROP in literature.

Symptoms

- *Cicatricial retinopathy of prematurity (ROP)*: decreased vision from myopia, astigmatism, retinal detachment and foveal distortion
- Glaucoma and cataract.

Signs

- *Leukokoria*: from retinal detachment
- *Pseudoexotropia*: from temporal displacement of the fovea
- Strabismus
- *Corneal clouding*: from glaucoma.

Investigations

- History including estimated gestational age (EGA) and birth weight
- Dilated stereoscopic fundus exam:
  - Dilated fundus exams for neonates 1,500 g or less, 28 weeks EGA or less, or any neonate 2,000 g or less felt to be at high risk.
  - First exam should be at 4–6 weeks of life, or at 31–33 weeks EGA, whichever is later.

Active Disease (Figs 1 to 7)

Stage 1: demarcation line between avascular and vascular retina.

Stage 2: ridge between avascular and vascular retina, becomes elevated and thickened.

Stage 3: neovascular tissue arising from ridge.

Stage 4: partial retinal detachment.

Stage 5: total retinal detachment.

Stages and Zones Used to Determine Need for Treatment (Fig. 8)

Zone I: area in posterior pole corresponding to a circle that encloses the disc and has a radius of twice the distance from the disc to the macula.

Zone II: area between zone I and a circle that is centered on the optic disc and that is tangential to the nasal ora serrata.

Zone III: area that includes the remaining temporal crescent of retina. This area is the last to be vascularized.

Differential Diagnosis

- Familial exudative vitreoretinopathy
- Retinoblastoma
- Incontinentia pigmenti
- Persistent fetal vasculature
- Norrie's disease.

Causes

- Prematurity is major cause. Smallest, sickest infants tend to have worst ROP, which is stimulated by removal from enriched O_2 source. No level of inspired O_2 is totally safe but is required by infants to prevent severe neurologic disease.
- Retinopathy of prematurity is associated with hypercarbia, multiple exchange transfusions, presence of intraventricular hemorrhage, respiratory distress syndrome and sepsis.
- Racial and familial tendencies may exist. Severe, vision-threatening ROP occurs more frequently in white infants of low birth weight than in black infants.

Pathology

- *Acute ROP:* true shunt at retinal ridge with obliteration of capillaries around arterioles and venules; neovascular tufting from ridge to vitreous and lens; with regression, neovascular buds develop from mesenchyme of ridge.
- *Progressive, severe, active ROP:* neovascular tissue develops from posterior border of the ridge.

Epidemiology

Thirteen hundred cases of vision loss from ROP each year In 1989, a fetus with weight of 700 g at 25 weeks of gestation had 50% chance of survival. In 1979, ROP blinded approximately 550 babies.

Incidence of ROP by Birth Weight:

- <1000 g: 80%
- 1001–1250 g: 60%
- 1251–1500 g: 20%
- >1501 g: 8%

Severity in infants more than *1501 g* (Plus disease is iris engorgement, retinal vascular tortuosity, and engorgement in infants with active ROP):

- No ROP: 50%
- <Stage 2+ ROP (ridge + disease): 36%
- >Stage 2+ ROP: 12%.

Diagnosis continued on p. 372

TREATMENT

Prevention of Prematurity

Compulsive, universal prenatal care should prevent some cases of prematurity.

Pharmacologic Treatment

- Recently, intravitreal injection (0.625 mg in 0.025 ml of solution) of bevacizumab for Stage 3. Zone I infants were shown to be statistically significant and beneficial. Vitamin E (alpha-tocopherol) at physiologic doses has been shown to decrease the incidence and severity of cicatricial ROP in infants with active ROP, but is less potent in the smallest premature infants. At higher doses, its use is associated with increased risk of necrotizing enterocolitis and *Escherichia coli* sepsis.

- Calf-lung surfactant treatment for acute respiratory distress syndrome in uncontrolled studies shows promise in decreasing the incidence and severity of active and cicatricial ROP.

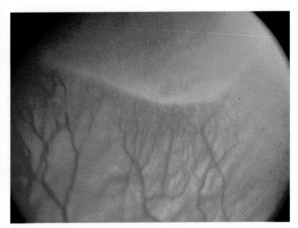

Fig. 1: Stage 1 retinopathy of prematurity. The flat, white border between avascular and vascular retina seen superiorly is called a demarcation line.
(*Source*: Earl A Palmer and the Multicenter Trial of Cryotherapy for Retinopathy of Prematurity).

Treatment Aims

- Help promote development of retina to the ora serrata
- To prevent and resolve retinal neovascularization
- To achieve the largest visual field without compromising or risking retinal detachment.

Prognosis

- After 3.5 years of cryogenic therapy for threshold ROP, letter acuity, grating acuity, and posterior-pole status were improved in treated versus untreated eyes.
- Treated eyes still had a 26% chance of unfavorable posterior-pole structural status, and patients who had active ROP in the posterior retina had poor outcomes even with cryogenic treatment.
- Few eyes undergoing retinal detachment repair with vitrectomy will have better than hand-motion vision.

Follow-up and Management

- Premature babies at risk for ROP with incomplete development should be examined every week until the vascular arcades have reached the ora serrata.
- Infants with active ROP should be examined weekly until the ROP regresses or they reach the threshold for laser/intravitreal therapy.

Treatment continued on p. 373

Retinopathy of Prematurity (362.21)

Complications

- Retinal detachment (at any stage in life)
- Strabismus
- Anisometropia
- Phthisis bulbi
- Band keratopathy
- Glaucoma, cataract, corneal clouding.

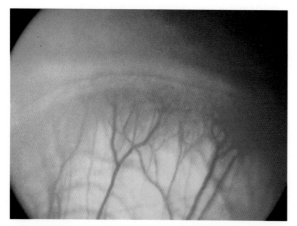

Fig. 2: Stage 2 retinopathy of prematurity. The elevated mesenchymal ridge has height. Highly arborized blood vessels from the vascularized retina dive into the ridge. (*Source*: Earl A Palmer and the Multicenter Trial of Cryotherapy for Retinopathy of Prematurity).

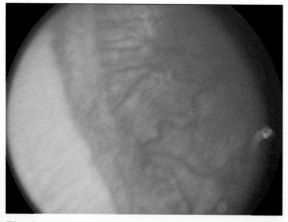

Fig. 3: Stage 3 retinopathy of prematurity. Vessels on top of the ridge project into the vitreous cavity. This extraretinal proliferation carries with it a fibrovascular membrane. Note the opalescent avascular retina anterior to the ridge.

Diagnosis continued on p. 374

TREATMENT—cont'd

Nonpharmacologic Treatment

Laser or Cryotherapy

Laser is the preferred method of treatment because of the ease of use and lack of external trauma, although cryotherapy can be used if laser is unavailable. The recommendation of the Early Treatment for Retinopathy of Prematurity Group is that earlier treatment ("prethreshold") has better outcomes than traditional timing of treatment ("threshold"). Retinal ablative therapy is recommended for:

- Retinopathy of prematurity any stage in Zone I with plus disease (dilation of posterior pole retinal vessels)
- Zone I Stage 3 ROP without plus disease
- Zone II Stages 2 or 3 ROP with plus disease
- Cryogenic or diode laser treatment to avascular retina in infants with prethreshold.

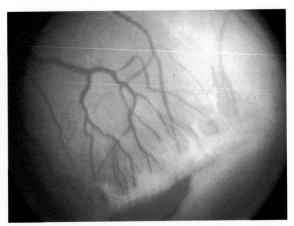

Fig. 4: Stage 3 retinopathy of prematurity. Note finger-like projections of extraretinal vessels into the vitreous cavity. Hemorrhage on the ridge is not uncommon.

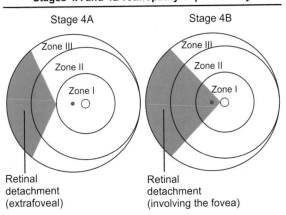

Stages 4A and 4B retinopathy of prematurity

Stage 4A	Stage 4B
Zone III	Zone III
Zone II	Zone II
Zone I	Zone I
Retinal detachment (extrafoveal)	Retinal detachment (involving the fovea)

Fig. 5: Stage 4. (A) Stage 4A detachment spares the fovea. (B) Stage 4B detachment involves the fovea.

Treatment continued on p. 375

Retinopathy of Prematurity (362.21)

DIAGNOSIS—cont'd

Pearls and Considerations

Many severe cases can lead to irreversible, total blindness.

Commonly Associated Conditions

- Myopia
- Strabismus
- Cataract
- Glaucoma
- Retinal detachment.

Referral Information

Management of lingering complications.

Stage 5 retinopathy of prematurity

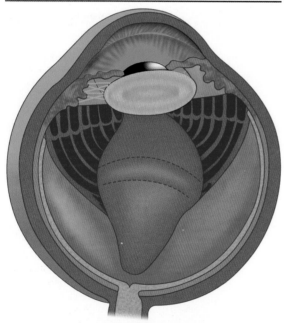

Fig. 6: Stage 5 retinal detachment. Depiction of an open anterior configuration secondary to fibrovascular proliferation that pulls the peripheral retina anteriorly.

TREATMENT—cont'd

- Retinopathy of prematurity has been shown to decrease incidence and severity of severe, blinding cicatricial ROP
- Ten years after treatment, eyes treated with laser had mean best-corrected visual acuity of 20/66, and eyes treated with cryotherapy had best-corrected visual acuity of 20/182, reflecting less retinal dragging in laser-treated eyes
- Retinal detachment repair is anatomically successful in approximately 50%, but reattached retina rarely functions, and the visual outcome is usually very poor (hand motions or light perception).

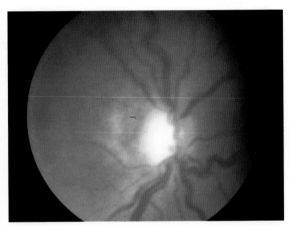

Fig. 7: An example of moderate plus disease. Dilated retinal veins and tortuous arteries in the posterior pole may be seen.

Classification of retinopathy of prematurity by zone

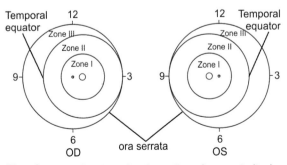

Fig. 8: Classification of retinopathy of prematurity by zone; The temporal edge of zone II coincides with the equator.

GENERAL REFERENCES

Binenbaum G, Ying GS, Quinn GE, et al. Premature Infants in Need of Transfusion Study Group. A clinical prediction model to stratify retinopathy of prematurity risk using postnatal weight gain. Pediatrics. 2011;127(3): e607-14. Epub 2011.

Chan CC, Roberge FG, Whitcup SM, et al. 32 cases of sympathetic ophthalmia. Arch Ophthalmol. 1995;113:597.

Cryotherapy for Retinopathy of Prematurity Cooperative Group. 31/2 year outcome: structure and function. Arch Ophthalmol. 1993;111:339-50.

Early Treatment for Retinopathy of Prematurity Cooperative Group. Revised indications for the treatment of retinopathy of prematurity: results of the early treatment for retinopathy of prematurity randomized trial. Arch Ophthalmol. 2003;121:1684-94.

Hartnett ME. Studies on the pathogenesis of avascular retina and neovascularization into the vitreous in peripheral severe retinopathy of prematurity (an american ophthalmological society thesis).Trans Am Ophthalmol Soc. 2010;108:96-119.

Higgins RD.(2006). Retinopathy of prematurity. [online] Available from www.emedicine.com.

Mintz-Hittner HA, Kennedy KA, Chuang AZ, et al. Efficacy of intravitreal bevacizumab for stage 3+ retinopathy of prematurity. N Engl J Med. 2011;364(7):603-15.

Ng EY, Connolly B, McNamara A, et al. A comparison of laser photocoagulation with cryotherapy for threshold retinopathy of prematurity at 10 years. Ophthalmology. 2002;109:928-35.

Palmer EA, et al. Retinopathy of prematurity. Retina, 4th edition. St Louis: Elsevier; 2006.

Shindo Y, Ohno S, Usi M, et al. Immunogenetic study of sympathetic ophthalmia. Tissue Antigens. 1997;49:111.

Rubeosis Iridis (364.42) and Neovascular Glaucoma (365.63)

DIAGNOSIS

Definition

Rubeosis iridis: neovascularization of the iris.

Neovascular glaucoma (NVG): increase in the intraocular pressure (IOP) secondary to blockage of aqueous outflow by neovascularization in the anterior-chamber angle.

Synonyms

None

Symptoms

Pain: a prominent feature in acute NVG; in early cases before the development of full-blown inflammatory NVG, patients may be relatively pain free.

Loss of vision: marked loss of vision is also prominent early in the course of NVG.

Signs

- *Hyperemia*: marked conjunctival and episcleral vessel engorgement is common
- Greatly elevated IOP
- *Corneal edema*: epithelial and sometimes stromal edema are seen in response to the rapid increase in IOP
- *Inflammation*: usually a marked inflammatory response with anterior-chamber flare and cells
- *Anterior-chamber hemorrhage*: red blood cells in the anterior chamber are often present; occasionally a spontaneous layered hyphema will occur
- *Neovascularization of the iris and angle*: abnormal new blood vessels are seen on the surface of the iris stroma and in the angle crossing the scleral spur and growing on the trabecular meshwork (Fig. 1); these vessels impart a red color to the iris and angle, thus the term "rubeosis iridis"; early in the course of the disease, fine tufts of vessels are barely visible in the peripupillary area; later, fine vessels are seen in the angle; as the disease advances, the entire iris and angle are involved; the vessels may become quite large.
- *Ectropion uveae*: often seen in NVG (Fig. 1)
- *Gonioscopic findings*: the angle may be open early in the course of disease; more typically, a nonpupillary block angle closure results from extensive peripheral anterior synechiae.

Differential Diagnosis

The differential diagnosis includes other acute inflammatory glaucomas:
- Acute angle-closure glaucoma
- Uveitic glaucoma
- Acute traumatic glaucoma and hyphema
- Neovascularization of the anterior segment resembling rubeosis may also be seen in Fuchs' heterochromic iridocyclitis and pseudoexfoliation syndrome.

Cause

Rubeosis is thought to result from the production of an intraocular angiogenic factor by ischemic retina. This factor provokes the growth of a fibrovascular membrane over the surface of the iris and trabecular meshwork. As the membrane contracts, it pulls the peripheral iris into the angle, causing peripheral anterior synechiae and progressive closure of the angle. As the ocular ischemia progresses, the pressure increases, and the abnormal blood vessels leak more; an inflammatory response occurs, leading to the complete clinical picture.

Classification

Rubeosis with NVG is seen in a variety of disease conditions that produce retinal ischemia. The most common causes are central retinal vein occlusion, proliferative diabetic retinopathy, carotid occlusive disease and ocular ischemic syndrome.

Associated Features

In susceptible eyes, the risk of NVG is increased after intraocular surgery, especially cataract surgery and pars plana vitrectomy.

Pathology

Proliferation of vascular endothelial cells and smooth muscle fibroblasts over the surface of the iris produces the fibrovascular membrane characteristic of rubeosis iridis.

Diagnosis continued on p. 378

TREATMENT

Diet and Lifestyle

Diabetic control: proliferative diabetic retinopathy is a common cause of NVG; the risk of developing this complication is significantly reduced if diabetes is well controlled with diet and medication.

Control of hypertension, cholesterol: other causes of NVG are often related to hypertension and arteriosclerosis; careful attention to dietary intake of fat and salt, as well as control of any existing hypertension, may reduce the risk of developing ocular vascular disease.

Pharmacologic Treatment

For Intraocular Pressure

During the acute phase, hyperosmotics and aqueous suppressants are useful to lower IOP, reduce pain, and reduce corneal edema to allow better visualization of the anterior segment and retina. After more definitive nonpharmacologic treatments, long-term treatment for glaucoma may be needed, as with any chronic glaucoma. Miotics should be avoided in NVG because of their effect on vascular permeability.

For Inflammation

Topical steroids and atropine are very useful for treating the associated inflammation and pain.

Analgesics

Patients with severe pain may require systemic analgesics.

Treatment Aims
- To adequately treat ischemic retina
- To control pain and inflammation
- To control IOP and preserve visual function.

Prognosis

The prognosis for patients with NVG is poor. Patients are often unresponsive to treatment. Complications of treatment (e.g. hypotony) are common. Vision rarely returns to normal and is often greatly reduced despite treatment. Early recognition and adequate treatment of retinal ischemic disease before the development of rubeosis is the best way to prevent NVG and preserve visual function.

Follow-up and Management

Because the underlying cause of NVG is often a systemic problem that affects both eyes, careful evaluation and prophylactic treatment of the fellow eye are important.

Treatment continued on p. 379

Rubeosis Iridis (364.42) and Neovascular Glaucoma (365.63)

DIAGNOSIS—cont'd

Investigations

Retinal evaluation: neovascular glaucoma is usually a manifestation of retinal vascular disease; occasionally it may be seen associated with intraocular neoplasms; careful examination of the posterior pole and peripheral retina is indicated; if the fundus cannot be seen, B-scan ultrasonography should be performed.

Carotid evaluation: some cases of NVG are seen in association with carotid occlusive disease; if a retinal cause is not apparent, noninvasive carotid flow and ultrasound studies are indicated.

Complications

Intraocular hemorrhage: anterior-chamber hemorrhage from the fragile rubeotic vessels is common; vitreous hemorrhages are also seen.

Pearls and Considerations

- Retinal ischemia is the most important factor leading to the development of NVG
- Generally, NVG is poorly responsive to treatment, and preserving vision is difficult.

Referral Information

- Refer to glaucoma specialist for immediate and aggressive care
- Refer to retinal specialist as needed for the treatment of underlying cause.

TREATMENT—cont'd

Nonpharmacologic Treatment

Panretinal Photocoagulation

Ischemic retina must be treated with panretinal photocoagulation to eliminate the angiogenic stimulus. Treatment should be initiated immediately and should be sufficiently extensive to destroy all ischemic retina. More than one session may be needed. If the retina cannot be seen, panretinal cryotherapy should be performed.

Filtering Surgery

Once the panretinal photocoagulation has been completed, filtering surgery is indicated if the IOP cannot be controlled medically. The failure rate with filtration is extremely high, and the use of antifibrotics (e.g. mitomycin-C or 5-fluorouracil) is usually indicated. In severe or recalcitrant cases, use of an aqueous tube-shunt device or cyclophotocoagulation may be useful. The results of treatment for NVG are generally among the worst for any common glaucoma.

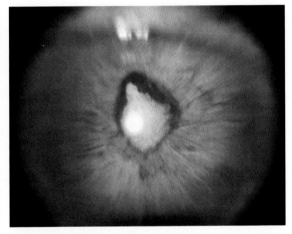

Fig. 1: Neovascular glaucoma showing neovascularization of the surface of the iris (rubeosis), ectropion uveae at the pupil, and cataract.

GENERAL REFERENCES

Eid TE, Katz LJ, Spaeth GL, et al. Tube shunt surgery versus neodymium:YAG cyclophotocoagulation in the management of neovascular glaucoma. Ophthalmology. 1997;104:1692-700.

Khan VA, Ahmed IIK. (2011). Neovascular glaucoma treatment and management. [online] Available from http://emedicine.medscape.com/article/1205736-treatment [Accessed April, 2013].

McGrath OJ, Ferguson JG, Sanborn GE. Neovascular glaucoma. In: Wolfley DE (Ed). Focal Points: Clinical Modules for Ophthalmologists. San Francisco: American Academy of Ophthalmology; 1997.

Shields MB (Ed). Glaucomas associated with disorders of the retina, vitreous, and choroid. Textbook of Glaucoma, 4th edition. Baltimore: Lippincott Williams & Wilkins; 1998. pp. 269-86.

Tsai JC, Feuer WJ, Parrish RK, et al. 5-Fluorouracil filtering surgery and neovascular glaucoma. Long-term follow-up of the original pilot study. Ophthalmology. 1995;102:887-92.

Wand M. Neovascular glaucoma: new approaches to inhibition of angiogenesis. J Glaucoma. 1994;3:178-80.

Seventh-Nerve Palsy (Facial) (351.0)

DIAGNOSIS

Definition

Loss of function of the seventh cranial (facial) nerve.

Synonyms

Bell's palsy

Symptoms

- Unable to hold food or liquid in mouth while eating
- Corner of mouth droops
- *Weak platysma*: makes shaving difficult
- Ipsilateral hyperacusis
- *Aguesia*: decreased taste to anterior two-thirds of tongue
- Aching pain around jaw or behind ear.

Signs

- Muscles of facial expression are paretic on side of lesion
- Eyebrow droops
- Palpebral fissure widens
- Eyelid does not close
- Punctum turns outward
- Forehead and nasolabial folds are lost
- Ala nasi is immobile on respiration.

Investigations

- Thorough cranial nerve testing on physical examination
- Complete blood count
- Erythrocyte sedimentation rate
- Two-hour postprandial blood sugar
- Thyroid function studies
- Rapid plasma reagin
- Fluorescent treponemal antibody absorption test
- Human immunodeficiency virus (HIV) screening by enzyme-linked immuno-sorbent assay (ELISA) and/or Western blot
- Herpes simplex virus serum titers (usually not helpful)
- Angiotensin-converting enzyme
- Lyme titer and cerebrospinal fluid analysis
- Neuroimaging [computed tomography (CT) and/or gadolinium-enhanced magnetic resonance imaging (MRI), with special attention to the temporal bones and pons]: if palsy not isolated, or in cases that do not improve, or worsen within 8–10 weeks.
- Schirmer's testing (abnormal tear flow in two-thirds of patients)
- Electrodiagnostic testing [e.g. stapedius reflex test, evoked facial-nerve electromyography (EMG), audiography].

Differential Diagnosis

- Acoustic neuroma/cerebellopontine angle tumor
- Geniculate ganglionitis (Ramsay-Hunt syndrome)
- Cerebral aneurysm
- Meningioma
- Cerebrovascular accident
- Guillain-Barré syndrome (GBS)
- Basilar meningitis.

Cause

Common
- Idiopathic (Bell's palsy)
- Trauma.

Rare
- Herpes simplex virus (HSV)
- Varicella-zoster virus (VZV)
- Cytomegalovirus (CMV)
- Epstein-Barr virus (EBV)
- Rubella
- Lyme disease
- Pregnancy (especially in third trimester)
- Syphilis
- Human immunodeficiency virus
- Sarcoid
- Tuberculosis
- Leprosy
- Wegener's vasculitis
- History of recent intervention along the facial nerve distribution (e.g. forceps delivery, nerve blocks, facial surgery).

Epidemiology

- 20:100,000 population per year
- 45.1:100,000 pregnant women per year.

Classification

Upper-motor-neuron seventh-nerve palsy: weakness of only the lower two-thirds of the face contralateral to a supranuclear lesion.

Lower-motor-neuron seventh-nerve palsy: all muscle actions of facial expression are lost on the side of the lesion.

Pathology

- Edema of the seventh nerve in the fallopian canal
- Infection
- Compression.

Diagnosis continued on p. 382

TREATMENT

Diet and Lifestyle

No special precautions are necessary.

Pharmacologic Treatment

Corticosteroids

Standard dosage: Prednisone, 60 mg for 5 days tapered within 14 days.

Special points: Administer during the first 48 hours; treatment is controversial.

Antivirals

- Acyclovir (Zovirax) 400 mg orally 5 times a day for 10 days
- Valacyclovir (Valtrex) 500 mg orally twice a day for 5 days, may be used instead of acyclovir. If VZV is the cause of Bell palsy, higher doses may be needed (1000 mg orally three times a day), which is associated with a higher rate of side effects.

Combination Therapy

- A recent Cochrane meta-analysis and systematic review has found no evidence for treatment with antivirals alone versus placebo; however, high quality evidence showed significant benefit from the combination of antivirals and corticosteroids compared with placebo
- The decision as to prednisone alone versus combination therapy is left up to the discretion of the individual physician.

Treatment Aims

To protect the cornea.

Other Treatments

- Facial massage
- Electrical stimulation.

Prognosis

- Untreated, about one person in five is left with permanent facial disfigurement or pain
- Facial-nerve conduction studies 3–5 days after onset can indicate prognosis
- Complete loss of conduction indicates Wallerian degeneration and poor prognosis
- Normal latencies and amplitudes at 5 days suggest excellent prognosis for recovery.

Treatment continued on p. 383

Seventh-Nerve Palsy (Facial) (351.0)

DIAGNOSIS—cont'd

Complications

- Filamentary keratitis
- Exposure keratopathy, corneal ulcer
- Aberrant regeneration of seventh nerve ("crocodile tears").

Pearls and Considerations

- The seventh cranial nerve carries parasympathetic fibers to the nose, palate, and lacrimal glands, as well as motor nerves to the facial muscles
- A diabetic patient's risk of Bell's palsy is up to 29% higher than that of the nondiabetic population
- Onset of symptoms are typically sudden, with symptoms peaking within less than 48 hours; patients often fear they have had a stroke. Gradual onset or progression of symptoms beyond 7–10 days should provoke evaluation for other causes
- If the paralysis involves only the lower portion of the face, a central cause should be suspected (i.e. supranuclear).

Referral Information

Refer to appropriate subspecialist (e.g. neurologist or otolaryngologist), depending on the suspected underlying etiology of paralysis.

TREATMENT—cont'd

Nonpharmacologic Treatment

- Artificial tears (may require gel or ointment formulation, e.g. Lacrilube ophthalmic ointment)
- Tape eyelids closed
- Moisture chamber patches
- Tarsorrhaphy (temporary versus permanent), to promote corneal healing and protection
- Decompression of facial nerve (controversial)
- Subocularis oculi fat lift with lateral tarsal strip procedure
- Eyelid implants (e.g. pretarsal gold or platinum weights)
- Transposition of temporalis
- Facial nerve grafting or hypoglossal-facial nerve anastomosis
- Direct brow lift (to correct brow ptosis; caution: can cause worsening of lagophthalmos and corneal decompensation).

GENERAL REFERENCES

Adour KK, Wingerd J. Idiopathic facial paralysis (Bell's palsy): factors affecting severity and ¬outcome in 446 patients. Neurology. 1974;24:1112-6.

Esslen E. The acute facial palsies. New York: Springer-Verlag; 1977.

Lockhart P, Daly F, Pitkethly M, et al. Antiviral treatment for Bell's palsy (idiopathic facial paralysis). Cochrane Database Syst Rev. 2009;(4):CD001869.

Morgan M, Nathurami D. Facial palsy and infection: the unfolding story. Clin Infect Dis. 1992;14:263-71.

Taylor DC. (2012). Bell palsy. [Online] Available from www.emedicine.com.

Sixth-Nerve Palsy (Abducens) (378.54)

DIAGNOSIS

Definition

Loss of function of the sixth cranial (abducens) nerve.

Synonyms

None

Symptoms

- *Horizonal diplopia*: greater at distance
- Some patients experience pain, others do not.

Signs

- Head turn
- Esodeviation increasing on ipsilateral gaze, often greater at distance
- Isolated abduction deficit
- Slowed ipsilateral saccades
- Papilledema (if increased intracranial pressure)
- Nystagmus (usually in children, i.e. secondary to pontine glioma)
- Otitis media
- Orbital wall fracture
- Tender, enlarged, nonpulsatile temporal arteries (in giant cell arteritis).

Investigations

- Thorough evaluation of all cranial nerves
- Complete blood count
- Erythrocyte sedimentation rate
- Two-hour postprandial blood sugar
- Rapid plasma reagin
- Fluorescent treponemal antibody absorption test
- Lyme titer
- Magnetic resonance imaging of brain and orbits
- Look for signs that distinguish a sixth-nerve palsy from mimicking conditions:
  - Greater abduction of the paretic eye with ductions than with versions
  - Slowed abducting saccades of the paretic eye
  - Negative forced ductions (Figs 1A and B)
  - Diminished abducting optokinetic nystagmus of the paretic eye
  - Antiacetylcholine antibody test, Tensilon (edrophonium) test to rule out myasthenia gravis
  - Thyroid function test
  - Forced-duction test to rule out Graves' disease
  - Lumbar puncture; increased intracranial pressure can cause nonlocalizing sixth-nerve palsy.

Differential Diagnosis

- Duane retraction syndrome Type I
- Medial wall fracture
- Spasm of the near reflex
- Graves' orbitopathy
- Myasthenia gravis
- Orbital tumor
- Loss of horizontal fusional reserves.

Cause

Adults

- Neoplasm
- Trauma
- Aneurysm
- Ischemic-vasculopathic
- Elevated intracranial pressure (can result in downward displacement of the brainstem, and stretching of the sixth nerve within Dorello's canal). About 30% of patients with pseudotumor cerebri have an isolated sixth cranial nerve palsy.

Children

- Neoplasm
- Trauma
- Febrile illness/postviral syndrome
- Congenital (rare).

By Age Group

- *From 1 to 15 years*: viral; febrile illnesses; postimmunization; Gradenigo syndrome; pontine glioma
- *From 15 to 35 years*: demyelinating
- *From 35 to 50 years*: nasopharyngeal carcinoma; meningioma
- *More than or equal to 55 years*: ischemic vascular; giant cell arteritis.

Classification

- Sixth-nerve palsy can be acute or chronic.
- Chronic sixth-nerve palsy is one that persists for more than or equal to 6 months and is usually a harbinger of serious intracranial disease.

Associated Features

See Table 1.

Diagnosis continued on p. 386

TREATMENT

Diet and Lifestyle

No special precautions are necessary.

Pharmacologic Treatment

Botulinum A (oculinum) injection

Nonpharmacologic Treatment

- Segment patch on glasses for distance
- Base-out prism for distance
- *Surgical intervention*: based on whether the patient can abduct beyond midline, can reach midline, or cannot achieve primary position
    - Generally, surgical intervention is held off unless the remaining deviation is unacceptable to the patient after 6 months of follow-up
    - *Graded recession/resection procedure*: if some residual function exists in the lateral rectus
    - *A transposition procedure (e.g. Hummelsheim or Jensen procedure)*: when little or no residual function is present, along with weakening the antagonist ipsilateral medial rectus (in appropriate patients).

Treatment Aims

To restore and maintain single, simultaneous, binocular vision in primary position at distance and near.

Prognosis

- Vasculopathic sixth-nerve palsies should resolve in 3 months
- Patients with traumatic sixth-nerve palsies may take up to 1 year to recover.

Follow-up and Management

Monitor patients every few weeks for secondary contracture during recovery period. Once the medial rectus muscle begins to contract, it is unlikely to relax.

Treatment continued on p. 387

Sixth-Nerve Palsy (Abducens) (378.54)

DIAGNOSIS—cont'd

Pearls and Considerations

See Table 1. In adults, the sixth cranial nerve is the most commonly affected of the ocular cranial nerves.

Referral Information

None

Table 1: Anatomic localization of a "complicated" sixth-nerve palsy: the checklist examination		
What to Look for	*Anatomic Location*	*Cause*
Sixth-nerve paresis plus contralateral hemiplegia (Raymond syndrome)	Pons	Infarction, demyelination, tumor, trauma
Sixth- and seventh-nerve paresis plus contralateral hemiplegia (Millard-Gubler syndrome)	Ventral pons	Infarction, demyelination, tumor, trauma
Gaze palsy, seventh- and eighth-nerve paresis, facial analgesia, and Horner's sign (Foville syndrome)	Dorsal pons	Infarction, demyelination, tumor, trauma
Bilateral sixth-nerve paresis	Clivus; subarach-noid space	Tumor (nonlocalizing)
Papilledema	Subarachnoid space	Nonlocalizing
Sixth-nerve paresis plus pain and decreased hearing (Gradenigo syndrome)	Petrous apex	Infection, thrombosis, compression fracture
Sixth-nerve paresis plus decreased tearing and hearing, and Horner's sign	Cavernous sinus	Tumor, thrombosis, fistula, infection, trauma, aneurysm
Sixth-nerve paresis plus third- and fourth-nerve paresis, VI, Horner's sign, and proptosis	Cavernous sinus	Tumor, thrombosis, fistula, infection, trauma, aneurysm
Sixth-nerve paresis plus second-never paresis and proptosis	Orbital apex/ superior orbital fissure	Tumor

TREATMENT—cont'd

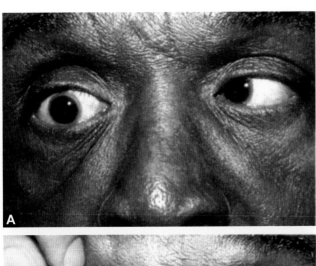

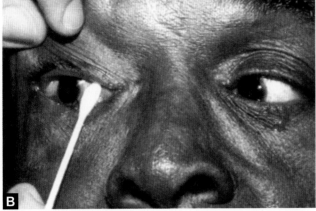

Figs 1A and B: (A) This man demonstrates a right abduction deficit in his attempt to look to the right; (B) Modified forced duction easily moves the right eye into abduction. He has a "negative" forced-duction test consistent with a right sixth-nerve palsy.

GENERAL REFERENCES

Anwar S, Nalla S, Fernando DJ. Abducens nerve palsy as a complication of lumbar puncture. Eur J Intern Med. 2008;19(8):636-7.

Bellusci C. Paralytic strabismus. Curr Opin Ophthalmol. 2001;12(5):368-72.

Ehrenhaus MP. (2012). Abducens nerve palsy. [Online] Available from www.emedicine.com.

Rucker JC, Tomsak RL. Binocular diplopia: a practical approach. Neurologist. 2005;11(2):98-110.

Skin Tumor, Benign (216.1)

DIAGNOSIS

Definition

Noncancerous growth or mass on the lid.

Synonyms

Benign neoplasm of eyelid, including canthus; dermoid cyst of eyelid; papilloma of eyelid.

Symptoms

- Growth or mass on lid
- Generally painless.

Signs

Seborrheic keratosis (702.19): waxy, sharply demarcated; appears stuck to surface.

Papilloma (skin tags): appear as skin-colored filiform lesions (Fig. 1).

Warts (078.1): firm growth with a papillomatous surface.

Inclusion cyst (374.84): single whitish nodule filled with keratin.

Xanthelasma (374.51): yellowish raised plaques (Fig. 2).

Molluscum (078.0): skin-colored, dome-shaped lesion with umbilicated center (Fig. 3).

Actinic keratosis (702.0): small erythematous lesions with overlying scales.

Investigations

History: duration of lesion, growth of lesion, previous type or similar lesions.

Biopsy: suspected lesion to rule out malignancy. Investigate similar lesions elsewhere on the body.

Complications

Some of the benign lesions (e.g. actinic keratosis) may have a premalignant potential and therefore should be excised.

Differential Diagnosis

Other benign lesions include:
- Verruca
- Keratosis
- Nevus
- Sebaceous adenoma
- Syringoma
- Hydrocystoma
- Hemangioma
- Lymphangioma
- Xanthelasma
- Chalazion
- Sarcoid
- Pyogenic granuloma
- Neurofibroma.

Cause

Warts: associated with human papillomavirus (HPV).
Xanthelasma: in one-third of people, associated with lipid abnormalities.
Molluscum: poxvirus.
Sebaceous adenoma: can rarely be associated with Muir-Torre syndrome.

Diagnosis continued on p. 390

TREATMENT

Diet and Lifestyle

Minimizing ultraviolet light exposure (e.g. actinic keratosis) and judicious sunscreen use.

Pharmacologic Treatment

Generally, no pharmacologic treatment is recommended.

Nonpharmacologic Treatment

- Most treatments are associated with biopsy of the lesion (incisional/excisional) to establish the diagnosis and remove the lesion
- Photodynamic therapy (PDT) with topical methyl aminolevulinate (Metvix cream, 16%; Photocure ASA, Oslo, Norway) has been used successfully by dermatologists for the treatment of lid margin papillomas and basal cell carcinomas, as well as nonmelanoma skin cancers elsewhere on the body.

Treatment Aims

To remove lesion and obtain tissue to confirm clinical diagnosis of benign neoplasm.

Other Treatments

Fulguration has been used for some benign lesions, but definitive diagnosis is not possible because of inability to obtain a specimen for microscopic examination.

Prognosis

Excision of lesions generally results in cure, although they may recur, which should be monitored for subsequent malignant transformation.

Follow-up and Management

As needed to ensure healing of incisional area and to verify suspected pathology so as not to overlook an occult malignant lesion, with subsequent observation for evidence of recurrence or new lesions.

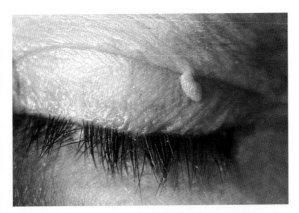

Fig. 1: Papilloma. Skin tag protrudes from the left upper lid. Histologically, this was a squamous cell papilloma.

Treatment continued on p. 391

DIAGNOSIS—cont'd

Pearls and Considerations

- Varied, and dependent on type of lesion
- In a recent large dermatopathology review of eyelid skin tumors, benign tumors largely predominated over malignant ones, representing 84% of cases, most frequently squamous cell papilloma (26%), seborrheic keratosis (21%), melanocytic nevus (20%), hidrocystoma (8%) and xanthoma/xanthelasma (6%). Basal cell carcinoma was the most frequent malignant tumor (86%), followed by squamous cell carcinoma (7%) and sebaceous carcinoma (3%).
- For several tumor subtypes, there is a poor correlation between clinical and histological diagnosis, particularly with sebaceous carcinoma presenting like inflammatory lesions, and for hair follicle tumors mimicking basal cell carcinoma.

Referral Information

Consider referral to an oculoplastics subspecialist for biopsy and excision.

TREATMENT—cont'd

Pathology

- *Seborrheic keratosis*: papillomatous lesion above the skin surface that contains basaloid-type cells and keratin cysts
- *Papilloma*: finger-like projection of hyperkeratosis with a fibrovascular core
- *Inclusion cysts*: cysts lined with squamous epithelium and keratin filling the lumen of the cyst
- *Xanthelasma*: dermal thickening with fat-filled macrophages
- *Molluscum*: key feature is intracytoplasmic molluscum bodies that appear eosinophilic in the deep layers and become basophilic in the superficial layers before breaking through and shedding into the tears
- *Actinic keratosis*: lesion above the skin surface that demonstrates hyperkeratosis and thickening.

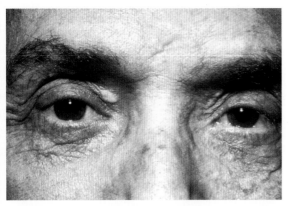

Fig. 2: Xanthelasma. Yellow placoid lid lesion is present superior nasally in each eye (larger in the right upper lid).

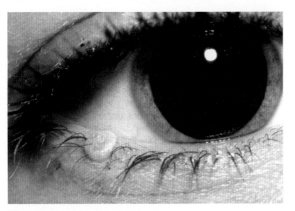

Fig. 3: Molluscum. Raised lesion with an umbilicated center is present temporally at the right lower lid margin. The lesion contains packets of molluscum bodies that are characteristic.

GENERAL REFERENCES

Baek SH, Chi MJ. Clinical analysis of benign eyelid and conjunctival tumors. Ophthalmologica. 2005;220(1):43-51.

Deprez M, Uffer S. Clinicopathological features of eyelid skin tumors: a retrospective study of 5504 cases and review of literature. Am J Dermatopathol. 2009;31:256-62.

Fraunfelder F, Roy F (Eds). Current Ocular Therapy. Philadelphia: Saunders; 2000.

Hornblass A, Hanig CJ. Oculoplastic, Orbital, and Reconstructive Surgery, Vol. 2. Baltimore: Lippincott Williams & Wilkins; 1990.

Neff AG, Carter KD. Benign eyelid lesions. In: Yanoff M, Duker JS (Eds). Ophthalmology, 3rd edition. St. Louis, MO: Mosby Elsevier; 2008. pp. 1422-33.

Older JJ (Ed). Eyelid Tumors: Clinical Diagnosis and Surgical Treatment. New York: Raven Press; 1987. pp. 27-45.

Tasman W, Jaeger E (Eds). Duane's Clinical Ophthalmology, Vol. 4. Philadelphia: Lippincott-Raven; 2006.

Togsverd-Bo K, Haedersdal M, Wulf HC. Photodynamic therapy for tumors on the eyelid margins. Arch Dermatol. 2009;145(8):944-7.

Yanoff M, Fine B. Ocular Pathology: A Color Atlas. Philadelphia: Lippincott; 2002.

Skin Tumor, Malignant (173.1)

DIAGNOSIS

Definition

Cancerous mass or growth on the eyelid.

Synonyms

None

Symptoms

Because of the slow growth and in many patients, lack of associated significant symptoms, patients may allow the lesion to grow to a fair size before seeking a medical opinion.

Basal Cell Carcinoma

Slow growing, painless lesion that may ulcerate, bleed or crust: *see* Figure 1.

Squamous Cell Carcinoma

Painless, enlarging mass: *see* Figure 2.

Sebaceous Gland Carcinoma

Simulates a benign lesion (especially a chalazion), but may present as chronic lid irritation or blepharoconjunctivitis; loss of lashes over lesion is common.

Madarosis has been found to be an important indicator of malignancy in eyelid lesions. In one recent study, presence of madarosis as a clinical finding in association with a suspicious lid lesion was associated with malignancy in nearly 70% of cases.

Signs

Basal Cell Carcinoma

Starts as discrete nodule (usually on lower lid, inner canthus), with the central area eventually becoming ulcerated.

Squamous Cell Carcinoma

Discrete, flat, slightly erythematous lesion with overlying vessels and scaling; frequently, loss of eyelashes.

Sebaceous Gland Carcinoma

Predilection for upper lid; lesion shows minimal ulceration; possible manifestations of unilateral chronic conjunctivitis, blepharoconjunctivitis, lid thickening; can often mimic blepharoconjunctivitis (25%), chronic chalazia (20%), basal cell carcinoma (13%) or squamous cell carcinoma (10%). Loss of cilia and of the normal anatomy of the eyelid margin is common.

Investigations

Basal Cell Carcinoma

If spread is suspected, consider computed tomography (CT) scan to rule out spread to globe, bone or sinuses.

Differential Diagnosis

Various benign or malignant tumors of the lid.

Cause

Basal Cell Carcinoma

Most often seen in patients aged 60–80 years.
- Approximately 5–15% of lesions occur in patients aged 20–40 years
- Although never proved, there is circumstantial evidence of increased occurrence from prolonged sun exposure.

Squamous Cell Carcinoma

One-tenth to four-tenths (0.1–0.4) as common as basal cell lesions; associated increased incidence with prolonged sun exposure.

Sebaceous Gland Carcinoma

Approximately the same frequency as squamous cell carcinoma; cause is unknown.

Epidemiology

Basal Cell Carcinoma

Most common malignancy of eyelid; accounts for 90% of all carcinomas.

Squamous Cell Carcinoma

Rare eyelid malignancy; accounts for about 7%; occurs more in fair-skinned and elderly individuals; thought to be sun related.

Sebaceous Gland Carcinoma

Rare malignancy; increased female predominance, with a mortality rate of ~22%.

Classification

Basal Cell Carcinoma Types

Nodular, ulcerative, syringoid, adenoid, basosquamous, multicentric, recurrent, morpheaform, sclerosing.

Pathology

Basal Cell Carcinoma

May take on several appearances: solid masses of uniform cells with basophilic nuclei, peripheral palisading of basal cells, or strands or cords of cells that appear in an "Indian file" pattern.

Squamous Cell Carcinoma

Deep dermal findings of keratin-producing squamous neoplastic cells.

Sebaceous Gland Carcinoma

Numerous cells resembling sebaceous elements with mitotic figures; the cells may stain positively for fat.

Diagnosis continued on p. 394

TREATMENT

Diet and Lifestyle

Because malignant skin tumors are most often seen on the most sun-exposed surfaces, it is believed that ultraviolet light may be a predisposing factor. Therefore, avoidance of intense sun exposure is recommended for patients with documented lesions.

Pharmacologic Treatment

For squamous cell carcinoma in situ (Bowen's disease, considered a premalignant condition), using 5% imiquimod topical cream as monotherapy has been successfully used instead of traditional complete surgical excision.

Squamous Cell Carcinoma

If distant metastases are present, chemotherapy may be warranted.

Nonpharmacologic Treatment

Basal Cell Carcinoma

- Mohs' surgery or complete surgical excision with frozen-section control of the margins offers the lowest tumor recurrence rate
- Irradiation/photodynamic therapy: effective only in early stages
- Excision: excision by frozen section, Mohs' technique or wide excision, with various types of reconstruction to ensure that clear margins are obtained
- Cryotherapy: freeze/thaw technique with use of thermocouple to ensure freezing to –25°C is effective for small lesions (< 1 cm).

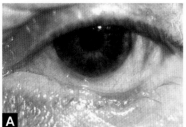 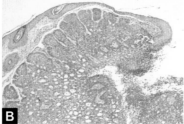

Figs 1A and B: Basal cell carcinoma. (A) Middle outer portion of the left lower lid contains an indurated, ulcerated, nontender lesion; (B) Histologically, basal cell carcinoma arises from the overlying surface epithelium and invades the dermis. Characteristically, the nests of basal cells demonstrate peripheral palisading.

Treatment Aims

To remove the malignant lesion to prevent local or systemic spread.

Other Treatments

For lesions that are nonresectable (particularly sebaceous cell carcinomas), orbital radiation may be warranted.

Prognosis

With wide excision and no evidence of metastasis, surgery results in a cure for the malignancies. However, sebaceous lesions have a high incidence of recurrence (~33%) and metastasis (~23%).

Follow-up and Management

Once a malignancy is found, ongoing monitoring for additional malignancies or metastatic sites is warranted. There is a marked increase in head-and-neck basal cell lesions found in patients with previous eyelid malignancies.

Treatment continued on p. 395

DIAGNOSIS—cont'd

Squamous Cell and Sebaceous Gland Carcinoma

- Biopsy lesion (map biopsy may be required for suspected sebaceous cell carcinoma diagnosis) to ensure the diagnosis; evaluate regional lymph nodes to rule out distant spread ($< 0.5\%$)
- Sebaceous cell carcinoma: pentagonal full-thickness eyelid excision or alternatively a punch biopsy is necessary to make the correct diagnosis. Multiple map biopsies of adjacent palpebral and bulbar conjunctiva should be obtained because of the potential for pagetoid spread and the multifocal origin of the tumor.

Complications

Basal Cell Carcinoma

Locally infiltrative; rarely metastasizes.

Squamous Cell Carcinoma

Small percentage shows distant metastasis.

Sebaceous Cell Carcinoma

Highly malignant, potentially lethal. Unlike basal cell carcinoma, squamous cell carcinoma has a potential for metastatic spread through direct extension or indirectly via lymphatic and hematogenous routes. Has a greater tendency to recur locally than basal cell carcinoma.

Merkel Cell Carcinoma

Rare but highly malignant, with two-thirds of patients presenting with lymph node metastasis at diagnosis or within 18 months from initial therapy, and one-third with local recurrences and satellite lesions.

Pearls and Considerations

- Varied, and dependent on the type of lesion
- Aside from general imaging with CT and magnetic resonance imaging (MRI), B-scan ultrasonography has been found to be useful in distinguishing a variety of benign and malignant periocular lesions.

Referral Information

Refer to oculoplastics specialist or dermatologist for biopsy and treatment. Referral to an ocular oncology subspecialist and a hematologist/oncologist in such patients is appropriate in many cases.

TREATMENT—cont'd

Squamous Cell Carcinoma

- Consider sentinel lymph-node biopsy as a standard procedure in patients with recurrent, large or invasive squamous cell carcinomas, with wide excision of lesion by techniques such as Mohs' and frozen section
- Successful use of photodynamic therapy with topical 5-aminolevulic acid after application of a Frost suture in order to protect the globe has also been reported.

Sebaceous Gland Carcinoma

- Wide excision of tumor, with lymph node evaluation and possible radical neck dissection
- Intraepithelial tumor growth is a peculiar feature of sebaceous gland carcinoma that seems to indicate an increased risk for orbital invasion; if there is periorbital involvement, exenteration is the treatment of choice.

Merkel Cell Carcinoma

- A wide surgical excision with 5 mm margins is recommended, with frozen-section control of the margins confirmed in definitive paraffin sections; this may reduce the incidence of lymph-node metastasis, hematogenous spread and local recurrences.
- Occult nodal involvement has been reported in up to a third of Merkel cell carcinoma cases; surgery plus local adjuvant irradiation, even in presence of free surgical margins, have been shown to be associated with significantly lower rates of local and regional recurrence than surgery alone.

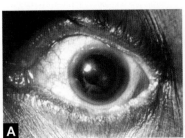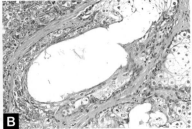

Figs 2A and B: Sebaceous gland carcinoma. (A) Eyelids are diffusely thickened, indurated and show some loss of eyelashes. Sebaceous carcinoma can present as a lesion simulating a chalazion or, as shown here, can masquerade as a chronic lid inflammation; (B) Histologically, the malignant sebaceous cells (left and upper left) can be seen arising from relatively normal sebaceous cells on the right.

GENERAL REFERENCES

Bajaj MS, Aalok L, Gupta V, et al. Ultrasound biomicroscopic appearances of eyelid lesions at 50 MHz. J Clin Ultrasound. 2007;35:424-9.

Bernardini FP. Management of malignant and benign eyelid lesions. Curr Opin Ophthalmol. 2006;17:480-4.

Fraunfelder F, Roy F (Eds). Current Ocular Therapy. Philadelphia: Saunders; 2000.

Groehler JM, Rose JG. Madarosis as an indicator for malignancy in eyelid margin lesions. Optom Vis Sci. 2012;89:350-2.

Hornblass A. Oculoplastic, Orbital, and Reconstructive Surgery, vol. 2. Baltimore: Lippincott Williams & Wilkins; 1990.

Older JJ (Ed). Eyelid Tumors: Clinical Diagnosis and Surgical Treatment. New York: Raven Press; 1987.

Patel GK, Goodwin R, Chawla M, et al. Imiquimod 5% cream monotherapy for cutaneous squamous cell carcinoma in situ (Bowen's disease): a randomized, double-blind, placebo-controlled trial. J Am Acad Dermatol. 2006; 54:1025-32.

Rossi R, Puccioni M, Mavilia L, et al. Squamous cell carcinoma of the eyelid treated with photodynamic therapy. J Chemother. 2004;16:306-9.

Shields JA, Demirci H, Marr BP, et al. Sebaceous carcinoma of the eyelids: personal experience with 60 cases. Ophthalmology. 2004;111:2151-7.

Tasman W, Jaeger E (Eds). Duane's Clinical Ophthalmology, vol. 4. Philadelphia: Lippincott-Raven; 2006.

Vaughn GJ, Dortzbach RK, Gayre GS. Eyelid malignancies. In: Yanoff M, Duker JS (Eds). Ophthalmology, 3rd edition. St. Louis, MO: Mosby Elsevier; 2008. pp. 1434-42.

Yanoff M, Fine B. Ocular pathology: A Color Atlas. Philadelphia: Lippincott Williams & Wilkins; 2002.

Third-Nerve Palsy (Oculomotor), Partial (378.51) and Complete (378.52)

DIAGNOSIS

Definition

Loss of function of the third cranial (oculomotor) nerve.

Synonyms

None

Symptoms

- Ptosis
- *Glare*: secondary to pupillary dilation
- Blurred near vision
- Vertical and horizontal diplopia
- *Pain*: present almost always with aneurysmal third-nerve palsy and pituitary apoplexy; variable with diabetic third-nerve palsy
- Acute onset suggests ischemic vascular disease and aneurysm
- Progressive implies compressive lesion.

Signs (Figs 1A to F)

- Ophthalmoparetic eye
- Eye unable to elevate, depress, or adduct (involved eye "down and out")
- *Ptosis*: subtle to profound
- Pupil may be spared or involved:
  - In adults, a painful, pupil-involving third-nerve paresis means an aneurysm at the junction of the internal carotid and posterior communicating arteries
  - A pupil-sparing third-nerve paresis can only be cited in a complete third-nerve palsy; usually vasculopathic in adults less than or equal to 50 years of age
  - A relative pupil-sparing third-nerve paresis means that the pupil is minimally reactive to light in the setting of a complete third-nerve palsy. Some physicians interpret this as being "pupil involving," whereas others interpret it as "pupil sparing".
- Loss of accommodation
- *Vitreous hemorrhage (Terson's syndrome)*: suggests an intracranial bleed from an aneurysm
- Signs of aberrant regeneration
- *Visual loss*: in pituitary apoplexy
- Pilocarpine 1% constricts pupil, unlike pupils dilated with other pharmacologic agents.

Differential Diagnosis

- Myasthenia gravis
- Graves' orbitopathy
- Inflammatory orbital pseudotumor
- Internuclear ophthalmoplegia
- Ocular skew torsion
- Anisocoria
- Chronic progressive external ophthalmoplegia
- Contact lens-associated complications
- Giant cell arteritis
- Complicated migraine
- Multiple sclerosis
- Trochlear nerve palsy.

Cause

Adults

Aneurysm, tumor (e.g. pituitary adenoma), infarction, idiopathic, trauma, infection (e.g. basilar meningitis, syphilis)

Children

Congenital, trauma, inflammation, neoplasm, aneurysm, ophthalmoplegic migraine and ischemia (rare)

Associated Features

Weber's Syndrome
- Third-nerve palsy
- Contralateral hemiparesis.

Benedikt's Syndrome
- Third-nerve palsy
- Contralateral hemiparesis
- Contralateral involuntary movements or tremor
- Lesion affects the third-nerve fascicle, cerebral peduncle, substantia nigra and red nucleus.

Claude's Syndrome
- Third-nerve palsy
- Contralateral ataxia
- Asynergy
- Dysdiadochokinesia
- Fourth-nerve palsy and sensory loss may be included. Lesion affects the third-nerve fascicle, red nucleus, superior cerebellar peduncle, and sometimes the fourth nerve, medial lemniscus, and medial longitudinal fasciculus.

Nothnagel's Syndrome
- Bilateral, asymmetric third-nerve palsies
- Gait ataxia
- Nystagmus
- Lesion affects both third-nerve fascicles and the superior and inferior colliculi.

Cavernous Sinus Syndrome
- Oculosympathetic paresis
- Sensory loss in V1, V2, sixth nerve, and fourth nerve; proptosis up to 4 mm
- The involvement of the optic nerve constitutes a superior orbital fissure/orbital apex syndrome.

Diagnosis continued on p. 398

TREATMENT

Diet and Lifestyle

Optimization of diet to alleviate vasculopathic status in "medical third nerve palsy".

Pharmacologic Treatment

- Botulinum toxin A (oculinum) injections
- Nonsteroidal anti-inflammatory agents (NSAIDs): to treat pain.

Nonpharmacologic Treatment

Prism lenses for persistent diplopia.

Surgical Intervention

- *For berry aneurysm*: clipping, gluing, coiling or wrapping of the berry aneurysm by a neurosurgeon in the acute stage. Aneurysm clipping is more likely to result in resolution than coiling, since the latter does not reliably remove the mass effect of the aneurysm on the nerve.
- May be considered for patient with persistent symptoms (> 6 months) uncorrected by conservative management (e.g. stable-angle diplopia, eye misalignment or torticollis).
- Factors related to poorer, more unpredictable surgical prognosis include prolonged delay to surgery (it is proposed that development of long-term secondary overactions are responsible) larger eye deviation. Factors associated with better prognosis include partial (pupil-sparing) and minor oculomotor palsy symptoms.
- Techniques include horizontal rectus muscle transposition procedures, superior oblique tenectomy, wall fixation procedures, augmented Hummelsheim technique, superior oblique anterior transposition, and palpebral fixation techniques.

Prognosis

- A vasculopathic third-nerve paresis resolves in 3 months, although a compressive etiology may persist.
- A compressive/inflammatory third-nerve paresis may develop signs of aberrant regeneration, including:
  - Pseudo-Graefe sign (eyelid fails to follow the eye downward)
  - Eyelid synkinesia (eyelid elevates in adduction and drops in abduction)
  - Light-gaze dissociation pupil (pupil fails to respond to light but constricts to adduction, elevation or depression)
  - Limitation of elevation and depression of the eye with occasional retraction of the globe on attempted vertical movement
  - Adduction of the involved eye on attempted elevation or depression
  - Monocular vertical optokinetic nystagmus.

Treatment Aims

To restore and maintain single, simultaneous, binocular vision in primary position at distance and near.

Prognosis

- Vasculopathic third-nerve palsies should resolve in 3 months
- Patients with compressive/inflammatory third-nerve paresis may develop signs of aberrant regeneration.

Follow-up and Management

Monitor patients every few weeks for secondary contracture during recovery period.

Treatment continued on p. 399

Third-Nerve Palsy (Oculomotor), Partial (378.51) and Complete (378.52)

DIAGNOSIS—cont'd

Investigations

- Immediately hospitalize patients with painful, pupil-involving third-nerve paresis
- Computed tomography (CT) and arteriography (CT more sensitive than magnetic resonance imaging to demonstrate subarachnoid hemorrhage, and also characteristic intralesional calcifications)
- Magnetic resonance imaging and arteriography (prefer 3-Tesla MRA with special attention to the circle of Willis)
- Cerebral angiography: definitive test for intracranial berry aneurysm. Small risk of complications including embolic stroke
- *Maddox rod or alternate cover testing*: in very mild cases, to elicit latent deviation or phoria during the examination
- Lumbar puncture
- Two-hour postprandial blood sugar
- Erythrocyte sedimentation rate
- Rapid plasma reagin.

Complications

- Subarachnoid bleed
- Coma
- Death.

Pearls and Considerations

- In a true isolated oculomotor palsy, the presumed location of the lesion is in the subarachnoid space
- Compression of the third nerve by an aneurysm at the junction of the internal carotid and posterior communicating arteries is considered a *true neuro-ophthalmologic emergency*. This is a life-threatening condition
- Angiography is indicated in a patient with third cranial nerve palsy and dilated, light-fixed pupil.

Referral Information

Refer to neuro-ophthalmologist and/or neurosurgeon as appropriate; medical optimization in vasculopathic third-nerve paresis.

TREATMENT—cont'd

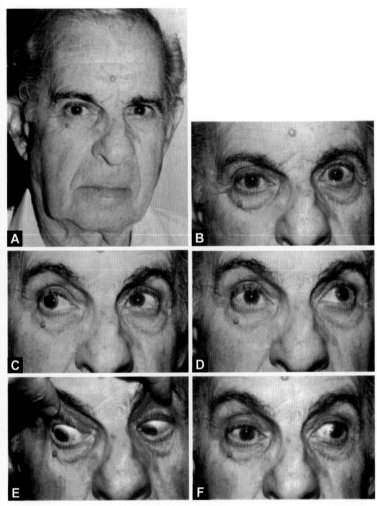

Figs 1A to F: (A) This man has an incomplete right third-nerve palsy. He turns his head to the left because of decreased innervation to the right medial rectus muscle; (B) The left eyelid is retracted to compensate for his partial right ptosis, and a small left hypertropia is measurable in primary gaze; (C and D) The left hypertropia is more pronounced in upgaze because of paretic right superior rectus and right inferior oblique muscle; (E) In downgaze the left hypertropia reverses to a right "hypertropia" because of a paretic right inferior rectus muscle; (F) The right exotropia increases in left gaze because of weak right medial rectus muscle.

GENERAL REFERENCES

Cabrejas L, Hurtado-Ceña FJ, Tejedor J. Predictive factors of surgical outcome in oculomotor nerve palsy. J Am Assoc Pediatr Ophthalmol Strabismus. 2009;13(5):481-4.

Flanders M, Hasan J, Al-Mujaini A. Partial third cranial nerve palsy: clinical characteristics and surgical management. Can J Ophthalmol (Journal Canadien d'Ophtalmologie). 2012;47(3):321-5.

Goodwin J. (2012). Oculomotor nerve palsy. [Online] Available from www.emedicine.com.

Johnston JL. Parasellar syndromes. Curr Neurol Neurosci Rep. 2002;2 (5):423-31.

Kau HC, Tsai CC, Ortube MC, et al. High-resolution magnetic resonance imaging of the extraocular muscles and nerves demonstrates various etiologies of third nerve palsy. Am J Ophthalmol. 2007;143(2):280-7.

Miller NR, Lee AG. Adult-onset acquired oculomotor nerve paresis with cyclic spasms: relationship to ocular neuromyotonia. Am J Ophthalmol. 2004;137(1):70-6.

Moster ML. Paresis of isolated multiple cranial nerves and painful ophthalmoplegia. In: Yanoff M, Duker JS (Eds). Ophthalmology. St Louis: Elsevier; 2006.

Tonic Pupil (379.46)

DIAGNOSIS

Definition

An enlarged, nonreactive pupil.

Synonym

Adie's tonic pupil

Symptoms

- Anisocoria
- "Funny looking" pupil
- Mid-dilated to small pupil
- *The larger pupil in bright illumination*: the same pupil is sometimes the smaller one in dim illumination
- *Blurred vision*: from accommodative paresis
- Difficulty reading
- Photophobia
- *"Brow ache"*: from ciliary spasm with near work.

Signs (Figs 1A to C)

- Attenuated and slow light reflex
- Light-near dissociation pupil, with exaggerated but tonic near response
- Sector iris sphincter palsy
- Stromal spread
- Stromal streaming
- Ectropion uvea
- Vermiform pupil movements.

Investigations

- Low-dose pilocarpine 0.1% yields constriction of pupils with cholinergic denervation sensitivity. Normal pupils do not constrict to such low concentration of pilocarpine
- *Microhemagglutination assay*: *Treponema pallidum* (MHA-TP) and rapid plasma reagin (RPR) to rule out syphilis
- Fasting blood glucose levels, hemoglobin A1c
- Lyme titers
- May need brain magnetic resonance imaging and computed tomography angiography (CTA)/magnetic resonance angiography (MRA) for patients with uncertain or high-risk findings.

Pearls and Considerations

- Typically, the affected pupil is larger than pupil in fellow eye
- Vermiform movements of the iris are often visible at the slit lamp
- The tonic pupil will typically react to 0.1% pilocarpine, whereas the normal pupil will not
- One-fifth of normal subjects will have unequal pupils of 0.4 mm or greater in dim light. When followed over time, the degree of anisocoria will vary, and occasionally switch sides. Physiologic anisocoria can be distinguished from pathologic anisocoria because of a normal light reaction and, generally, no change in the degree of anisocoria in light or dark conditions.

Referral Information

None

Differential Diagnosis

- Toxic (pharmacologic) pupil
- Posterior synechia
- Traumatic iridoplegia
- Iris structural abnormalities
- Oculomotor nerve compression ("Hutchinson pupil")
- Physiologic anisocoria
- Aberrant regeneration of the third nerve
- Horner's syndrome/oculosympathetic paresis
- Angle closure
- Tectal pupils (dorsal midbrain syndrome)
- Argyll-Robertson pupils.

Cause

Damage to the ciliary ganglion and/or short posterior ciliary nerves.

Epidemiology

Idiopathic Tonic Pupil
- Female/male ratio is 2.6:1
- Age of onset is 20–40 years
- Ninety percent of patients present unilaterally
- Involvement of the fellow eye is common.

Classification

Local Tonic Pupil
- Ophthalmic laser procedures (e.g. laser peripheral iridotomy, argon laser panretinal photocoagulation)
- Varicella
- Retrobulbar injection
- Orbital tumor
- Orbital surgery.

Neuropathic Tonic Pupil (Bilateral)
- Diabetes
- Syphilis
- Connective tissue diseases (e.g. rheumatoid arthritis, Sjögren's syndrome)
- Sarcoid
- Human immunodeficiency virus (HIV) neuropathy
- Paraneoplastic neuropathy.

Idiopathic (Adie's Tonic Pupil)
Harlequin Syndrome: along with ipsilateral asymmetric sweating and flushing on the upper thoracic region of the chest, the neck, and the face. Poorly understood.
Ross Syndrome: tonic pupil, hyporeflexia and segmental anhidrosis.

Associated Features

Accommodative paresis, tonicity and induced astigmatism at near gaze

Idiopathic Tonic Pupil
- Decreased corneal sensation
- *Holmes-Adie Syndrome:* tonic pupil in association with diminished deep tendon reflexes.

TREATMENT

Diet and Lifestyle

No special precautions are necessary.

Pharmacologic Treatment

Cycloplegia: for the tonic pupil with a tonicity cramp; prescribe reading glasses to match the near point between the two eyes.

Nonpharmacologic Treatment

- Patch
- Cosmetic contact lens.

Treatment Aims

- To normalize appearance of pupil
- To synchronize near points between the two eyes with reading lenses
- To relieve cramping with tropine medication.

Prognosis

- Mid-dilated pupil tends to become more miotic over time and may actually become smaller than normal
- Bilateral cases are fairly common; there may be no "control eye" for comparison
- Direct light reflex remains impaired
- Fellow eye will become involved at a rate of 4%/year, so at the end of 20 years, 50% of patients will have bilateral involvement.

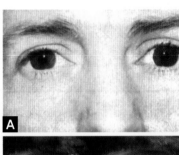
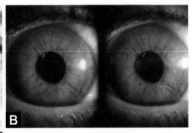
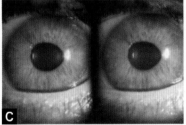

Figs 1A to C: (A) This woman has bilateral Adie's tonic pupils; (B) Stereophotograph of the right eye in which a segmental paralysis of the pupillary sphincter from the 6 o'clock to the 9 o'clock positions is associated with a spreading of the iris stroma; (C) Stereophotograph of the left eye in which the pupil assumes a polygonal appearance with segmental paresis from the 3 o'clock to the 6 o'clock positions.

GENERAL REFERENCES

Bremner F. Pupil evaluation as a test for autonomic disorders. Clin Auton Res. 2009;19(2):88-101.

Cheshire WP, Low PA. Harlequin syndrome: still only half understood. J Neuro-ophthalmol. 2008;28(3):169-70.

Foroozan R, Buono LM, Savino PJ, et al. Tonic pupils from giant cell arteritis. Br J Ophthalmol. 2003;87(4):510-2.

Kawasaki A. Physiology, assessment, and disorders of the pupil. Curr Opin Ophthalmol. 1999;10(6):394-400.

Kelly-Sell M, Liu GT. "Tonic" but not "Adie" pupils. J Neuro-ophthalmol. 2011; 31(4):393-5.

Lobes LA, Bourgon P. Pupillary abnormalities induced by argon laser photocoagulation. Ophthalmology. 1985;92(2): 234-6.

Moeller JJ, Maxner CE. The dilated pupil: an update. Curr Neurol Neurosci Rep. 2007;7(5):417-22.

Wilhelm H. Neuro-ophthalmology of pupillary function: practical guidelines. J Neurol. 1998;245(9):573-83.

Toxic Retinopathies (362.55)

DIAGNOSIS

Definition

Drug toxicity of the posterior segment.

Synonyms

None

Symptoms

- Chloroquine and hydroxychloroquine (Plaquenil, commonly used to treat rheumatoid arthritis and lupus)
- Often asymptomatic; photophobia, nyctalopia, photopsias
- Phenothiazines (a class of antipsychotic medications)
- Blurry vision, decreased night vision, brown color to vision
- Methanol ("wood alcohol")
- White, blurry vision, blindness.

Signs

- Chloroquine and hydroxychloroquine
- Corneal whorls, poliosis, irregular macular pigmentation, loss of foveal reflex, classic bull's-eye maculopathy (Figs 1A and B)
- *Peripheral pigmentation*: gives pseudoretinitis pigmentosa appearance; bone spicule formation, arteriolar attenuation, optic nerve pallor
- Phenothiazines
- *Granularity to postequatorial fundus*: found early, although early on fundus may be normal
- Transient edema of optic nerve and retina
- *Large patches of increased pigmentation*: may give appearance of bone spiculization
- Large areas of depigmentation and atrophy
- Methanol
- Nystagmus, poorly reactive dilated pupils
- *Edema of optic nerve and retina*: retinal edema spreads out along major arcades
- Central or cecocentral scotomas.

Differential Diagnosis

Chloroquine and Hydroxychloroquine
Retinitis and pseudoretinitis pigmentosa.
Phenothiazines
Retinitis pigmentosa, syphilis, rubella.
Methanol
Increased intracranial pressure, causing papilledema.

Causes

Chloroquine and Hydroxychloroquine
Have an affinity for pigmented structures in the eye; half-lives also increase as the dosage increases.
Phenothiazines
The mechanism of injury is unknown.
Methanol
Methanol is converted to formic acid after ingestion; formic acid is a mitochondrial toxin and is felt to be responsible for the toxicity.

Epidemiology

Toxic retinopathy affects approximately 10% of unmonitored patients receiving chloroquine and 3–4% of patients taking hydroxychloroquine. Incidence increases with both dose and duration.

Classification

Chloroquine and hydroxychloroquine are members of quinolone drug family.

Associated Features

Chloroquine and Hydroxychloroquine
Hydroxychloroquine used to treat rheumatoid arthritis, systemic lupus erythematosus; chloroquine used to treat malaria.
Methanol
Metabolic acidosis, depressed level of consciousness, respiratory distress, coma, death.

Pathology

Chloroquine and Hydroxychloroquine
- Outer segments of the retina degenerate, often sparing the fovea
- Pigment migrates to the retina
- Ganglion cells develop membranous cytoplasmic bodies within 1 week of treatment.

Methanol
It is believed that the damage is caused by axoplasmic stasis, and that permanent damage is caused by secondary swelling of the optic nerve and retina.

Diagnosis continued on p. 404

TREATMENT

Diet and Lifestyle

No special precautions are necessary.

Pharmacologic Treatment

Chloroquine and Hydroxychloroquine

Discontinue the drug when symptoms begin.

Phenothiazines

- Discontinue the drug when symptoms of decreased vision begin will allow reversal of the symptoms
- *Standard dosage*: thioridazine, 300 mg/day (maximum 800 mg/day).

Methanol

Intravenous ethanol acts as a competitive inhibitor of the metabolism of methanol.

Nonpharmacologic Treatment

Chloroquine, Hydroxychloroquine, and Phenothiazines

No nonpharmacologic treatment is recommended.

Methanol

- Respiratory support
- Treatment of the metabolic acidosis
- Dialysis
- Intravenous ethanol.

Complications

Chloroquine and Hydroxychloroquine

- Most severe toxic retinal findings are due to chloroquine. Hydroxychloroquine infrequently causes a maculopathy.
- If found early, functional and fundus changes should return to normal with discontinuation of the chloroquine or hydroxychloroquine. If not, irreversible visual damage can occur.

Treatment Aims

Chloroquine and Hydroxychloroquine

To discontinue use once maculopathy has started.

Phenothiazines

- To discontinue the use of the phenothiazine once symptoms start
- To titrate the dosage of the medication to stay within the guidelines.

Prognosis

Chloroquine and Hydroxychloroquine

Good, if doses are monitored and patients are followed carefully.

Phenothiazines

Good, if caught early.

Methanol

Usually, vision should improve within 6 days; if not, improvement is unlikely.

Follow-up and Management

Chloroquine and Hydroxychloroquine

- *Amsler grid*: for patient home monitoring; look for central scotomas or paracentral scotomas
- *Macular visual field*: annually during the first 3 years, when most of the toxicity generally develops
- Color vision monitoring.

Phenothiazines

All patients on this type of medication should have a baseline eye examination and should be followed periodically if symptoms begin.

Methanol

Optic atrophy and excavation usually occurs after 1–2 months.

Treatment continued on p. 405

Toxic Retinopathies (362.55)

DIAGNOSIS—cont'd

Investigations

Chloroquine and Hydroxychloroquine

- *Amsler grid*: screening to look for central and paracentral scotomas
- *Goldmann perimetry*: small paracentral scotomas sparing fixation superiorly
- *Electroretinography*: abnormal in advanced retinopathy
- *Electro-oculogram*: reduced with more retinopathy
- *Fluorescein angiography*: highlights the pigmentation changes (Fig. 1)
- *Fundus autofluoresence (FAF)*: loss of central FAF early. Advanced cases also have concentric peripheral increases in FAF.

Phenothiazines

- *Careful history*: to determine the use of antipsychotic medication
- Slit-lamp and dilated fundus examination
- *Fluorescein angiography*: demonstrates window-defect changes in pigment layer
- Reduction in the photopic and scotopic electroretinogram
- Abnormal dark adaptation.

Methanol

Careful history: to determine if the patient had been drinking solvents or home-made liquors; although the usual method of poisoning is through ingestion, patients may also develop toxicity from vapors or skin contact.

Pearls and Considerations

An open line of communication with the patient's prescribing physician is the key to effective management of toxic retinopathies.

Referral Information

Refer/co-manage these cases with the prescribing physician.

TREATMENT—cont'd

Phenothiazines

The risk of retinopathy is dose-related. Even if the medication is discontinued, the pigmentary changes can continue.

Methanol

Severe visual loss: can occur from ingesting as little as 1 oz of methanol; the more severe the retinal findings, the more severe the eye damage.

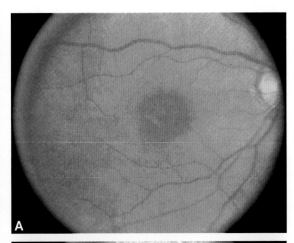

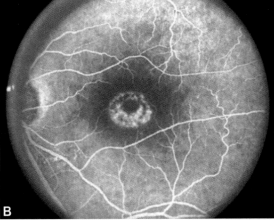

Figs 1A and B: Retinopathy caused by chloroquine and hydroxychloroquine. (A) Color photograph of the right eye of a patient with increasing pigmentation in the macula; (B) Fluorescein angiogram of the same patient's left eye showing window-defect hyperfluorescence corresponding to the area of pigment alteration.

GENERAL REFERENCES

Baumbach GL, Cancilla PA, Martin-Amat G, et al. Methyl alcohol poisoning. IV. Alterations in morphological findings of the retina and optic nerve. Arch Ophthalmol. 1977;95:1859-65.

Fishman GA. Retinal toxicity with the use of chloroquine or hydroxychloroquine. In: Heckenlively JR, Aden GB (Eds). Principles and Practice of Electrophysiology of Vision. St Louis: Mosby; 1991. pp. 594-9.

Hayrah MS, Hayreh SS, Baumbach GL, et al. Methyl alcohol poisoning. III. Ocular toxicity. Arch Ophthalmol. 1977;95:1851-9.

Marmor MF, Kellner U, Lai TY, et al. American Academy of Ophthalmology: Revised recommendations on screening for chloroquine and hydroxychloroquine retinopathy. Ophthalmol. 2011;118:415-22.

Uveal Malignant Melanoma, Primary (190.6)

DIAGNOSIS

Definition

A malignant lesion occurring in the uveal tract.

Synonyms

None

Symptoms

- Patients can be asymptomatic
- *Blurry or decreased vision*: from extension of tumor into fovea, fluid in fovea, or tumor contact with lens
- Photopsias, visual field defects, dark spot on iris.

Signs

- Elevated pigmented lesion of iris, ciliary body, or choroid
- *Iris melanomas*: usually arise from an existing iris nevus; will have an elevated nodular area; prominent vessels may be present in the lesion; pigmentation may vary (Fig. 1)
- *Ciliary body and choroidal tumors*: often takes on characteristic collar-button appearance when the tumor breaks through Bruch's membrane; pigmentation may vary; may have associated orange lipofuscin pigment on the surface; often associated with serous retinal detachment when tumor exceeds 4 mm in height; although most tumors are pigmented, approximately 20% are amelanotic; anterior tumors extending to involve ciliary body will have prominent episcleral vessels (Figs 2 and 3).

Investigations

- *Clinical history*: not useful when trying to differentiate choroidal melanoma from other simulating lesions, except for metastasis
- *Gonioscopy*: for iris and ciliary body lesions, to look for pigment dispersion in the angle and to determine if lesion is arising from iris or extending anteriorly from ciliary body
- *Dilated fundus examination*: usually makes the diagnosis in more than 95% of cases of ciliary body and choroidal malignant melanoma.

Differential Diagnosis

- *Choroidal nevus*: usually asymptomatic; flat or less than 1.5 mm in thickness; sharply defined borders; drusen on surface; fluorescein angiography shows early hypofluorescence; serous detachment and secondary hemorrhage are rare (Fig. 4).
- *Choroidal melanocytoma*: often jet black in appearance, does not enlarge, and usually develops around the optic disc (Fig. 5).
- *Subretinal hemorrhage*: secondary to age-related macular degeneration, macroaneurysm, or choroidal hemorrhage.
- *Metastatic disease*: usually more than one lesion in the choroid; these tumors are usually less pigmented, are more likely found in the posterior pole, and often involve the macula; serous retinal detachment is also possible (Fig. 6).
- *Choroidal osteoma*: cream-colored, calcified macular or peripapillary lesion; relatively flat; more common in women; bilateral in 10–20%; calcification can be documented by ultrasound or CT scan (Fig. 7).
- Choroidal hemangioma
- Retinal pigment epithelial tumors
- Congenital hypertrophy of the pigment epithelium (CHRPE).

Cause

Controversial; some believe primary ocular melanoma arises from a pre-existing nevus; others believe they develop de novo.

Epidemiology

- Iris melanomas are rare. Late metastasis is possible, occurring 20–30 years after diagnosis despite excision of the original ocular lesion.
- Ciliary body melanomas have the highest rate of metastasis and are thought to develop because of the anterior location and relatively high blood flow rate through the ciliary body.
- Choroidal melanoma has a 50% mortality rate after enucleation at 10–15 years, with a peak incidence at 3 years.

Pathology

Melanomas can be spindle A, spindle B, epithelioid, or mixed tumors. Epithelioid and mixed cell tumors carry a worse prognosis.

Diagnosis continued on p. 408

TREATMENT

Diet and Lifestyle

No special precautions are necessary.

Pharmacologic Treatment

If metastatic disease, then patient may need to refer for systemic chemotherapy. Extremely poor prognosis if becomes metastatic.

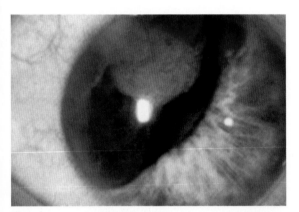

Fig. 1: Iris melanoma showing the elevated amelanotic nodule with a pigmented base. Note the prominent vasculature.

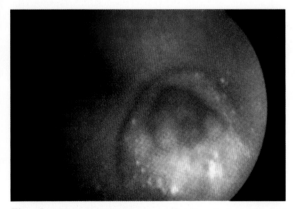

Fig. 2: Choroidal melanoma with elevated pigmented lesion and surface pigmentation. Yellow dots in the vitreous represent asteroid hyalosis.

Treatment Aims

To decrease the risk of tumor growth and metastasis while trying to maintain vision in the eye.

Prognosis

• Cell type is important for determining prognosis in all types of uveal melanoma.
• Iris melanomas are rare and have a better prognosis, but metastasis can occur 20–30 years after excision of the tumor.
• For choroidal melanoma, three important factors that imply a worse prognosis are anterior location of tumor margin, cellular pleomorphism, and presence of extrascleral extension.

Follow-up and Management

• Fundus photographs and ultrasound measurements should be taken of all lesions. This allows the physician to study the tumor margins carefully on subsequent visits.
• Follow-up management largely depends on the site, location, and associated features of the tumor, which is beyond the scope of this book. Most patients with uveal melanoma are followed by retina specialists or ocular oncologists, who have a better understanding of these lesions.

Treatment continued on p. 409

DIAGNOSIS—cont'd

- *Fluorescein angiography*: may have a characteristic "double circulation" in choroidal malignant melanoma; scleral transillumination is usually blocked by the ciliary body and choroidal tumor.
- *Ultrasonography*: of ciliary body and choroidal melanoma; B mode: acoustically silent zone within the tumor, choroidal excavation, orbital shadowing; A mode: medium-to-low internal reflectivity. Ultrasound is the most useful diagnostic tool to determine response to treatment.
- *Computed tomography (CT), magnetic resonance imaging (MRI)*: not always necessary; expensive to perform; increased uptake of the tumor on T1-weighted MR images for larger tumors; most useful to determine extraocular extension of tumor.
- *Fine-needle biopsy*: useful when diagnosis is difficult and chance of metastatic disease exists, although interpretation of the tissue is difficult.

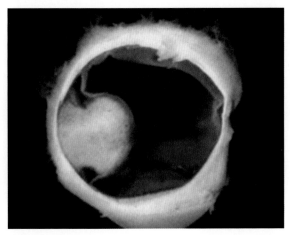

Fig. 3: Gross specimen of a choroidal melanoma showing the mushroom-shape configuration.

Diagnosis continued on p. 410

TREATMENT—cont'd

Nonpharmacologic Treatment

For Iris Melanoma

Most pigmented iris lesions are benign, so observation is recommended. If there is documented evidence of growth, local excision through an iridectomy or irido-cyclectomy should be performed.

For Ciliary Body and Choroidal Melanoma

- *Enucleation*: least common treatment modality; collaborative ocular mela-noma study showed that enucleation and plaque radiation therapy were equally effective for the prevention of metastatic disease.
- *Radiation therapy*: two methods are in use:
  - *Brachytherapy*: a plaque containing radioactive seeds is applied directly to episcleral surface of eye directly exterior to the tumor; common isotopes used are ^{60}Co, ^{106}Ru, and ^{125}I; plaque remains in place to deliver 80-100 Gy to the tumor apex.
  - *Charged particle (proton or helium) beam radiotherapy*: tumor base is located, and tantalum buttons are surgically sewn to the sclera; radia-tion is administered while monitoring position of the eye and tumor by fluoroscopy.

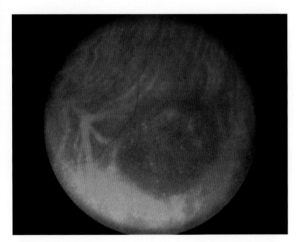

Fig. 4: Choroidal nevus. Note the feathery borders, flat appearance, and drusen on the surface.

Treatment continued on p. 411

Uveal Malignant Melanoma, Primary (190.6)

DIAGNOSIS—cont'd

Complications

- *Intraocular*: Glaucoma, decreased vision, loss of vision, cataract, pain and discomfort, serous retinal detachment, hemorrhage into the anterior chamber and vitreous.
- Systemic
- *Metastasis*: usually occurs in the liver and then in the lungs, bone, and skin.
- Death.

Pearls and Considerations

- Uveal tract melanoma is the most common ocular tumor in adults
- Can metastasize through the bloodstream to other parts of the body, especially the liver
- Patients with increasing astigmatic refractive changes need to have a thorough peripheral retinal examination to rule out a ciliary body melanoma as the cause of the astigmatism.

Referral Information

Refer to ocular oncologist as appropriate.

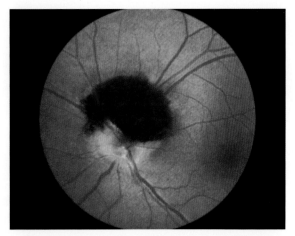

Fig. 5: Melanocytoma. Note the jet-black color with feathery borders.

TREATMENT—cont'd

- *Laser photocoagulation*: reserved for tumors less than 3 mm in thickness and 7 mm in largest basal dimension. This is used infrequently. This has mostly been replaced by transpupillary thermal therapy (TTT).
- *Surgical resection*: reserved for anterior choroidal and ciliary body tumors; tedious and complicated surgery; done infrequently.
- *Observation*: a suspicious nevus may be observed to document growth before instituting therapy. Not all nevi that grow are melanomas.
- *Transpupillary thermal therapy (TTT)*: commonly used for small- to medium-sized tumors; uses infrared laser light with a large spot size to induce hyperthermia; results in regression of tumor and is done in the office.

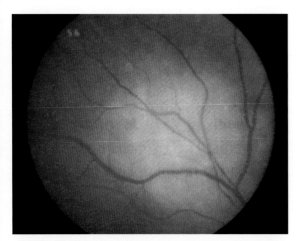

Fig. 6: Choroidal metastasis with creamy-yellow choroidal infiltrate located superior to the optic nerve in a patient with metastatic nasopharyngeal carcinoma.

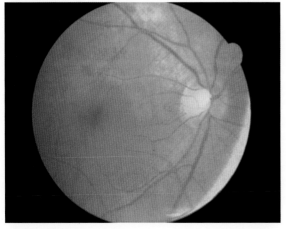

Fig. 7: Choroidal osteoma with areas of retinal pigment epithelium atrophy located supratemporally to the optic nerve.

GENERAL REFERENCES

Augsberger JJ, Damato BE, Bornfeld N. Uveal melanoma. In: Yanoff M, Duker JS (Eds). Ophthalmology. St Louis: Elsevier; 2006.

Augsburger JJ. Intraocular neoplasms. In: Podos SM, Yanoff M (Eds). Textbook of Ophthalmology, vol. 2; 1992. pp. 11.1-11.19.

Mukai S, Gragoudas ES. Diagnosis of choroidal melanoma. In: Albert DM, Jakobiec FA (Eds). Principles and Practice of Ophthalmology. Philadelphia: Saunders; 1994. pp. 3209-17.

Sahel JA, Marcus DM, Albert DM. Nevus and melanocytoma. In: Albert DM, Jakobiec FA (Eds). Principles and Practice of Ophthalmology. Philadelphia: Saunders; 1994. pp. 3244-51.

Uveitis Sympathetic (360.11)

DIAGNOSIS

Definition

Inflammation of the uveal tract after a penetrating ocular injury.

Synonym

Sympathetic ophthalmia

Symptoms

Sympathetic uveitis always follows a penetrating ocular injury to one eye (the "exciting" eye) and is characterized by a bilateral granulomatous uveal inflammatory reaction with the following symptoms:

- Photophobia in the noninjured ("sympathizing") eye: see Fig. 1
- Ocular irritation or pain
- Blurred vision in the noninjured (sympathizing) eye
- Trouble with near vision (difficulty with accommodation).

Signs

- Red eye secondary to ciliary injection
- *Evidence of previous ocular injury*: in rare cases, the injury occurred years before the onset of uveitis, and the patient does not remember
- Bilateral mutton-fat keratic precipitates (Fig. 2)
- *Bilateral uveitis*: the presentation of sympathetic uveitis has a wide spectrum, from an anterior uveitis or focal choroiditis to a severe panuveitis; Dalen-Fuchs nodules are tiny areas of focal choroidal inflammation most often seen in the midperiphery but also in the posterior pole (Fig. 3).
- Papillitis (inflammation of optic nerve head)
- Exudative retinal detachment.

Investigations

- *History*: a penetrating ocular injury, usually with uveal prolapse; generally after a 2-week "safe period"; most cases (80%) occur 3 weeks to 3 months after the injury, and both eyes are affected; rarely, sympathetic uveitis can occur years after a penetrating ocular injury.
- Visual acuity test
- Refraction
- Complete external examination
- Intraocular pressure
- Undilated and dilated slit-lamp examination
- Dilated fundus examination
- *Fluorescein angiography*: can be helpful; characteristically, multiple tiny areas of fluorescein hyperfluorescence that spread with time (leakage) are noted.

Differential Diagnosis

- Vogt-Koyanangi-Harada syndrome
- Bilateral phacoanaphylactic endophthalmitis
- Multifocal choroiditis
- Other causes of bilateral uvulitis.

Cause

Appears to be a delayed type of hypersensitivity reaction of the uvea to antigens located along the retinal pigment epithelium or uveal melanocytes.

Epidemiology

- Sympathetic uveitis occurs after intraocular surgical trauma (>0.200%)
- The incidence is higher in men than women, because men sustain penetrating ocular injuries more than women.

Two peaks of frequency occur:

- *Children less than 10 years*: Most likely because of the increased to occurrence of nonsurgical penetrating ocular injuries in this age group.
- *Adults more than 60 years*: Most likely because of the increased occurrence of intraocular surgery in this age group.

Associated Features

Cutaneous and neurological findings, similar to those found in Vogt-Koyanangi-Harada syndrome (alopecia, poliosis, vitiligo, dysacousia, tinnitus, vertigo, cerebrospinal fluid pleocytosis) trauma rarely accompany sympathetic uveitis.

Immunology

Lymphocytic choroidal infiltrate is composed almost exclusively of T lymphocytes.

Pathology

Histologic hallmarks of coronal inflammatory infiltrate include bilateral granulomatous (epithelioid cells) uveal reaction, sparing of the choriocapillaris, epithelioid cells containing phagocytosed uveal pigment, and Dalen-Fuchs nodules (epithelioid cells between retinal pigment epithelium and Bruch's membrane).

Diagnosis continued on p. 414

TREATMENT

Diet and Lifestyle

No special precautions are necessary.

Pharmacologic Treatment

Intensive topical and systemic corticosteroids should be started as soon as possible.

Standard Dosage

Prednisone, 1.0–1.5 mg/kg daily.

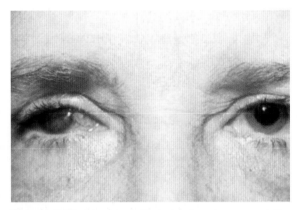

Fig. 1: Patient had complicated cataract surgery. Inflammation of the right eye and photophobia in the left eye occurred a few months later.

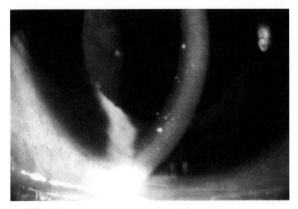

Fig. 2: Mutton-fat, keratic precipitates are present on the posterior corneal surface.

Treatment Aims

- To preserve vision in both eyes
- Even though sympathetic uveitis is rare, it can be (and often is) a blinding disease. Therefore, aggressive, rapid therapy is necessary if any chance exists of preserving visual function.

Other Treatments

Therapy aimed at T-cell subsets is being investigated. Most investigation of alternate therapy focus on patients who do not respond (or only partially respond) to high-dose corticosteroid therapy.

Prognosis

Approximately 60% of patients will retain visual acuity of more than or equal to 20/60; however, ~33% will have useful visual acuity of less than 20/200.

Follow-up and Management

Long-term follow-up is indicated to treat the entity and to protect against recurrence. Relapses occur in more than 50% of patients and may not occur for a few years after seemingly successful therapy.

Treatment continued on p. 415

Uveitis Sympathetic (360.11)

DIAGNOSIS—cont'd

Complications

- *Decreased visual acuity*: worst case is bilateral blindness; approximately one-third of patients are left with a visual acuity of less than 20/200 (legal blindness); the exciting (injured) eye may have better vision than the sympathizing eye.
- Band keratopathy
- Hypotony
- Glaucoma
- Cataract
- *Chorioretinal scarring*: after the inflammation resolves, chorioretinal scarring occurs and may be severe in the peripheral retina and macula in approximately one-third of patients; chorioretinal scarring in the region of the macula may be responsible for central visual loss in some patients.
- Macular edema
- Retinal detachment
- *Phthisis bulbi*: the end stage of ocular disease—a shrunken, functionless eye.

Pearls and Considerations

- If pain in nontraumatized eye is out of proportion to ocular findings, early sympathetic ophthalmia needs to be considered as the cause
- Sympathetic ophthalmia is a bilateral disease, so both eyes will have evidence of uveitis.

Referral Information

Needs immediate referral to ophthalmologist for aggressive immunosuppressive therapy.

TREATMENT—cont'd

Special Points

- After control of the inflammation, taper the systemic corticosteroid and institute alternate-day therapy until the inflammation has cleared. After the inflammation has cleared, treatment should be continued for 3–6 months with alternate-day therapy in the range of 10–20 mg of oral prednisone.
- In patients who are intolerant or do not respond to corticosteroids, periocular or immunosuppressive therapy (e.g. cyclosporine, methotrexate, chlorambucil, or azathioprine) along with reduced dosage of oral corticosteroid therapy may be indicated.

Nonpharmacologic Treatment

Enucleation

- Enucleation of the injured eye before the second eye becomes involved protects against the development of sympathetic uveitis
- Prophylactic corticosteroids do not prevent sympathetic uveitis
- In general, after a penetrating ocular injury with uveal prolapse, if no potential for useful vision exists, the injured eye should be enucleated within 2 weeks of injury. Enucleation of an injured eye that has a potential for navigational (i.e. "getting around") visual function is not justified, because the injured eye may ultimately turn out to have a better visual acuity than the sympathizing eye.
- Because of the 2-week safe period, every effort should be made to salvage the injured eye as soon as possible after the injury. The surgery often consists of immediate repair of the laceration of the ocular coats, often accompanied (at the same time or shortly thereafter) by vitreous surgery, which includes evacuation of any hemorrhage in the vitreous compartment and repair of any retinal tears or detachment.

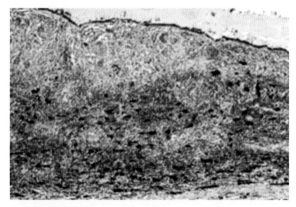

Fig. 3: A granulomatous inflammatory reaction diffusely involves the choroid. The choriocappilaris is spared.

GENERAL REFERENCES

Chan CC, Roberge RG, Whitcup SM, et al. 32 cases of sympathetic ophthalmia. Arch Ophthalmol. 1995;113:597.

Galor A, Davis JL, Flynn WW, et al. Sympathetic ophthalmia: incidence of ocular complications and vision loss in the sympathizing eye. Am J Ophthalmol. 2009;148:704.

Sen HN, Nussenblatt RB. Sympathetic ophthalmia: what have we learned? Am J Ophthalmol. 2009;148:632.

Yanoff M, Sassani JW. Ocular Pathology, 6th edition. Philadelphia: Mosby; 2009. pp. 73-5.

Vitreous Detachment, Posterior (379.21)

DIAGNOSIS

Definition

Separation of the vitreous gel from the retina.

Synonyms

None; usually abbreviated as PVD (posterior vitreous detachment).

Symptoms

* Flashing lights
* Floaters.

Signs

Free-floating ring of formed vitreous in front of optic nerve, also known as a *Weiss ring*.

Investigations

* History
* Slit-lamp and dilated eye examination
* 360° scleral depression: should be performed to rule out retinal tears.

Complications

* Vitreous hemorrhage
* Retinal tears
* Retinal detachment.

Pearls and Considerations

Vitreous detachment is a normal degenerative process in the aging eye, and most people will develop it in time. The vast majority of patients require no treatment.

Referral Information

Needs to be referred to an ophthalmologist within 24 hours of onset of symptoms to rule out associated pathologies such as retinal tear or retinal detachment.

Differential Diagnosis

* Ocular migraine can cause swirling or "zigzag" flashing lights
* Vitritis can cause floaters.

Cause

Age-related vitreous changes lead to synchysis and vacuolization of the vitreous.

Epidemiology

* Thirty-seven percent of myopic patients have had a posterior vitreous detachment at an earlier age
* The prevalence of posterior vitreous detachment formation increases with age and greater axial length
* Approximately 10% of patients with a symptomatic posterior vitreous detachment will have a retinal tear.

Pathology

Vacuolization and synchysis of the vitreous

TREATMENT

Diet and Lifestyle

No special precautions are necessary.

Pharmacologic Treatment

No pharmacologic treatment is recommended.

Nonpharmacologic Treatment

No nonpharmacologic treatment is recommended.

Treatment Aims

- To reassure the patient
- To teach the signs and symptoms of a retinal detachment to the patient.

Prognosis

Good

Follow-up and Management

Symptomatic patients with acute posterior vitreous detachment associated with flashes and floaters should be seen at first week, then at first month. If the dilated eye examination with scleral depression is normal, an annual follow-up examination is appropriate.

GENERAL REFERENCES

Tasman WS. Posterior vitreous detachment and peripheral retinal breaks. Trans Am Acad Ophthalmol Otolaryngol. 1968;72:217-24.

Yonemoto J, Noda Y, Mashara N, et al. Age of onset of posterior vitreous detachment. Curr Opin Ophthalmol. 1996;7:73-9.

Vitreous Hemorrhage (379.23)

DIAGNOSIS

Definition

Blood in the vitreous cavity.

Synonyms

None; usually abbreviated as VH (vitreous hemorrhage).

Symptoms

- Sudden, painless loss of vision
- *Sudden appearance of floaters and black spots*: with or without flashing lights.

Signs

The amount of blood in the vitreous cavity often determines the presenting visual acuity and the ability to examine the retina to determine the cause. The amount of blood, however, offers no help in determining the cause. Longstanding hemorrhage may take on a yellow appearance as the blood cells lose their hemoglobin.

Investigations

- History of preceding symptoms
- *Careful medical history*: to rule out diabetes, hypertension, trauma, sickle cell disease, anticoagulation therapy, and previous eye surgery
- *Careful slit-lamp and dilated fundus examination of both eyes*: even if the fundus is obscured by blood, often the fellow eye can provide clues on the possible cause
- *B-scan ultrasound*: to help rule out a retinal break or detachment if the retina cannot be visualized.

Complications

Secondary or "ghost cell" glaucoma: if the erythrocytes enter the anterior chamber, they can block the trabecular meshwork, causing a secondary elevation in intraocular pressure.

Pearls and Considerations

Causes loss of red reflex.

Referral Information

Usually needs to be referred to an ophthalmologist within 24 hours. If the patient is known to have diabetes with a history of proliferative disease, may be referred within several days.

Differential Diagnosis

- Spontaneous posterior vitreous detachment (PVD)
- Proliferative diabetic retinopathy
- Retinal break with or without detachment
- Retinal vein occlusion
- Macroaneurysm
- Age-related macular degeneration
- Sickle cell hemoglobinopathies
- Trauma
- Tumors and vascular anomalies
- Postoperative hemorrhage.

Cause

Avulsion of a retinal blood vessel is the most common cause. Shearing effect on the ciliary body or damage to the iris can also cause blood to leak into the vitreous cavity.

Epidemiology

Most common causes are as follows:
- Posterior vitreous detachment with a retinal tear (29%)
- Proliferative diabetic retinopathy (20%)
- Retinal vein occlusion (16%)
- Vitreous detachment without a tear (12%).

Associated Features

Neovascularization of the iris may be seen in patients with diabetes and vascular occlusion. Drusen in the fellow eye may help with the diagnosis of age-related macular degeneration.

TREATMENT

Diet and Lifestyle

- Avoid heavy lifting
- Sleep with head elevated on two pillows
- Avoid contact sports and forms of exercise that would cause the hemorrhage to remain suspended in the vitreous cavity.

Pharmacologic Treatment

- Usually can continue use of prophylactic baby aspirin therapy without worsening vitreous hemorrhage
- No pharmacologic treatment is recommended.

Nonpharmacologic Treatment

- Treat the underlying cause
- *Pars plana vitrectomy*: if the view remains cloudy for more than 2 months, or much sooner if there is a high level of suspicion for a retinal tear or detachment
- *Panretinal photocoagulation*: for proliferative diabetic retinopathy, vascular occlusive disease, or sickle cell retinopathy.

Treatment Aims

- To treat underlying cause
- To restore visual acuity
- To prevent visual loss
- To avoid secondary complications (e.g. glaucoma).

Prognosis

Depends on the cause of the hemorrhage.

Follow-up and Management

Patients should be followed on a weekly basis. It is hoped the blood will clear, allowing a view of the fundus. If not, sequential B-scan ultrasound should be performed, looking for a retinal detachment.

GENERAL REFERENCES

Lingren G, Sjodell L, Lindblom B. A prospective study of dense spontaneous vitreous hemorrhage. Am J Ophthalmol. 1995;119:458-65.

Schweitzer KD, Eneh AA, Hurst J, et al. Predicting retinal tears in posterior vitreous detachment. Can J Ophthalmol. 2011;46:481-5.

Index

Note: Page number followed by *f* and *t* indicates figure and table respectively.